Perioperative Drug Manual

SECOND EDITION

Perioperative Drug Manual

Paul F. White, PhD, MD
Professor and Holder of the Margaret Milam McDermott
Distinguished Chair in Anesthesiology
Department of Anesthesiology and Pain Management
University of Texas Southwestern Medical Center
Dallas, Texas

**Cover illustration courtesy of
Pablo McClure, Santiago, Chile
(www.pablomcclure.com)**

**ELSEVIER
SAUNDERS**

ELSEVIER
SAUNDERS

QV
39
P445
2005

The Curtis Center
170 S. Independence Mall W 300 E
Philadelphia, Pennsylvania 19106

PERIOPERATIVE DRUG MANUAL, Second E   ISBN 0-7216-0538-9

NOTICE

The editor has carefully checked the generic and trade drug names and verified drug
dosages to ensure that the drug information in this work is accurate and in accord with
the standards accepted at the time of publication. Readers are advised, however, to
check the product information currently provided by the manufacturer of each drug to
be administered to be certain that changes have not been made in the recommended dose
or in the contraindications for administration. This is of particular importance in regard
to new or infrequently used drugs. It is the responsibility of the treating physician,
relying on experience and knowledge of the patient, to determine dosages and the best
treatment for the patient. The editors cannot be responsible for misuse or misapplication
of the material in this work.

The Publisher

Library of Congress Cataloging-in-Publication Data

Perioperative drug manual / [authored by] Paul F. White.—2nd ed.
    p. ; cm.
Rev. ed. of: Anesthesia drug manual. ©1996.
ISBN 0-7216-0538-9
    1. Drug interactions—Handbooks, manuals, etc. 2. Anesthesiology—Handbooks,
manuals, etc. 3. Drugs—Handbooks, manuals, etc. I. White, Paul F. II. Anesthesia drug
manual.
    [DNLM: 1. Pharmaceutical Preparations—Handbooks. 2. Anesthesia—Handbooks.
3. Perioperative Care—Handbooks. QV 39 P445 2005]
RD82.7.D78A54 2005
617.9′6—dc22   2004051058

Printed in the United States of America

Last digit is the print number: 9   8   7   6   5   4   3   2   1

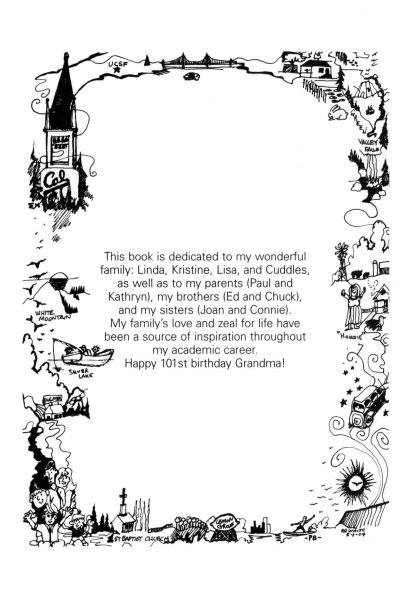

This book is dedicated to my wonderful family: Linda, Kristine, Lisa, and Cuddles, as well as to my parents (Paul and Kathryn), my brothers (Ed and Chuck), and my sisters (Joan and Connie). My family's love and zeal for life have been a source of inspiration throughout my academic career.
Happy 101st birthday Grandma!

Foreword

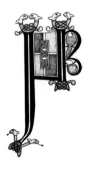

I arise today
Through the strength of heaven,
Light of sun,
Radiance of moon,
Splendour of fire,
Speed of lightning,
Swiftness of wind,
Depth of sea,
Stability of earth,
Firmness of rock.

From the novel *The Princes of Ireland*
by Edward Rutherfurd.
© 2004 Random House, Inc.

When I chose anesthesiology over internal medicine 32 years ago, I had the hope I would master the five "big" textbooks in the field. I am amazed as I look at the anesthetic library today. With anesthesiology sitting at the crossroads of several medical specialties and requiring operational speed to make important patient care decisions, we are in need of accurate summaries of pharmacologic interactions to guide these decisions.

Paul F. White is one of the foremost pharmacologists that anesthesiology has ever produced. He has dedicated himself to an enormously important endeavor—compiling the new edition of *Perioperative Drug Manual,* a comprehensive yet concise handbook that lists all the drugs that affect the practice of anesthesiology and perioperative medicine.

Thanks to his experience and dedication, Dr. White has produced an efficient and essential book with a PDA companion that instantly provides the anesthesiologist with critically important information. This handbook will, I believe, become not only essential but also mandatory in operating and recovery rooms, diagnostic suites, and critical care units around the world.

Michael B. Howie, MD
Professor and Chairman
Department of Anesthesiology
Ohio State University
Columbus, Ohio

Preface

As the number of drugs that our patients receive during the perioperative period continues to increase at a rapid rate, it has become more difficult for busy practitioners to keep abreast of the dosages and pharmacologic properties of the new compounds and their potential interactions with existing drugs. Many more patients are using alternative medications (e.g., herbals and dietary supplements), and these can exert effects during the perioperative period. From the clinician's perspective, the problem has been compounded by the dramatic shift in health care delivery from the hospital to the ambulatory setting. Currently, more than 90% of all patients undergoing elective surgery are admitted on the day of the operation. The difficulty in assessing the potential implications of chronic medications on their perioperative course is further complicated by the fact that many more elderly patients with complex medical problems, as well as immunosuppressed patients, are now routinely undergoing surgery.

The inability to casually evaluate patients awaiting surgery in a hospital setting has necessitated a more efficient process for identifying potential adverse drug interactions during the perioperative period and for having more rapid access to key pharmacologic and drug dosage information. The availability of a pocket-size drug reference manual would allow the practitioner to quickly review essential pharmacokinetics, pharmacodynamics, drug dosage, and interactions. The concept in writing the *Perioperative Drug Manual* was to develop a concise template containing key information on the pharmacology of virtually all drugs in the *Physicians' Desk Reference (PDR)* for busy physicians and nurses caring for surgical patients in both the hospital and clinic setting.

The drugs in this book are grouped according to the pharmacologic classification system utilized by the PDR and the *United States Pharmacopeia (USP)*. Within each of the 40 drug classes, the drugs are arranged alphabetically according to their generic name. The properties listed include the generic and trade names, clinical indications, principal pharmacokinetic and dynamic features, dosages (and/or concentrations), contraindications, and adverse drug interactions. Finally, key points relevant to the management of patients during the perioperative period have been provided. The concept was to allow practitioners to quickly identify the salient pharmacologic properties of an unfamiliar drug without having to wade through a voluminous amount of text material or locate one of the large reference sources. Hopefully, this goal has been realized in the Second Edition of this manual.

Paul F. White

Acknowledgments

As the complexity of medical care has grown and the number of medications being prescribed to surgical patients has increased dramatically over the past 10 years, it has become necessary to greatly expand the original concept for this drug manual to include virtually all currently available pharmaceutical products. To complete this lengthy literature review in a timely fashion, I enlisted the expert assistance of Linda D. White, MS, and Irina Gasanova, MD, PhD. Both these individuals were incredibly helpful with this "in-depth" analysis of the pharmacologic properties of the important drugs in medicine. Without the tireless efforts of my administrative assistant, Dolly Tutton, this project would not have been completed. The gracious assistance of Publisher Natasha Andjelkovic at Elsevier in facilitating the publication of this drug manual is also deeply appreciated. Finally, I would like to acknowledge my family, friends, and colleagues in anesthesia, surgery, critical care, and pain management, who have provided loving support and encouragement during this labor-intensive project. I would like to express a special thanks to Pablo McClure, a fantastic artist and a "muy bien amigo" from Santiago, Chile, who generously allowed me to use one of his beautiful paintings on the book's cover; Mike Howie, a special friend and colleague who shares my passion for scientific knowledge and the arts, for the kind words and the beautiful Celtic poem; and my brother "Big Ed," a gentle giant whose creative talents never cease to amaze me, for creating the lovely artwork on the dedication page. Hopefully, the "rebirth" of my **White Mountain Institute** from the ashes of the Cedar fire in Julian, California, will serve to advance both art and science in the future. Finally, I would like to express my most sincere appreciation to a very special Texan, Margaret Milam McDermott, who has generously supported both the arts and medicine through a lifetime of giving. In addition to being extremely generous in her support of the University of Texas Southwestern Medical Center and our local museums, she has been a wonderful friend to me and my daughters. I am indeed honored and privileged to hold the Margaret Milam McDermott Distinguished Chair in Anesthesiology, which was established by her late husband, Eugene McDermott. Without the unfailing support of Mrs. Eugene McDermott, I would not have had the time necessary to complete this project!

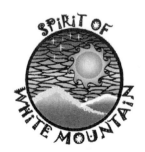

Contents

1

Adrenergic Agonists and Antagonists

Adrenergic Agonists

CLONIDINE

Trade Name:	**Catapres**
Indications:	Hypertension, anesthetic and analgesic adjuvant, vasomotor menopausal symptoms, opioid withdrawal, nicotine withdrawal, migraine (vascular) headache, ulcerative colitis, diabetic diarrhea, postoperative shivering
Pharmacokinetics:	Onset: 60–90 min (TTS 12–24 h); bioavailability: 100%; peak: 1–3 h; protein binding: 30%; Cl: 3.1 mL/min/kg; duration: 12–24 h (TTS 7–8 d); Vd: 2.1 L/kg; $T_{1/2}$ β: 12–16 h; hepatic metabolism (40%) and urinary excretion

Pharmacodynamics: Centrally acting α_2-adrenergic receptor agonist/antagonist
- *CNS:*   Drowsiness, dizziness, depression
- *CV:*   ↓ BP, ↓ SVR, ↓ HR, pedal edema, ↓ renin activity
- *GI:*   Dry mouth, constipation, nausea, vomiting, ↑ LFTs
- *Other:*   Fluid retention, pruritus, ↓ libido, diaphoresis

Dosage:	0.2–0.8 mg/d in divided doses; 3–5 µg/kg (IV); 150 µg (IT); 0.1–0.3 mg/72 h (TTS)
Contraindications:	Porphyria, Raynaud's phenomenon, breast-feeding
Drug Interactions:	Abrupt withdrawal causes rebound ↑ BP, antagonized by MAOIs and TCAs, cimetidine ↑ CNS toxicity, β-blockers enhance ↓ HR
Key Points:	↓ Anesthetic and analgesic requirements, produces sedation during perioperative period; TTS patch should be applied the day prior to surgery and removed 2–3 d prior to elective cardioversion

DEXMEDETOMIDINE

Trade Name:	**Precedex**
Indications:	Anesthetic and analgesic adjuvant, sedative/analgesic in ICU
Pharmacokinetics:	Onset: <5 min; peak: 20–30 min; protein binding: 94%; Vd_{ss}: 2.2 L/kg; Cl: 0.75 L/kg/h; $T_{1/2}$ β: 2 h; extensively metabolized and excreted in urine

Pharmacodynamics: Centrally acting α_2-receptor agonist
- *CNS:*   Sedation, dizziness, headache, confusion, neuralgias
- *CV:*   Sympatholysis (↓ catecholamines), ↓ HR, sinus arrest, ↓ BP, oliguria

DEXMEDETOMIDINE *continued*

GI:	Dry mouth, nausea, vomiting, thirst, diarrhea
Pulmonary:	Hypoxia, pleural effusion, edema
Other:	↓ ACTH, ↓ ADH, ↓ insulin, ↑ growth hormone, anemia, leukocytosis, ↓ shivering, impaired wound healing

Dosage: 0.25–1.0 µg/kg IV (boluses), 0.5–2.5 µg/kg IM (↓ in elderly); 0.2–0.7 µg/kg/h infusion (<24 h)

Contraindications: Sick sinus syndrome, 1st- and 2nd-degree AV, hypovolemia

Drug Interactions: ↑ Sedation with CNS-depressant drugs

Key Points: ↑ Bradycardia with opioid analgesics and/or β-blockers; use as adjuvant to ↓ anesthetic and analgesic requirements, improves control of perioperative hypertension

DOBUTAMINE

Trade Name: **Dobutrex**

Indications: Low cardiac output states after cardiac surgery, CHF and acute MI, pulmonary hypertension

Pharmacokinetics: Onset: 1–2 min; peak: <10 min; duration <5 min (after infusion); Vd: 0.25 L/kg; Cl: 2.35 L/min/m²; $T_{1/2}$ β: 3 min; metabolized in liver, excreted in urine

Pharmacodynamics: β_1-adrenergic receptor agonist, weak effect on β_2 and α_1 receptors

CNS:	↑ CBF, headaches
CV:	↓ BP, ↑ contractility, ↑ SV, ↑ CO, ↑ HR, ↓ SVR, ↓ atrial filling pressure, arrhythmias, palpitations, ↑ RBF, thrombophlebitis
GI:	Nausea, vomiting
Pulmonary:	↓ Pulmonary vascular resistance, wheezing

Dosage: 2–20 µg/kg/min IV infusion (do *not* mix with alkaline solutions)

Contraindications: Idiopathic hypertrophic subaortic stenosis (IHSS), pregnancy

Drug Interactions: ↑ α-adrenergic effects with β-blockers, bretylium, guanadrel, guanethidine, oxytocic drugs

Key Points: ↑ Arrhythmias with volatile anesthetics, β-blockers may antagonize ↑ CO, correct hypovolemia using volume expanders, incompatible with alkaline solutions, heparin, steroids, antibiotics

DOPAMINE

Trade Name:	**Intropin**
Indications:	Shock, acute cardiac failure, acute renal failure, ↓ HR
Pharmacokinetics:	Onset: <5 min; peak: 5–10 min; duration: <10 min (after infusion); Vd: 0.25 L/kg; $T_{1/2}$ β: 2 min; does not cross blood-brain barrier; metabolized in kidney and plasma by MAO and COMT, excreted in urine
Pharmacodynamics:	Endogenous catecholamine
CNS:	Intracerebral vasodilation; headache
CV:	↑ CO, coronary dilation, vasoconstriction (at high doses), ventricular arrhythmias, palpitations, angina, ↑ RBF
GI:	Nausea, vomiting, mesenteric vasodilation
Pulmonary:	↑ Pulmonary artery pressure, ↓ hypoxic drive, dyspnea, wheezing
Other:	Tissue necrosis, piloerection, hyperglycemia, ↑ Na excretion, azotemia
Dosage:	0.5–2 µg/kg/min (renal); 2–10 µg/kg/min (cardiac); 10–20 µg/kg/min (vascular)
Contraindications:	Pheochromocytoma, tachyarrhythmias
Drug Interactions:	Effects prolonged and intensified by MAOIs; phenytoin can cause seizures, ↓ BP, and ↓ HR; butyrophenones ↓ vascular vasodilation
Key Points:	Volatile anesthetics can ↑ HR and/or ↑ arrhythmias; abrupt withdrawal can result in severe hypotension during perioperative period

EPHEDRINE

Trade Name:	**Same**
Indications:	Bronchospasm, nasal decongestant, orthostatic hypotension, enuresis, myasthenia gravis
Pharmacokinetics:	Onset: <5–10 min (IV/IM), 30–60 min (oral); duration: 30–60 min (parenteral), 3–5 h (oral); $T_{1/2}$ β: 3–6 h; crosses placenta; metabolized in liver (oxidative deamination), excreted in urine
Pharmacodynamics:	Noncatecholamine sympathomimetic with both direct and indirect α- and β-adrenergic stimulation
CNS:	Restlessness, insomnia, tremor, confusion, dizziness
CV:	↑ CO, ↑ BP, ↑ HR, arrhythmias, palpitations, angina, ↓ RBF
GI:	Nausea, vomiting, anorexia
GU:	↑ Uterine blood flow, dysuria, urinary retention
Pulmonary:	Bronchodilation, pulmonary edema (rare)

EPHEDRINE *continued*

Other:	Constricts vessels in skin and mucous membranes; muscle weakness, diaphoresis, hyperglycemia
Dosage:	5–20 mg IV q 5–10 min (<150 mg/d), 25–50 mg SC/IM; 3 mg/kg IV qd (children)
Contraindications:	Angle-closure glaucoma, heart disease, hypertension, diabetes, hyperthyroidism, benign prostatic hypertrophy (BPH)
Drug Interactions:	↑ Effects with other sympathomimetics; MAOIs and TCAs ↑ pressor effects, α- and β-blockers effects
Key Points:	Anticholinergics and theophylline attenuate ↑ HR and BP; volatile anesthetics ↑ arrhythmias

EPINEPHRINE

Trade Name:	**Adrenaline**
Indications:	Bronchospasm, anaphylaxis, cardiac arrest, ↑ myocardial contractility, prolong local anesthetics, open-angle glaucoma
Pharmacokinetics:	Onset: <15 min; peak: <30 min; duration: 1–4 h; Cl: 62 mL/kg/min; $T_{1/2}$ β: 2 min (IV); crosses blood-brain barrier, but not placenta; terminated by uptake and metabolism in sympathetic nerve ending; hepatic metabolism, excreted in urine
Pharmacodynamics:	Endogenous catecholamine, activates α- and β-adrenergic receptors
CNS:	Restlessness, tremor, headache, disorientation, dizziness, weakness, cerebral hemorrhage
CV:	↑ CO, ↑ MVO_2, ↑ SV, ↑ HR, ↑ contractility, ↑ BP, ↑ arrhythmias, ↑ coronary blood flow, vasoconstriction, ↓ RBF, ↑ renin, angina
GI:	↑ Splanchnic blood flow, nausea, vomiting
Other:	Hypokalemia, ↑ temperature, uterine relaxant, hyperglycemia, lipolysis
Dosages:	*For bronchospasm:* 0.1–0.5 mg SC/IM q 0.5–4 h (0.1–0.5 mL of 1:1000 solution), followed by 0.1–1 µg/kg/min infusion (inotropic support); 0.01 mg/kg SC q 0.5–4 h (children) *For anaphylaxis:* 0.5–1 mg IV q 3–5 min (5–10 mL of 1:10,000 solution) (anaphylaxis); 0.01–0.03 mg/kg IV q 3–5 min (children) *For local anesthesia:* 1:100,000 (10 µg/mL); 1:200,000 (5 µg/mL)
Contraindications:	Angle-closure glaucoma, β-blocker therapy, hyperthyroidism

EPINEPHRINE *continued*

Drug Interactions:	↓ Effects with α- and β-blockers; ↑ insulin requirements in diabetics; MAOIs, TCAs, antihistamine, oxytocics, thyroid supplements ↑ risk of hypertensive crisis
Key Points:	Potential CV toxicity when combined with other sympathomimetics; limit dose to <5 µg/kg with volatile anesthesia to ↓ risk of arrhythmias

GUANABENZ

Trade Name:	**Wytensin**
Indications:	Hypertension, opioid withdrawal syndrome
Pharmacokinetics:	Onset: <60 min; peak: 2–4 h; protein binding: 90%; duration: 6–8 h; Vd: 100 L/kg; Cl: 1.3 mL/min/kg; $T_{1/2}$ β: 6–12 h; extensive 1st-pass metabolism, excreted 1° in urine
Pharmacodynamics:	Centrally acting $α_2$-adrenergic receptor agonist
CNS:	Drowsiness, dizziness, headache
CV:	↓ BP, ↓ SVR, ↓ HR
GI:	Dry mouth
Dosage:	4–8 mg PO bid (max. 32 mg/d)
Contraindications:	None known
Drug Interactions:	Withdrawal produces rebound ↑ BP; ↑ effect with other antihypertensives (e.g., β-blockers); naloxone precipitates rebound hypertension
Key Points:	↑ Sedative effects of IV and volatile anesthetics, possesses both anesthetic and analgesic-sparing effects

GUANFACINE

Trade Name:	**Tenex**
Indications:	Hypertension, opioid withdrawal symptoms, migraine headaches
Pharmacokinetics:	Onset: 30 min; bioavailability: 80%; peak: 1–4 h; protein binding: 70%; duration: 24 h; Vd: 6.5 L/kg; Cl: 2.6–5.2 mL/min/kg; $T_{1/2}$ β: 12–22 h; hepatic metabolism with urinary excretion
Pharmacodynamics:	Centrally acting $α_2$-adrenergic receptor agonist
CNS:	Dizziness, somnolence, confusion, fatigue, insomnia
CV:	↓ HR, ↓BP, ↓ SVR
GI:	Dry mouth, nausea, constipation
Other:	Impotence, ↑ growth hormone levels, pruritus

GUANFACINE *continued*

Dosage:	0.5–3 mg/d PO
Contraindications:	None known
Drug Interactions:	Withdrawal syndrome (rebound ↑ BP), estrogens, NSAIDs, TCAs ↓ antihypertensive effect; effects antagonized with naloxone (with ↑ BP)
Key Points:	Opioid-sparing and ↑ CNS depressant effects of anesthetic drugs; withdrawal ↑ postoperative hypertension

ISOPROTERENOL

Trade Name:	**Isuprel**
Indications:	Bronchodilation, bradyarrhythmias, heart block, shock
Pharmacokinetics:	Onset: <1 min; peak: <5 min; duration: <10 min (IV), 1–2 h (SC/inhaler); metabolized in liver, excreted in urine
Pharmacodynamics:	Synthetic sympathomimetic amine, direct β_1 and β_2 stimulant
CNS:	Nervousness, insomnia, dizziness, headache
CV:	↑ HR, ↑ contractility, ↑ CO, ↑ automaticity, ↓ conduction time, ↓ SVR
GI:	Nausea, vomiting, dyspepsia
Pulmonary:	Bronchodilation, ↓ PVR, pulmonary edema, ↑ sputum
Other:	Diaphoresis, hyperglycemia, parotid swelling
Dosages:	*For bronchospasm:* 1–2 puffs (80 µg/metered spray) 4–6 times/d; 0.5% for nebulization, 5–15 puffs (max. 5 times/d) *For hypotension:* 0.2 mg IM/SC; 0.5–5 µg/min IV (adult); 0.05–0.1 µg/kg/min (children) *For heart block:* 0.02–0.06 mg IV (adult); 0.01–0.03 mg IV (children) followed by 0.02–0.15 µg/kg/min infusion
Contraindications:	Cardiac arrhythmias, angina, advanced heart block, tachycardia 2° to glycoside intoxication
Drug Interactions:	↑ Cardiotoxicity with other sympathomimetics or theophylline; effects antagonized by β-blockers, ↑ arrhythmias with glycosides and K^+-depleting diuretics; ↑ pressor response with TCAs, bretylium, oxytocics, guanethidine
Key Points:	Potential CV toxicity when combined with other bronchodilators, arrhythmias with volatile anesthetics and sympathomimetic drugs

MEPHENTERMINE

Trade Name:	**Wyamine**
Indications:	Hypotension (during spinal anesthesia), ganglionic blockade
Pharmacokinetics:	Onset: <2 min (IV), <15 min (IM); duration: 15–30 min (IV) and 1–4 h (IM); metabolized in liver, excreted in urine
Pharmacodynamics:	Synthetic sympathomimetic, stimulates α- and β-receptors
CNS:	Restlessness, ↑ CBF
CV:	↑ Contractility, ↑ BP
Dosage:	0.5 mg/kg IM; 20–60 mg IV, then infusion at 1–5 mg/min; 0.4 mg/kg IM (children)
Contraindications:	Hypertension, hyperthyroidism, hemorrhagic shock
Drug Interactions:	Digitalis ↑ arrhythmias; MAOIs ↑ CV effects; phenothiazine, reserpine, guanethidine ↓ hypertensive response
Key Points:	↑ Volatile anesthetic requirement; may produce arrhythmias during general anesthesia with volatile agents

METAPROTERENOL

Trade Names:	**Alupent, Metaprel**
	See Chapter 18, "Bronchodilators"

METARAMINOL

Trade Name:	**Aramine**
Indications:	Intraoperative hypotension, paroxysmal atrial tachycardia (PAT)
Pharmacokinetics:	Onset: <2 min (IV), <10 min (IM), <20 min (SC); peak: 20–90 min; does not cross blood-brain barrier; effect terminated by uptake of drug into tissues
Pharmacodynamics:	Synthetic sympathomimetic amine, stimulates both β- and α-adrenergic receptors
CNS:	Restlessness, ↑ CBF, ↓ $CMRO_2$
CV:	↑ BP, reflex, ↓ HR, (+) inotrope, ↓ RBF
GI:	↓ Hepatic and mesenteric blood flow
GU:	Uterine stimulant
Other:	Glycogenolysis, ↓ insulin release, lipolysis, ↑ body temperature

METARAMINOL *continued*

Dosage:

2–10 mg IM/SC q 10 min, or 0.5–5 mg IV, followed by 1 mg/kg SC/IM q 10 min; 0.01 mg/kg IV, then 0.4 mg/kg (children)

Contraindications:

Sulfite allergic, peripheral/mesenteric thrombosis

Drug Interactions:

α- and β-blockers, ↓ CV effects; MAOIs, TCAs, guanethidine, ergot alkaloids ↑ pressor effects

Key Points:

Severe vasoconstriction diminishes hepatic and renal function in shocklike states, risk of arrhythmias with volatile anesthetics

METHOXAMINE

Trade Name:

Vasoxyl

Indications:

Hypotension (shock), paroxysmal SVT

Pharmacokinetics:

Onset: <2 min (IV), <20 min (IM); duration: 5–15 min (IV) and 60–90 min (IM); hepatic metabolism, excreted in urine

Pharmacodynamics:
CNS:
CV:
GI:
GU:
Pulmonary:
Other:

Selective α_1-adrenergic agonist
Nervousness, restlessness, ↑ CBF
↑ BP, reflex, ↓ HR, ↑ PVR, ↓ RBF
Projectile vomiting, ↓ splanchnic and hepatic blood flow
Bladder contractions, ↓ uterine blood flow
↑ Pulmonary artery pressure
Extravasation causes tissue sloughing

Dosages:

For shock: 5–20 mg IM or 2–5 mg IV q 15 min
For PSVT: 10 mg IV over 3–5 min or 10–20 mg IM; 0.25 mg/kg IV, then 0.08 mg/kg IV (children)

Contraindications:

Sulfite allergic, severe hypertension

Drug Interactions:

Phenothiazine and furosemide ↓ pressor effect; MAOIs, TCAs, vasopressin and ergot alkaloids ↑ CV effects

Key Points:

Hypotensive-prone anesthetic technique (e.g., central neuroaxis blockade) should be avoided

METHYLDOPA

Trade Name:

Aldomet

Indications:

Hypertension

Pharmacokinetics:

Onset: 1–2 h; bioavailability 25%; peak: 4–6 h; protein binding: 15%; duration: 10–24 h; Vd: 0.60 L/kg; Cl: 3.1 mL/min/kg; $T_{1/2}$ β: 1.4 h; metabolized to α_2-methyl-norepinephrine and epinephrine, excreted in urine

METHYLDOPA *continued*

Pharmacodynamics:	Centrally acting α_2-adrenergic receptor agonist
CNS:	Sedation, headache, dizziness, paresthesia, parkinsonism, $\downarrow$ mental acuity, movement disorders
CV:	$\downarrow$ HR, $\downarrow$ BP, $\downarrow$ SVR, orthostatic hypotension, myocarditis, angina
GI:	Dry mouth, colitis, diarrhea, nausea, vomiting, $\uparrow$ LFTs
Other:	(+) Coombs' test, hemolytic anemia, bone marrow depression, impotence, arthralgias, gynecomastia, galactorrhea, rash, $\uparrow$ BUN, amenorrhea, pedal edema
Dosage:	250–2000 mg/d PO in divided doses ($\downarrow$ dose in elderly)
Contraindications:	Acute hepatitis, cirrhosis, porphyria, use of MAOIs, breast-feeding
Drug Interactions:	MAOIs can cause hyperexcitability and $\uparrow$ BP; $\downarrow$ response to ephedrine; sympathomimetics $\uparrow$ pressor effects; haloperidol produces confusion, $\uparrow$ lithium levels; $\uparrow$ antihypertensives and diuretics
Key Points:	$\uparrow$ Opioid analgesia, $\downarrow$ volatile anesthetic requirement, may cause acute hypertension after dialysis

NOREPINEPHRINE

Trade Name:	**Levophed**
Indications:	Hypotension, GI bleeding, CPR
Pharmacokinetics:	Onset: <1 min; peak: <2 min; duration: <5 min; $T_{1/2}\,\beta$: 2 min; localizes mainly in sympathetic tissue; crosses placenta but not blood-brain barrier; uptake and metabolism in nerve endings; hepatic metabolism via COMT and MAO, excreted in urine
Pharmacodynamics:	Endogenous catecholamine, direct-acting adrenergic agonist
CNS:	$\downarrow$ CBF, headache, restlessness, weakness, insomnia
CV:	$\uparrow$ SVR, $\uparrow$ BP, $\downarrow$ RBF, (+) inotrope, $\downarrow$ HR, arrhythmias
GI:	$\downarrow$ Hepatic and splanchnic blood flow
Metabolic:	$\uparrow$ Glycogenolysis, $\downarrow$ insulin release, $\uparrow$ lipolysis, $\uparrow$ body temperature
Pulmonary:	$\uparrow$ Pulmonary artery pressure, wheezing
Other:	Extravasation causes necrosis and sloughing, uterine stimulant
Dosages:	*For hypotension:* 8–12 µg/min IV initially, followed by 2–4 µg/min; 2 µg/min IV (children) *For CPR:* 0.1 µg/kg/min (to max. 2 µg/kg/min)
Contraindications:	Pregnancy, sulfite allergic, mesenteric/peripheral vascular thrombosis, profound hypovolemia, hypoxia

NOREPINEPHRINE *continued*

Drug Interactions:	α- and β-adrenergic blockers ↓ pressor effect; TCAs, MAOIs, antihistamines, guanethidine, methyldopa may cause hypertensive crisis
Key Points:	Avoid hypotensive-prone anesthetic technique (e.g., central neuroxis block) and halothane due to arrhythmias, general anesthetics can ↑ hypotension in the presence of volume depletion

OXYMETAZOLINE

Trade Names:	**Afrin, Allerest**
Indications:	Nasal congestion, eye redness
Pharmacokinetics:	Onset: 5–10 min; peak: 6 h; duration: <12 h
Pharmacodynamics:	Direct-acting α-adrenergic sympathomimetic agonist, mucosal vasoconstriction
CNS:	Headache, insomnia, drowsiness, dizziness, nervousness, ↑ IOP
CV:	Palpitations, ↑ HR, ↑ BP
GI:	Dry mucous membranes, rebound nasal congestion
Other:	Blurred vision, lacrimation, keratitis
Dosage:	0.025% and 0.05% spray, 2–3 metered doses into each nostril q 10–12 h; 1–2 drops in each eye qid
Contraindications:	Severe hypertension, angle-closure glaucoma, BPH
Drug Interactions:	β-blockers ↑ CV toxicity; TCAs ↑ pressor effects
Key Points:	Use with volatile anesthetics and sympathomimetics ↑ dysrhythmias in patients with cardiac disease; local anesthetics ↑ absorption

PHENYLEPHRINE

Trade Name:	**Neo-Synephrine**
Indications:	Hypotension (during spinal anesthesia), shock, paroxysmal SVT, prolong local anesthetics, nasal decongestion, mydriasis
Pharmacokinetics:	Onset: <2 min (IV/mucosal); duration: 15–20 min (IV), 0.5–2 h (SC/IM), 0.5–4 h (nasal), 3–7 h (ophthalmic); effects terminated by uptake into tissues; metabolized in liver and intestine by MAOIs
Pharmacodynamics:	Synthetic sympathomimetic with direct α-adrenergic receptor activity
CNS:	Headache, restlessness, tremor, dizziness

PHENYLEPHRINE *continued*

CV:	Vasoconstriction, ↑ BP, ↓ HR (reflex); ↑ coronary blood flow, arrhythmias
GI:	Nausea, ↑ splanchnic and hepatic blood flow
Pulmonary:	Wheezing, ↑ pulmonary artery pressure
Other:	Pallor, dermatitis, diaphoresis, tissue sloughing with extravasation, uterine stimulant
Dosages:	0.1–0.5 mg IV (boluses), or 2–5 mg IM; 0.1–0.4 mg/kg IM/SC (children) *For PSVT:* 0.5–1 mg IV, then ↑ 0.1–0.2 mg increments
Contraindications:	Severe hypertension, ventricular tachycardia, mesenteric vascular thrombosis, injections into end arteries, angle-closure glaucoma
Drug Interactions:	↑ Pressor effects with oxytocin, MAOIs, TCAs, guanethidine; ↓ pressor response with phenothiazines
Key Points:	↑ Arrhythmias with volatile anesthetics and sympathomimetic adjuvants

PSEUDOEPHEDRINE

Trade Name:	**Sudafed**
Indications:	Nasal and eustachian tube congestion
Pharmacokinetics:	Onset: <30 min; peak: 0.5–1 h; Vd: 3 L/kg; duration: 4–12 h; $T_{1/2}$ β: 6 h; hepatic *N*-demethylation, excreted in urine
Pharmacodynamics:	Synthetic sympathomimetic amine, directly stimulates α- and β-adrenergic receptors, indirectly releases norepinephrine
CNS:	Restlessness, agitation, headache, tremor, dizziness, insomnia
CV:	↑ HR, arrhythmia, palpitations
GI:	Anorexia, nausea, vomiting, dry mouth
Other:	Dysuria
Dosage:	50 mg PO q 4–6 h; 15–30 mg PO q 4–6 h (children)
Contraindications:	Severe hypertension, CAD, MAOI therapy, breast-feeding
Drug Interactions:	MAO and β-adrenergic blockers ↑ pressor effect; ↓ effects of methyldopa, mecamylamine, reserpine, TCAs antagonize effects
Key Points:	Use with volatile anesthetics may predispose to ↑ HR and arrhythmias

RITODRINE

Trade Name:	**Yutopar**
Indications:	Preterm labor (to inhibit uterine contractions)
Pharmacokinetics:	Onset: 15 min (SC), 30 min (oral); bioavailability: 40% (oral); peak: 30 min (SC), 2–3 h (oral); duration: 2–4 h (SC), 4–8 h (oral); $T_{1/2}$ β: 10 h (IV), 20 h (oral); crosses placenta and blood-brain barrier; metabolized in liver, excreted in urine
Pharmacodynamics:	Synthetic sympathomimetic amine, $β_2$-selective stimulant
CNS:	Headache, anxiety, tremor, nervousness, dizziness, diaphoresis
CV:	↑ HR, ↑ CO, ↑ BP, arrhythmias, palpitations, flushing
GI:	Nausea, vomiting, dyspepsia
GU:	Uterine smooth muscle relaxant (tocolytic)
Metabolic:	↑ Maternal/fetal glucose, ↑ insulin, hypokalemia, ketoacidosis
Pulmonary:	Bronchodilation, dyspnea, pulmonary edema
Dosage:	50–100 µg/min for 12 h (to cessation of uterine contractions), followed by 10 mg PO q 2 h for 24 h, then 10–20 mg q 4–6 h
Contraindications:	Pulmonary edema, sulfite allergic, <20 wk gestation, eclampsia, uterine hemorrhage, fetal death, abruptio placentae, placenta previa, arrhythmia, pulmonary hypertension, pheochromocytoma, hyperthyroidism, uncontrolled diabetes
Drug Interactions:	Corticosteroids can ↑ pulmonary edema; sympathomimetics, meperidine, anticholinergics, $MgSO_4$, ↑ CV effects and β-adrenergic blockers ↓ CV effect
Key Points:	Volatile anesthetics should be avoided because ↑ risk of arrhythmias and potentiation of CV depression

Adrenergic Antagonists

ALFUZOSIN

Trade Name:	**Uroxatral**
Indications:	BPH
Pharmacokinetics:	Onset: 1 h; bioavailability: 49%; peak: 2–3 h; protein binding: 86%; duration: 24 h; Vd: 3.2 L/kg; Cl: 80 mL/min; $T_{1/2}$ β: 10 h; extensive hepatic metabolism
Pharmacodynamics:	Selectively blocks α_1-adrenergic receptors in the lower urinary tract; relaxes smooth muscle in bladder neck
CNS:	Dizziness, headache, tiredness (fatigue)
CV:	↓ BP, syncope, angina
Pulmonary:	URI
Dosage:	10 mg/d
Contraindications:	Hepatic insufficiency, potent CYP3A4 inhibitors, women/children, other α-blocking drugs
Drug Interactions:	Diltiazem, atenolol ↑ antihypertensive effect; ketoconazole, itraconazole, ritonavir ↑ effect
Key Points:	May enhance hypotensive effects of anesthetic drugs

DOXAZOSIN

Trade Name:	**Cardura**
Indications:	Hypertension, BPH
Pharmacokinetics:	Onset: 1–2 h; bioavailability: 65%; peak: 2–3 h; protein binding: 98%; duration: 24 h; $T_{1/2}$ β: 22 h; metabolized in liver, excreted 1° in the feces
Pharmacodynamics:	Selective α_1-adrenergic blocker
CNS:	Somnolence, fatigue, headache, vertigo
CV:	Orthostatic hypotension, angina, edema, arrhythmia, ↑ HR
GI:	Nausea, vomiting
GU:	Sexual dysfunction, polyuria, incontinence
Pulmonary:	Dyspnea
Other:	Arthralgias, myalgias, fluid retention, skin rash
Dosage:	1–8 mg/d (max. 16 mg)
Contraindications:	Sensitivity to quinazolines (i.e., prazocin, terazosin), breast-feeding
Drug Interactions:	β-blockers ↑ hypotension, ↓ effect of clonidine
Key Points:	Use with volatile anesthetics and central neuroaxic blocks accentuate hypotensive responses

GUANADREL

Trade Name:	**Hylorel**
Indications:	Hypertension
Pharmacokinetics:	Onset: <30 min; peak: 1.5–2.0 h; protein binding: 20%; Cl: 38 mL/min/kg; Vd: 11.5 L/kg; T$_{1/2}$ β: 5–45 h; urinary excretion (85%)
Pharmacodynamics:	Peripheral-acting adrenergic blocker
CNS:	Dizziness, faintness, paresthesias
CV:	↓ BP, ↓ SVR, orthostatic hypotension, ↑ HR
GI:	Diarrhea
Pulmonary:	Cough, dyspnea, ↑ wheezing
Other:	Retrograde ejaculation, pedal edema, fluid retention
Dosage:	20–75 mg/d PO in divided doses
Drug Interactions:	↑ Sensitivity to catecholamines; antagonized by TCAs and phenothiazines; MAOIs ↑ BP (discontinue >2 wk)
Key Points:	Adequate hydration before induction of anesthesia ↓ risk of acute intraoperative hypotension

GUANETHIDINE

Trade Name:	**Ismelin**
Indications:	Hypertension, thyrotoxicosis
Pharmacokinetics:	Onset: 1–3 h; bioavailability: 20%; peak: 8 h (max. 1–3 wk); protein binding: <10%; duration: 3–4 d; Cl: high; T$_{1/2}$ β: 43 h; hepatic metabolism, urinary excretion
Pharmacodynamics:	Peripheral-acting adrenergic blocker, inhibits norephinephrine release and depletes norephinephrine in adrenergic nerves
CNS:	Fatigue, headache, paresthesia, confusion, depression
CV:	↓ BP, ↓ SVR, ↓ cardiac output, fluid retention, orthostatic hypotension, ↓ HR, angina, syncope
GI:	Diarrhea, dry mouth, peptic ulceration, dyspepsia, anorexia
Pulmonary:	Nasal congestion, dyspnea, cough, ↑ wheezing
Other:	Delayed ejaculation, myalgia (cramps), urinary incontinence
Dosage:	10–50 mg/d PO
Contraindications:	Pheochromocytoma, MAOI therapy, CHF, acute MI, asthma

GUANETHIDINE *continued*

Drug Interactions:
Antagonized by TCAs, phenothiazines, oral contraceptives, indirect sympathomimetics; MAOIs ↑ BP, ↑ oral hypoglycemic agents, dopamine, phenylephrine

Key Points:
Preoperative use can ↑ hypotensive effect of general anesthetics, discontinue 2–3 wk before elective surgery

PHENOXYBENZAMINE

Trade Name:
Dibenzyline

Indications:
Hypertension (2° to pheochromocytoma), vasospastic disorders (Raynaud's)

Pharmacokinetics:
Onset: 2–3 h; duration: 3–4 d; $T_{1/2}$ β: 24 h; metabolized in liver, excreted in urine and feces

Pharmacodynamics:
α-adrenergic receptor antagonist
CNS: Sedation
CV: ↓ BP, reflex ↑ HR, ↑ CO, ↑ RBF
GI: ↑ Splanchnic blood flow, nausea, vomiting, dry mouth

Dosage:
10 mg PO bid (max. 40 mg); 0.2–0.4 mg/kg/d (max. 10 mg), then 0.4–1.2 mg/kg/d (children)

Contraindications:
Severe hypotension (shock)

Drug Interactions:
Antagonist-stimulating drugs, α- and β-agonists (e.g., epinephrine) cause ↓ BP and ↑ HR

Key Points:
↓ Absorption of local anesthetic following regional nerve block; adequate preoperative hydration prevents anesthesia-induced hypotension

PHENTOLAMINE

Trade Name:
Regitine

Indications:
Hypertension (2° to pheochromocytoma), autonomic hyperreflexia, dermal necrosis and sloughing (due to drug extravasation)

Pharmacokinetics:
Onset: <2 min; duration: 10–15 min; hepatic metabolism, excreted in feces

Pharmacodynamics:
α-adrenergic receptor antagonist
CNS: Dizziness, weakness, cerebrovascular spasm
CV: ↓ BP, (+) inotrope and chronotrope, ↑ CO, ↑ HR, arrhythmias, angina, orthostatic hypotension, shock, flushing
GI: Hyperperistalsis, abdominal pain, diarrhea, ↑ gastric acid and pepsin secretion, nausea, vomiting, nasal congestion

PHENTOLAMINE *continued*

GU:	Uterine relaxant
Pulmonary:	↓ Pulmonary artery pressure, bronchodilation
Dosage:	5 mg IM/IV 1–2 h preoperatively, infusion 0.1–1 mg/min (10–20 µg/kg/min), 5 mg during surgery; 0.1 mg/kg IM/IV (children)
Contraindications:	Gastritis/peptic ulcer, CAD, acute MI, severe hypotension
Drug Interactions:	Antagonizes effects of epinephrine and ephedrine, ↑ β_2-adrenergic vasodilatation
Key Points:	Adequate hydration required to prevent hypotension during induction of general anesthesia (or after spinal block); avoid nasal intubation due to nasal mucosal vasodilation

PRAZOSIN

Trade Name:	**Minipress**
Indications:	Hypertension, BPH
Pharmacokinetics:	Onset: 0.5–1.5 h; peak: 2–4 h (max. 4–6 wk); duration: 7–10 h; $T_{1/2}$ β: 2–3 h; metabolized in liver, excreted in feces
Pharmacodynamics:	Selective, reversible α-adrenergic receptor antagonist
CNS:	Dizziness, headache, drowsiness, nervousness, paresthesia, weakness
CV:	Postural hypotension, syncope, edema, palpitations
GI:	Vomiting, nausea, abdominal cramps, ↑ LFTs
GU:	Priapism, impotence, urinary frequency/incontinence
Other:	Arthralgia, myalgia, pruritus, diaphoresis, fever
Dosage:	1–2 mg PO bid (max. 20 mg/d)
Contraindications:	Chronic antihypertensive therapy, chronic renal failure
Drug Interactions:	Diuretics ↑ hypotensive effect
Key Points:	Use with volatile anesthetic or spinal block techniques accentuates hypotensive effect

TERAZOSIN

Trade Name:	**Hytrin**
Indications:	Hypertension, BPH
Pharmacokinetics:	Onset: 15 min; bioavailability: 90%; peak: 2–3 h; protein binding: 94%; duration: 24 h; $T_{1/2}$ β: 12 h; hepatic metabolism, excreted in urine and feces

TERAZOSIN *continued*

Pharmacodynamics:	Selective α_1-adrenergic receptor antagonist
CNS:	Paresthesias, somnolence, headache, nervousness, asthenia
CV:	Orthostatic hypotension, arrhythmias, palpitations, pedal edema
GI:	Nausea, nasal congestion, sinusitis
GU:	Impotence, priapism, UTI
Pulmonary:	Dyspnea
Other:	Thrombocytopenia, blurred vision, muscle pain
Dosage:	1–2 mg/d PO (max. 10 mg/d)
Contraindications:	Sensitivity to quinazoline derivatives
Drug Interactions:	Antihypertensive and α-blocker ↑ hypotension, ↓ clonidine effect
Key Points:	↑ Volatile anesthetic or spinal-induced hypotension; avoid nasal intubation

TOLAZOLINE

Trade Name:	**Priscoline**
Indications:	Pulmonary hypertension, vasospastic disorders (Raynaud's)
Pharmacokinetics:	Onset: <2 min; peak: 1 h; duration: 2–4 h
Pharmacodynamics:	Mixed α-adrenergic blocker, pulmonary and systemic vasodilator
CV:	↓ PVR, ↓ BP, ↑ HR
GI:	↑ Gastric secretion, mucosal ulcers
Dosage:	0.5–1.0 mg/kg IV
Contraindications:	Severe hypotension (shock)
Drug Interactions:	H_2-blocker ↓ acute CV effects
Key Points:	Premedication with an H_2-blocker is recommended; use with volatile anesthetics and spinal blockade accentuates hypotensive response

2

Angiotensin-Converting
Enzyme (ACE) Inhibitors
and Receptor
Antagonists

BENAZEPRIL, FOSINOPRIL, PERINDOPRIL

Trade Names:	**Lotensin (benazepril), Monopril (fosinopril), Aceon (perindopril)**
Indications:	Hypertension, CHF
Pharmacokinetics:	Onset: 1 h; peak: 2–4 h; protein binding: 95%; duration: 24 h; metabolized in liver to active metabolites (i.e., benazeprilat, fosinoprilat, perindroprilat), excreted 1° in urine
Pharmacodynamics:	Inhibits conversion of angiotensin I to angiotensin II
CNS:	Headache, dizziness, fatigue, paresthesia, nervousness
CV:	↓ BP, ↓ SVR, palpitation, angina, arrhythmias
GI:	Nausea, vomiting, ↑ salivation, constipation, abdominal pain
GU:	Impotence, ↓ libido, ↑ BUN/Cr, proteinuria
Pulmonary:	Dry cough, dyspnea, laryngeal edema, sinusitis
Other:	Dysphagia, diaphoresis, angioedema, rash, arthralgia, bone marrow suppression, myalgia, ↑ K^+
Dosages:	*Benazepril:* 10 mg/d PO (max. 40 mg/d) *Fosinopril:* 10 mg/d PO (max. 80 mg/d) *Perindopril:* 4 mg/d PO (max. 16 mg/d)
Contraindications:	Breast-feeding, pregnancy
Drug Interactions:	Antihypertensives ↑ hypotension; K^+-sparing diuretics ↑ ↑ K^+; ↑ digoxin and lithium levels; antacids ↓ absorption; capsicum ↑ coughing
Key Points:	Adequate hydration during general anesthesia minimizes hypotension; ↑ K^+ occurs with concomitant use of K^+-containing solutions

CANDESARTAN, OLMESARTAN-MEDOXOMIL

Trade Names:	**Atacand (candesartan), Benicar (olmesartan-medoxomil)**
Indications:	Hypertension
Pharmacokinetics:	Onset: <1 h; bioavailability: 26%; peak: 1–2 h; protein binding: 99%; duration: 24 h; Vd: 17 L; Cl: 1.3 L/h; $T_{1/2}$ β: 9–13 h; prodrug metabolized to olmesartan during GI absorption; minimal hepatic metabolism, excreted 1° in feces
Pharmacodynamics:	Selectively blocks binding of angiotensin II to angiotensin I receptor in vascular smooth muscle and adrenal gland

CANDESARTAN, OLMESARTAN-MEDOXOMIL *continued*

CNS:	Dizziness, fatigue, headache
CV:	Peripheral edema, orthostatic hypotension ($\downarrow$ SVR)
GI:	Nausea, vomiting, diarrhea, abdominal pain
GU:	Albuminuria, hematuria, hyperuricemia
Pulmonary:	Cough, URI
Other:	Back pain, flulike symptoms, hyperglycemia, myalgia
Dosages:	*Candesartan:* 8–16 mg/d PO (max. 32 mg/d)
	Olmesartan: 20–40 mg/d PO
Contraindications:	Chronic renal failure, sulfonamide-type allergies
Drug Interactions:	Thiazide diuretics enhance salt and water excretion; $\uparrow$ antihypertensives; $\uparrow$ lithium toxicity
Key Points:	$\uparrow$ Hypotensive effects of anesthetic and analgesic drugs; $\uparrow$ neuromuscular block with curare-like muscle relaxants

CAPTOPRIL, MOEXIPRIL

Trade Names:	**Capoten (captopril), Univasc (moexipril)**
Indications:	Hypertension, CHF, diabetic nephropathy, Raynaud's syndrome
Pharmacokinetics:	Onset: 30 min; bioavailability: 65% ($\downarrow$ with food); peak: 1–2 h; protein binding: 30%; duration: 6–12 h; Vd: 0.7 L/kg; Cl: 13 mL/min/kg; $T_{1/2}$ β: 2 h; 1° urinary excretion
Pharmacodynamics:	Competitive inhibitor of ACE, $\downarrow$ formation of angiotensin II
CNS:	Headache, fatigue
CV:	$\downarrow$ BP, $\downarrow$ SVR, angina, CHF
GI:	$\downarrow$ Taste, cholestatic jaundice, $\uparrow$ LFTs
Pulmonary:	Dry cough (with capsaicin), airway edema
Renal:	$\uparrow$ BUN/Cr, proteinuria
Other:	Rash, pruritus, blood dyscrasias, $\uparrow$ K$^+$, angioedema
Dosages:	*Captopril:* 12.5–25 mg tid, $\uparrow$ to 100 tid (max. 450 mg/d); 100 mg/d; $\downarrow$ dose if sodium-depleted (e.g., diuretics), $\downarrow$ renal function in elderly
	Moexipril: 7.5 mg/d, $\uparrow$ to 30 mg/d (max. 60 mg)
Contraindications:	Porphyria, renovascular disease, SLE, pregnancy, valvular stenosis
Drug Interactions:	Diuretics $\uparrow$ hypotensive effect; NSAIDs $\downarrow$ antihypertensive effect; antacids $\downarrow$ absorption; $\uparrow$ lithium and digoxin levels
Key Points:	Intraoperative $\downarrow$ BP should be treated with volume replacement

ENALAPRIL/ENALAPRILAT

Trade Names:	**Vasotec (enalapril), Vasotec IV (enalaprilat)**
Indications:	Hypertension (with diuretic), CHF, LV dysfunction
Pharmacokinetics:	Onset: 15 min (IV), 1 h (oral); bioavailability: 40%; peak: 1–4 h (IV), 4–6 h (oral); protein binding: 50%; duration: 6 h (IV), 24 h (oral); Vd: 1.7 L/kg; Cl: 4.9 mL/min/kg; $T_{1/2}$ β: 35 h; enalapril is a prodrug with an active metabolite (enalaprilat [IV]); extensively metabolized, excreted 1° in urine
Pharmacodynamics:	ACE inhibitor, ↓ angiotensin II, ↓ aldosterone
CNS:	Headache, fatigue, somnolence, paresthesia, vertigo
CV:	↓ BP, ↓ SVR, angina, ↓ HR, angioedema, ↑ CO
GI:	Loss of taste, nausea, diarrhea, abdominal pain
Pulmonary:	Wheezing, dry cough (with capsaicin), dyspnea
Renal:	↑ BUN/Cr (with renal artery stenosis), proteinuria
Other:	Rash, bone marrow suppression, blurred vision
Dosages:	*Enalapril:* 2.5–5.0 mg PO (max. 40 mg/d) *Enalaprilat:* 0.625–1.25 mg IV q 6 h IV
Contraindications:	Porphyria, pregnancy
Drug Interactions:	↑ Hypotensive effects of vasodilators, phenothiazines, diuretics; ASA, NSAIDs ↓ hypotensive effect; ↑ risk of hypoglycemia; ↑ lithium level; ↓ rifampin level
Key Points:	Hypotension in patients under general anesthesia should be treated with vasopressin agonists; risk of ↑ K^+ with K^+-containing solutions

EPLERENONE

Trade Name:	**Inspra**
Indications:	Hypertension
Pharmacokinetics:	Onset: rapid; peak: 1.5 h; protein binding: 50%; duration: 12 h; Vd: 65 L; Cl: 10 L/h; $T_{1/2}$ β: 4–6 h; metabolized by CYP_{450} 3A4, excreted in urine and feces
Pharmacodynamics:	Blocks aldosterone binding at the mineralocorticoid receptor
CNS:	Headache, dizziness, fatigue
CV:	Angina, hypotension
GI:	Diarrhea, abdominal pain, ↑ GGT
GU:	Albuminuria, vaginal bleeding, ↑ BUN/Cr, ↑ K^+
Pulmonary:	Coughing
Other:	Flulike symptoms, ↑ renin, ↑ aldosterone, gynecomastia

EPLERENONE *continued*

Dosages: 25–50 mg PO bid

Contraindications: ↑ K+ (>5.5 mEq/L); type 2 diabetes with microalbumin-
                             uria; Cr >2 mg/dL or CrCl <50 mL/min

Drug Interactions: Use with other cytochrome P_{450} 3A4 inhibitors
                             (e.g., ketoconazole, fluconazole) ↑ effect; ACE
                             inhibitors ↑ K

Key Points: Careful monitoring of ECG when administering
                             anesthetic drugs that can acutely ↑ K+ (e.g.,
                             succinylcholine)

EPROSARTAN, IRBESARTAN, TELMISARTAN

Trade Names: **Teveten (eprosartan), Avapro (irbesartan),
                             Micardis (telmisartan)**

Indications: Hypertension, diabetic nephropathy

Pharmacokinetics: Onset: 1–2 h; bioavailability: 25%; peak: 0.5–3 h;
                             protein binding: >95%; duration: 24 h; $T_{1/2}$ β: 5–24 h;
                             metabolized in liver, excreted in bile and feces

Pharmacodynamics: Selectively blocks binding of angiotensin II,
                             ↓ aldosterone
  CNS: Dizziness, headache, fatigue, anxiety, depression
  CV: Peripheral edema, ↑ HR, orthostatic hypotension
  GI: Nausea, vomiting, diarrhea, dyspepsia, ↑ LFTs
  GU: UTI, ↑ BUN/Cr
  Pulmonary: Dry cough, pharyngitis, sinusitis
  Other: Neutropenia, myalgias, arthralgias, angioedema

Dosages: *Eprosartan:* 400–800 mg/d PO
                             Irbesartan: 75–300 mg/d PO
                             Telmisartan: 40–80 mg/d PO

Contraindications: Pregnancy, severe CHF, volume depleted, renal failure

Drug Interactions: ↑ Digoxin level; ↑ lithium toxicity; ↓ warfarin levels;
                             ACTH, steroids ↑ hypokalemia

Key Points: CNS depressants ↑ risk of intraoperative hypotension
                             in type 2 diabetics and with end-stage renal disease;
                             ↑ response to muscle relaxants

LISINOPRIL

Trade Names: **Zestril, Prinivil**

Indications: Hypertension (with diuretic), CHF, acute MI

LISINOPRIL *continued*

Pharmacokinetics:	Onset: 1 h; bioavailability: 30%; peak: 7 h; minimal protein binding; duration: 24 h; Vd: 1.8 L/kg; Cl: 1.5 mL/min/kg; $T_{1/2}$ β: 12 h; not metabolized, excreted unchanged in urine
Pharmacodynamics:	ACE inhibitor, ↓ aldosterone secretion
CNS:	Headache, fatigue, dizziness, paresthesias, syncope
CV:	Orthostatic hypotension, ↓ SVR, ↓ BP (if sodium-depleted)
GI:	Nausea, diarrhea, ↑ LFTs
Pulmonary:	Dry cough (with capsaicin), airway edema, dyspnea
Renal:	↑ BUN/Cr, ↑ K^+
Other:	Impotence, ↑ K^+, ↓ WBC, rash, angioedema
Dosage:	2.5–5 mg, ↑ to 5–40 mg/d (↓ dose if sodium-depleted, ↓ renal function in elderly)
Contraindications:	Porphyria, hypotension, renovascular disease, pregnancy
Drug Interactions:	↑ Hypotensive effects with vasodilators; indomethacin attenuates ↓ BP; ↑ lithium levels
Key Points:	↑ Hypotensive effects of anesthetic drugs, ↑ muscle relaxant effects of curare-like neuromuscular blockers

LOSARTAN

Trade Name:	**Cozaar**
Indications:	Hypertension, diabetic nephropathy
Pharmacokinetics:	Onset: <30 min; peak: 1 h; high protein binding; duration: 8–12 h; Vd: 34 L; Cl: 600 mL/min; $T_{1/2}$ β: 2 h; hepatic metabolism via cytochrome P_{450} to form an active metabolite, excreted 1° in feces
Pharmacodynamics:	Angiotensin II receptor antagonist, ↓ aldosterone
CNS:	Dizziness, insomnia, asthenia, fatigue, headache
CV:	↓ BP, ↓ SVR, arrhythmias, angina, pedal edema
GI:	Dyspepsia, diarrhea, abdominal pain, nausea
Pulmonary:	Nasal congestion, dry cough, sinusitis, pharyngitis, URI
Other:	Angioedema, ↑ K^+, hypoglycemia, cramps, myalgia
Dosage:	25–50 mg PO bid (or 50–100 mg/d)
Contraindications:	Pregnancy, breast-feeding, hepatorenal dysfunction
Drug Interactions:	None known
Key Points:	With volume depletion, marked hypotension may occur during anesthesia

QUINAPRIL, RAMIPRIL, TRANDOLAPRIL

Trade Names:	**Accupril (quinapril), Altace (ramipril), Mavik (trandolapril)**
Indications:	Hypertension, CHF
Pharmacokinetics:	Onset: 1–4 h; peak: 1–10 h; protein binding: 85%; duration: 24 h; $T_{1/2}$ β: 6–25 h; metabolized in liver to active metabolites (e.g., quinaprilat, ramiprilat, trandolaprilat), excreted 1° in urine
Pharmacodynamics:	ACE inhibitors, ↓ angiotensin II, ↓ aldosterone
CNS:	Somnolence, headache, dizziness, seizures
CV:	Orthostatic hypotension, ↓ HR, arrhythmia, angina, flushing
GI:	Dry mouth, nausea, vomiting, abdominal pain
GU:	Urinary frequency, impotence, ↓ libido
Pulmonary:	Dry cough (with capsaicin), tickling sensation
Other:	↑ K^+, neutropenia/agranulocytosis, ↓ platelets, pruritus, exfoliative dermatitis, photosensitivity, angioedema
Dosages:	*Quinapril:* 5 mg PO bid (max. 40 mg/d) (heart failure); 10–20 mg/d (max. 80 mg/d) (hypertension) *Ramipril:* 2.5 mg/d (max. 20 mg/d) *Trandolapril:* 1–2 mg/d (max. 8 mg/d)
Contraindications:	Cardiogenic shock, renal failure; pregnancy, breast-feeding
Drug Interactions:	Antacids and fatty food ↓ bioavailability, ↑ digoxin and lithium levels; ↓ tetracycline absorption; K^+-sparing diuretics ↑ risk of ↑ K^+; antihypertensives and diuretics ↑ risk of hypotension; sun exposure ↑ risk of photosensitivity; licorice ↓ effect
Key Points:	IV and volatile anesthetics ↑ risk of intraoperative hypotension; K^+-containing solutions ↑ risk of ↑ K^+

VALSARTAN

Trade Name:	**Diovan**
Indications:	Hypertension, CHF
Pharmacokinetics:	Onset: <2 h; bioavailability: 25%; peak: 2–4 h; highly protein bound; Cl: 2 L/h; duration: 24 h; Vd: 17 L; $T_{1/2}$ β: 6 h; minimally metabolized, excreted 1° in feces
Pharmacodynamics:	Angiotensin II receptor antagonist, ↓ aldosterone
CNS:	Anxiety, insomnia, somnolence, paresthesia, tinnitis, vertigo
CV:	Syncope, ↑ HR, edema, orthostatic hypotension, flushing
GI:	Dyspepsia, dry mouth, abdominal pain, nausea

VALSARTAN *continued*

GU:	Dysuria, impotence, UTI, micturition, ↑ BUN/Cr
Pulmonary:	Dyspnea, bronchospasm, pharyngitis, sinusitis
Other:	Rash, diaphoresis, hyperuricemia, blurred vision, angioedema
Dosage:	40 mg PO bid, ↑ to 80 mg bid (max. 320 mg/d)
Contraindications:	None known
Drug Interactions:	Diuretics ↑ hypotensive response
Key Points:	Risk of ↑ K⁺ with CHF; volatile anesthetics may cause marked hypotension with volume depletion

3

Antacids and Antisecretories

ALUMINUM CARBONATE, ALUMINUM HYDROXIDE, MAGNESIUM HYDROXIDE, MAGNESIUM TRISILICATE, CALCIUM CARBONATE

Trade Names:	**Basaljel, Amphojel, Milk of Magnesia, Alamag, Maalox, Almacone, Gelusil, Aludrox, Mylanta, Magnatril, Calcilac**
Indications:	Hyperacidity, gastric/duodenal ulcer, gastroesophageal reflux, gastric aspiration prophylaxis, postoperative gas pain, hyperphosphatemia
Pharmacokinetics:	Onset: <10 min ($CaCO_3$, MgOH), 20 min ($AlCO_2$, AlOH, Mg trisilicate); minimally absorbed; duration: 20–180 min (on empty stomach), 2–3 h (after meal); crosses placenta; excreted in breast milk
Pharmacodynamics:	Particulate antacids neutralize acid in GI tract, binds phosphate (Al)
CNS:	Neurotoxicity, encephalopathy
GI:	↑ Gastric pH, inhibits pepsin, ↑ gastric volume, ↑ lower esophageal sphincter tone, laxative effect (Mg), constipation (Al), intestinal obstruction (Al), rebound hyperacidity (Ca)
Pulmonary:	Lung damage (if aspirated)
Other:	Metabolic alkalosis, Al intoxication, osteomalacia, osteoporosis, hypophosphatemia (Al), inhibited precipitation of calcium oxalate (MgOH), hypermagnesemia, milk-alkali syndrome ($CaCO_3$)
Dosage:	15–45 mL PO q 2–3 h; 5–15 mL q 3–6 h (children)
Contraindications:	Severe renal disease, Alzheimer's disease
Drug Interactions:	↓ Absorption of digoxin, phenytoin, chlorpromazine, isoniazid; oral tetracycline and cimetidine; ↑ absorption of psuedophedrine and levodopa; ↑ urinary pH ↓ quinidine and amphetamine excretion; ↑ salicylate excretion; Al and Mg intoxication with renal impairment; renal calculi with prolonged use of Ca antacids
Key Points:	Administration prior to induction of anesthesia ↑ residual gastric volume, should be combined with metoclopramide

CIMETIDINE

Trade Name:	**Tagamet**
Indications:	Gastric aspiration prophylaxis (e.g., parturients, hiatal hernia, esophageal dysfunction), duodenal ulcer, Zollinger-Ellison syndrome

CIMETIDINE *continued*

Pharmacokinetics:
Onset: <30 min; bioavailability: 69%; peak: 45–90 min (oral); protein binding: 18%; duration: 4–5 h; $T_{1/2}$ β: 2 h (PO), parenteral, 1–2 h (IV); hepatic metabolism (30–40%); renal elimination: (parenteral) 75% unchanged, (oral) 48% unchanged, crosses placenta, excreted in breast milk

Pharmacodynamics:
Inhibits histamine at gastric H_2 receptors
CNS: Dizziness, confusion, agitation, headache, somnolence
CV: Arrhythmias, ↓ HR, ↓ BP, ↓ RBF
GI: ↓ Gastric acid/volume, diarrhea, ↑ LFTs
Pulmonary: Wheezing
Other: Gynecomastia, impotence, neutropenia, myalgias, skin rash

Dosage:
200–800 mg PO 60–90 min before anesthesia or 150–300 mg IV 30–60 min before anesthesia

Contraindications:
Breast-feeding, hepatic dysfunction

Drug Interactions:
↓ Metabolism of lidocaine, xanthines, phenytoin, phenothiazines, metronidazole, triamterene, quinidine, propranolol, coumarin, TCAs, alcohol, procainamide, nifedipine, dobutamine, α-methyldopa, clonidine; ↑ effects of antihypertensive drugs; antacids ↓ absorption

Key Points:
Dilute parenteral solution with D_5W, may prolong clinical effects of benzodiazepines and potent opioid analgesics

ESOMEPRAZOLE

Trade Name:
Nexium

Indications:
GERD, erosive esophagitis, *Helicobacter pylori* eradication

Pharmacokinetics:
Onset: <1 h; bioavailability: 64–90% (↓ with food); peak: 1.5 h; protein binding: 97%; duration: 13–17 h; Vd: 16 L; $T_{1/2}$ β: 1–1.5; metabolized in liver by cytochrome P_{450}, excreted 1° in urine

Pharmacodynamics:
Proton pump inhibition, ↓ gastric acid secretion
CNS: Headache
GI: Diarrhea, nausea, flatulence, dry mouth, vomiting

Dosage:
20–40 mg/d for 4–8 wk (GERD); 20 mg/d for 6 mo (erosive esophagitis); 40 mg/d with amoxicillin (1 g bid) and clarithromycin (500 mg bid) for 10 d (*H. pylori*)

Contraindications:
Pregnancy, breast-feeding, hepatic dysfunction

ESOMEPRAZOLE *continued*

Drug Interactions:	Amoxicillin and clarithromycin ↑ levels
Key Points:	May prolong effect of benzodiazepines due to ↓ hepatic clearance

FAMOTIDINE

Trade Name:	**Pepcid**
Indications:	GERD, gastric aspiration prophylaxis, Zollinger-Ellison syndrome
Pharmacokinetics:	Onset: <1 h; bioavailability: 42%; peak: 0.5–4 h; protein binding: 15%; duration: 10–15 h; $T_{1/2}$ β: 2.5–4 h; hepatic metabolism, excreted 1° in urine; crosses placenta, excreted in breast milk
Pharmacodynamics:	Inhibits histamine at gastric H_2 receptors
CNS:	Dizziness, headache, confusion, tinnitis, malaise, paresthesias
CV:	Arrhythmias, palpitations, flushing
GI:	Constipation, nausea, vomiting, ↓ appetite, ↓ gastric acid/volume, dry mouth, taste disorder, jaundice, ↑ LFTs
Pulmonary:	Bronchospasm
Other:	Rash, acne, thrombocytopenia, orbital edema, arthralgias, myalgias
Dosage:	20–40 mg PO prior to surgery (↓ dosage with renal disease)
Contraindications:	Breast-feeding
Drug Interactions:	Weak inhibitor of hepatic drug metabolism; antacids ↓ absorption; ↓ ketoconazole absorption
Key Points:	Tolerance develops to ↓ gastric acid secretion with prolonged use (>4 wk); fewer side effects than cimetidine

LANSOPRAZOLE

Trade Name:	**Prevacid**
Indications:	Erosive esophagitis, duodenal and gastric ulcer, GERD, *H. pylori* eradications, Zollinger-Ellison syndrome
Pharmacokinetics:	Onset: <30 min; bioavailability: >80%; peak: 1–2 h; plasma protein binding 97%; metabolized in liver, excreted 1° in feces
Pharmacodynamics:	Inhibits proton pump activity at gastric parietal cells
CNS:	Asthenia, headache, agitation, paresthesia, fever, tinnitus

LANSOPRAZOLE *continued*

CV:	Angina, pedal edema, palpitations, vasodilation
GI:	Diarrhea, halitosis, dyspepsia, eructation, abdominal pain
GU:	Impotence, candidiasis, renal calculus, gynecomastia
Pulmonary:	Bronchitis, cough, URI
Other:	Acne, rash, pruritus, arthritis, myalgia, diabetes, gout
Dosage:	15–30 mg/d before meals for 4–8 wk (ulcers and GERD); 30 mg tid with amoxicillin 1 g tid for 14 d (*H. pylori*); 60 mg/d (Zollinger-Ellison)
Contraindications:	Sensitivity to proton pump inhibitors (PPIs)
Drug Interactions:	Sucralfate ↓ absorption; ↓ absorption of ampicillin, iron, salts, ketoconazole; ↑ theophylline excretion
Key Points:	No known adverse interactions with anesthetic drugs

MAGALDRATE (ALUMINUM MAGNESIUM HYDROXIDE)

Trade Names:	**Iosopan, Riopan**
Indications:	Indigestion, hyperacidity
Pharmacokinetics:	Onset: 20 min; peak: 30–60 min; duration: 120–180 min; no metabolism; excreted in feces
Pharmacodynamics:	Reduces direct acid irritant effect; ↑ gastric pH inactivates pepsin; ↑ GE sphincter tone
GI:	Mild constipation, diarrhea
Other:	Hypokalemia
Dosage:	0.5–1 g PO between meals and at bedtime
Contraindications:	Severe renal disease
Drug Interactions:	↓ Drug absorption (e.g., anticoagulants, benzodiazepines, phenothiazines), ↓ NMDA receptor activity
Key Points:	Check renal function and electrolyte levels preoperatively

MISOPROSTOL

Trade Name:	**Cytotec**
Indications:	Gastric ulcers, hyperacidity conditions
Pharmacokinetics:	Onset: <30 min; protein binding: 90%; peak: 14–20 min; duration: 3–6 h; $T_{1/2}$ β: 20–40 min; rapidly de-esterified in liver to active metabolites; excreted 1° in urine

MISOPROSTOL *continued*

Pharmacodynamics:	Synthetic PGE_1 analogue, $\downarrow$ gastric acid, $\uparrow$ bicarbonate secretion
CNS:	Headache, fatigue, anxiety
CV:	Arrhythmias
GI:	Diarrhea, dyspepsia, nausea, flatulence
Respiratory:	Wheezing, depression
Other:	Uterine cramps, hypermenorrhea, postmenopausal bleeding
Dosage:	100–200 µg PO qid with meal ($\downarrow$ dosage with renal disease)
Contraindications:	Pregnancy, breast-feeding
Drug Interactions:	Blocks cyclosporine-induced $\downarrow$ renal function
Key Points:	In women with child-bearing potential, do pregnancy test <2 wk of initiating therapy for NSAID-induced gastritis

NIZATIDINE

Trade Name:	**Axid**
Indications:	Gastric acid aspiration prophylaxis, duodenal ulcer, GERD
Pharmacokinetics:	Onset: 0.5 h; bioavailability: >90%; peak effect: 1–3 h; protein binding: 35%; duration: 6–12 h; $T_{1/2}\beta$: 1–2 h; hepatic metabolism; excreted 1° in urine; crosses placenta, excreted in breast milk
Pharmacodynamics:	Competitive, reversible gastric H_2 receptor antagonist
CNS:	Dizziness, somnolence, confusion
CV:	Arrhythmias
GI:	Constipation, nausea, vomiting, $\downarrow$ gastric acid/volume, $\uparrow$ LFTs
Other:	Rash, diaphoresis, thrombocytopenia, gynecomastia, gout
Dosage:	150–300 mg PO prior to surgery (1.5–2 mg/kg in children)
Contraindications:	Severe renal impairment
Drug Interactions:	Weak inhibitor of hepatic drug metabolism; antacids $\downarrow$ absorption; $\uparrow$ salicylate level
Key Points:	Tolerance to effects on gastric acid secretion with prolonged use; cholinergic side effects with overdosage

OMEPRAZOLE

Trade Names:	**Prilosec, Losec**
Indications:	Gastroesophageal reflux, gastric acid hypersecretion (Zollinger-Ellison syndrome), active duodenal and gastric ulcers, *H. pylori* eradication
Pharmacokinetics:	Onset: <1 h; peak: 1–4 h; protein binding: 95%; duration: >72 h; $T_{1/2}$ β: 0.5–1 h; metabolized by liver, excreted 1° in urine
Pharmacodynamics:	Inhibits activity of acid (proton) pump; ↓ H^+/K^+ ATPase activity at the secretory surface of gastric parietal cell; ↓ gastric acid formation
CNS:	Dizziness, headache, asthenia
GI:	Abdominal pain, colic
GU:	Hematuria, UTI
Pulmonary:	Cough, URI
Other:	Bone marrow suppression, rash, Stevens-Johnson syndrome, erythema multiforma, myalgias
Dosage:	20–60 mg/d for 2–8 wk
Contraindications:	Severe hepatic impairment
Drug Interactions:	↓ Absorption of ampicillin, iron salts, itraconazole, ketoconazole; ↓ metabolism of drugs dependent on hepatic cytochrome P_{450} metabolism (e.g., anticoagulants, diazepam, propranolol, theophylline, phenytoin); ↑ leukopenia or thrombocytopenia with chemotherapy
Key Points:	May prolong CNS depressant and cardiovascular effect of anesthetic drugs dependent on hepatic clearance for early recovery

PANTOPRAZOLE

Trade Name:	**Protonix**
Indications:	Erosive esophagitis, GERD, gastric hypersecretion (Zollinger-Ellison)
Pharmacokinetics:	Onset: <30 min (IV); bioavailability: 77%; peak: 2–3 h; protein binding: 99%; duration: 24 h; metabolized in liver via cytochrome P_{450}; excreted 1° in urine
Pharmacodynamics:	Inhibits proton pump by binding to hydrogen-potassium ATPase on surface of gastric parietal cells
CNS:	Migraine headache, insomnia, asthenia, dizziness
CV:	Angina
GI:	Abdominal pain (cramps), gastroenteritis
GU:	Urinary frequency, UTI
Pulmonary:	Bronchitis, cough, dyspnea, URI
Other:	Hyperglycemia, hyperlipidemia, rash

PANTOPRAZOLE *continued*

Dosage:	40 mg/d IV for 7–10 d (GERD and hypersecretion); 80 mg IV bid for 6 d (Zollinger-Ellison); 40 mg/d PO (chronic antacid)
Contraindications:	None known
Drug Interactions:	↓ Absorption of ampicillin, iron salts, ketoconazole
Key Points:	Rapid oral absorption on empty stomach in the preoperative period

RABEPRAZOLE

Trade Name:	**Aciphex**
Indications:	GERD, erosive esophagitis, duodenal ulcer, gastric hypersecretion (Zollinger-Ellison syndrome)
Pharmacokinetics:	Onset: <1 h; peak: 2–5 h; protein binding: 96%; duration: 24 h; $T_{1/2}$ β: 1–2 h; hepatic metabolism, excreted 1° in urine
Pharmacodynamics:	Inhibits H^+-K^+ ATPase (proton) pump on gastric parietal cells
CNS:	Headache, asthenia
GI:	Dyspepsia, flatulence
Dosage:	20 mg/d (GERD, duodenal ulcer); 60 mg/d (max. 100 mg/d) (Zollinger-Ellison)
Contraindications:	Severe hepatic impairment
Drug Interactions:	Inhibits cyclosporin metabolism; ↓ absorption of digoxin, ketoconazole, low pH–dependent drugs
Key Points:	No interactions with anesthetic drugs have been reported

RANITIDINE

Trade Name:	**Zantac**
Indications:	Gastric acid aspiration prophylaxis (e.g., parturients, hiatal hernia, esophageal dysfunction), duodenal ulcer, hypersecretory conditions
Pharmacokinetics:	Onset: 1 h; bioavailability: 50%; peak: 1–3 h; protein binding: 15%; duration: 13 h; $T_{1/2}$ β: 2–3 h; hepatic metabolism, excreted 1° in urine, crosses placenta, excreted in breast milk

RANITIDINE *continued*

Pharmacodynamics:	Competitively inhibits gastric H_2 receptor antagonist
CNS:	Dizziness, malaise, confusion, blurred vision
CV:	Arrhythmias, angioedema
GI:	↓ Gastric acid/volume, constipation, nausea, vomiting, ↑ LFTs
Other:	Gynecomastia, skin rash, reversible pancytopenia, arthralgias
Dosage:	150 mg PO or 50 mg IV 60–90 min before surgery; (1.5–2 mg/kg PO in children)
Contraindications:	Breast-feeding; hepatic dysfunction
Drug Interactions:	Antacids ↓ absorption; ↓ metabolism of coumarin, nifedipine, phenytoin, theophylline, midazolam, alcohol metaprolol; ↓ elimination of procainamide; ↓ diazepam absorption
Key Points:	Tolerance develops to antisecretory effect (>4 wk); the H_2-blocker least likely to interfere with anesthetic and analgesic drugs

SODIUM CITRATE

Trade Names:	Bicitra, Polycitra, Alka-Seltzer
Indications:	Neutralize gastric fluid (pH), cystitis
Pharmacokinetics:	Onset: rapid (mixing with gastric acid <1 h); duration: 1–3 h
Pharmacodynamics:	Nonparticulate antacid, metabolized to Na^+ and water to bicarbonate (Na^+ bicarbonate)
GI:	↑ Gastric acid/gastric volume, ↑ gastric distention, flatulence, unpleasant taste
Pulmonary:	↓ Pulmonary damage if aspirate gastric contents
Other:	Metabolic alkalosis, hypernatremia, hypocalcemia, ↑ K^+
Dosage:	10–20 mL; 10–15 mL (<30 min prior to anesthesia)
Contraindications:	Gastric obstruction, hypertension, hepatorenal impairment
Drug Interactions:	↑ Toxicity with K^+-containing medications and K^+-sparing diuretics
Key Points:	Use with metoclopramide to minimize ↑ residual gastric volume when given immediately prior to induction of anesthesia

4

Antiarrhythmics

ACEBUTOLOL

Trade Name:	Sectral
Indications:	Hypertension, ventricular arrhythmias, angina
Pharmacokinetics:	Onset: 1.5 h; bioavailability: 40%; peak: 2–3 h; protein binding: 26%; duration: 24 h; Vd: 1.6–3 L/kg; Cl: 7–11 mL/min/kg; $T_{1/2}$ β: 3–4 h (8–13 h diacetolol); crosses placenta and breast milk; extensive 1st-pass metabolism to active metabolite (diacetolol); excreted 1° in feces
Pharmacodynamics:	Cardioselective $β_1$ antagonist, AV nodal conduction velocity
CNS:	Fatigue, dizziness, headaches, depression, anxiety
CV:	↓ BP, ↓ HR, membrane-stabilizing effect on heart, antiarrhythmic activity (class II), ↑ RBF, heart failure
GI:	Dyspepsia, nausea, vomiting, abdominal pain
Pulmonary:	Wheezing (in asthmatics/COPD)
Other:	Impotence, pruritis, dysuria, SLE
Dosage:	200–400 mg/d (hypertension and angina); 200 mg bid (arrhythmias)
Contraindications:	Severe myocardial dysfunction, 2nd or 3rd AV block, breast-feeding, active bronchospastic disease
Drug Interactions:	Antihypertensives ↑ hypotensive effect, NSAIDs and α-adrenergic stimulants ↓ hypotensive effect; acute withdrawal causes rebound ↑ HR and ↑ BP, masks signs of hyperthyroidism and hypoglycemia; antagonizes bronchodilation produced by β agonists; ↑ hypoglycemia with glyburide
Key Points:	Masks signs of intraoperative blood loss; use with volatile anesthetics causes dose-dependent cardiac depression

ADENOSINE

Trade Name:	Adenocard
Indications:	Paroxysmal SVT, Wolff-Parkinson-White syndrome, controlled hypotension, thallium stress testing
Pharmacokinetics:	Onset: <2 min; peak: <2 min; $T_{1/2}$ β: 10 sec; biotransformation: immediate; deamination, phosphorylation, and cellular uptake
Pharmacodynamics:	Class IV antiarrhythmic, naturally occurring nucleoside, slows conduction through A-V node, inhibits reentry pathways

ADENOSINE *continued*

CNS:	Dizziness, numbness, blurred vision, headaches, irritability
CV:	↓ HR, ↓ BP, arrhythmias, chest pain, palpitations, facial flushing
GI:	Nausea, metallic taste
Pulmonary:	Dyspnea, wheezing, chest tightness, cough
Dosage:	3–6 mg IV over 1–2 min (max. 12 mg over 5 min); 0.05–0.25 mg/kg IV (children)
Contraindications:	Advanced heart block, sick sinus syndrome, asthma
Drug Interactions:	Methylxanthines, caffeine, CCBs ↓ effect; dipyridamole, carbamazepine ↑ effect
Key Points:	↑ Hypotensive effects of volatile anesthetics and opioid analgesics; transient asystole may occur with rapid IV administration; ↓ opioid analgesic requirement

AMIODARONE

Trade Names:	**Cordarone, Pacerone**
Indications:	Ventricular tachycardia and SVT
Pharmacokinetics:	Onset: 1–2 h; bioavailability: 22–86%; peak: 3–7 h; protein binding: 96%; duration: 40–50 d; Vd: 66 L/kg; Cl: 1.9 mL/min/kg; $T_{1/2}$ β: 25–110 d; metabolized in liver (active metabolite desethylamiodarone), excreted in bile
Pharmacodynamics:	Class III antiarrhythmic; inhibits repolarization; ↑ PR, RR, QT intervals; ↑ nodal refractoriness; blocks β-adrenergic receptors
CNS:	Fatigue, peripheral neuropathy, ataxia, tremor, headache, insomnia
CV:	↓ HR, cardiac arrest, ↓ BP, CHF, ventricular arrhythmias
GI:	Nausea, vomiting, ↑ LFTs, constipation, abdominal pain, anorexia
Pulmonary:	Interstitial pneumonitis, hemoptysis, pleuritis, wheezing
Other:	Parotitis, hyperthermia, thyroid dysfunction, skin discoloration, visual disturbance (corneal deposits), myopathy, pancytopenia
Dosage:	400–800 mg q 8–12 h for 10–14 d, then 600–800 mg/d for 4–8 wk, followed by 200–600 mg/d
Contraindications:	SA node disease, 2nd- and 3rd-degree AV blockade (without pacemaker), concomitant use of ritonavir

AMIODARONE *continued*

Drug Interactions:
↑ Effects of digoxin, warfarin, metoprodol, quinidine, procainamide, phenytoin, encainide, lidocaine, precainide, diltiazem (↓ dosages by 50%); ↑ bradycardia and AV block with β-adrenergic antagonists and CCBs; cholestyramine ↑ elimination; cimetidine ↑ levels; disopyramide, phenothiazines, sparfloxacin TCAs ↑ QT interval (torsades de pointes)

Key Points:
↑ Myocardial depressant effects of volatile anesthetics

BRETYLIUM

Trade Name:
Bretylol

Indications:
Ventricular tachycardia or fibrillation (VT)

Pharmacokinetics:
Onset: 3–40 min; protein binding: 1–10%; duration: 6–24 h; Vd: 8 L/kg; Cl: 10 mL/min/kg; $T_{1/2}$ β: 5–10 h; excreted unchanged in urine

Pharmacodynamics:
Class III antiarrhythmic, inhibits repolarization (↑ APD, ↑ ERP), transient catecholamine release

CNS:
Dizziness, syncope

CV:
↓ HR, ↓ BP, ↓ PVR (vasodilation), orthostatic hypotension

GI:
Nausea, vomiting, diarrhea

Other:
Rash, hyperthermia, renal impairment, respiratory depression

Dosage:
5–10 mg/kg IV over 10–30 min, repeat in 1–2 h (max. 30 mg/kg); 1–2 mg/min infusion

Contraindications:
Digitalis toxic, aortic stenosis, pulmonary hypertension

Drug Interactions:
↑ Effects of lidocaine, procainamide β-blockers; MAOIs ↑ catecholamine release; TCAs block drug uptake in adrenergic nerve

Key Points:
↑ Toxicity of local anesthetics and hypotensive effects of general anesthetics, ↑ neuromuscular blockers

DIGOXIN

Trade Names:
Lanoxin, Lanoxicaps, Digitek

Indications:
CHF, ↓ ventricular response to atrial fibrillation/flutter, PAT

DIGOXIN *continued*

Pharmacokinetics:
: Onset: 5–30 min (IV), <30 min (IM/IV), 1.5–2 h (oral); bioavailability: 72%; peak: 1–6 h; protein binding: 25%; duration: 3–4 d; Vd: 3.12 L/kg; Cl: 0.88 mL/min/kg (therapeutic level: 0.5–2 ng/mL); $T_{1/2}$ β: 39 h; metabolized in liver, excreted 1° unchanged in urine

Pharmacodynamics:
: Class IV antiarrhythmic inhibits membrane-bound Na^+/K^+-activated ATPase, ↓ inward Ca^{2+} current during action potential, ↑ vagal (cholinergic) and sympatholytic effects at SA node, ↑ AV node refractory period, ↓ AV node conduction, ↓ SA nodal automaticity, (+) inotropic effect, ↑ PVR, ↑ sympathetic outflow

CNS:
: Headache, fatigue, psychosis, confusion, vertigo, paresthesias, blurred vision, photophobia

CV:
: Arrhythmias (AVB, PVCs), ↓ BP

GI:
: Anorexia, nausea, vomiting, diarrhea, abdominal pain

Other:
: Gynecomastia, hypokalemia, myalgias

Dosages:
: 0.75–1.25 mg/d PO (initially), 0.125–0.5 PO mg/d; 10–35 µg/kg/d PO (children); 0.4–0.6 IV (initially), 0.1–0.3 mg IV q 4–8 h; 8–12 µg/kg/d (children)

Contraindications:
: Ventricular fibrillation/tachycardia, beri-beri

Drug Interactions:
: Diuretics, amphotericin B, amiodarone, anticholinergics, aminoglycosides, benzodiazepines, erythromycin, esmolol, verapamil, quinidine, laxatives, ibuprofen, indomethacin, nifedipine captophil ↑ effect; amiloride, ASA, antacids, St. John's Wort, kaolin-pectin, magnesium, sulfasalazine, cytotoxic drugs, cholestyramine, colestipol, metoclopramide ↓ effect

Key Points:
: Use of succinylcholine can precipitate cardiac arrhythmias; hypokalemia can also ↑ digoxin toxicity during perioperative period

DISOPYRAMIDE

Trade Name:
: Norpace

Indications:
: PVCs, ventricular tachycardia, PAT, atrial flutter, atrial fibrillation

Pharmacokinetics:
: Onset: 1–3 h; bioavailability: 60–80%; peak: 2–3 h; protein binding: 50–70%; duration: 2–8 h; Vd: 0.6 L/kg; therapeutic level: 2–6 µg/mL; Cl: 1.2 mL/min/kg; $T_{1/2}$ β: 5–7 h; ↑ in renal failure; metabolized in liver, excreted 1° in urine as unchanged drug

Pharmacodynamics:
: Class IA antiarrhythmic, ↓ diastolic depolarization, ↓ CV, ↑ ERP, ↓ myocardial excitability, ↓ conduction velocity, anticholinergic activity

DISOPYRAMIDE *continued*

CNS:	Dizziness, confusion, peripheral neuropathy, headache, depression, nervousness, fatigue, syncope
CV:	↑ HR, (−) inotropic effect (↓ CO), ↓ BP, heart block, ↑ QT interval, arrhythmias, angina, pedal edema, palpitations
GI:	Dry mouth, bloating, anorexia, nausea, cramps, vomiting, jaundice
Pulmonary:	Dyspnea
Other:	Blurred vision, urinary hesitancy, impotence, myalgias, pruritus, hypokalemia, hypoglycemia, agranulocytosis, gynecomastia
Dosage:	200–300 mg PO (initially), then 150 mg q 6 h
Contraindications:	Cardiogenic shock, 2nd or 3rd heart block (in absence of pacemaker), sick sinus syndrome, prolonged QT interval
Drug Interactions:	Glycopyrrolate, atropine, erythromycin can ↑ effects; hydantoins ↓ effects; β-blockers ↑ CV effects (↓ BP, ↓ HR); ↑ anticoagulant effect of warfarin
Key Points:	Prolongs neuromuscular blockade produced by nondepolarizing relaxants; use with volatile anesthetics ↑ CV depressant effect; neostigmine used to treat anticholinergic effects

DOFETILIDE

Trade Name:	Tikosyn
Indications:	Atrial fibrillation, atrial flutter
Pharmacokinetics:	Oral: <1 h; bioavailability: 90%; peak: 2–3 h; protein binding: 65%; Vd: 3 L/kg; metabolized in liver, excreted 1° in urine
Pharmacodynamics:	Class III antiarrhythmic, prolongs repolarization without affecting conduction velocity by blocking cardiac K⁺ ion channel
CNS:	Headache, dizziness, syncope, paresthesia, cerebral ischemia, CVA
CV:	Ventricular arrhythmias, torsades de pointes, AV block, ↑ BP, angina
GI:	Nausea, diarrhea, abdominal pain, ↑ LFTs
Pulmonary:	Dyspnea, cough, URI
Other:	Facial paralysis, myalgias, arthralgias, angioedema, UTI
Dosage:	500 µg bid (if CrCl >60 mL/min); 250 µg bid (if CrCl 40–60 mL/min); 150 µg bid (if CrCl 20–40 mL/min)
Contraindications:	Renal failure; prolonged QT interval syndrome

DOFETILIDE *continued*

Drug Interactions:
Digoxin, phenothiazines, TCAs, K^+-wasting diuretics ↑ QT interval and risk of torsades; amiloride, amiodarone, diltriazem, macrolides, metformin, protease inhibitors, SSRIs, triamterene, grapefruit juice ↑ effect

Key Points:
Anesthetic drugs that prolong the QT interval (e.g., antiemetics, sevoflurane) should be administered with ECG monitoring

ENCAINIDE

Trade Name:
Enkaid

Indications:
Wolff-Parkinson-White syndrome, ventricular arrhythmias

Pharmacokinetics:
Onset: <30 min; bioavailability: 85%; peak: 1–2 h; protein binding: 70%; Vd: 1.3–2.6 L/kg; Cl: 4–13 mL/min/kg; $T_{1/2}$ β: <2 h; metabolized in liver (active metabolite), excreted in urine

Pharmacodynamics:
Class IC antiarrhythmic, ↓ conduction velocity through SA node, AV node, and His bundle, ↑ APD and ↑ ERP

CNS: Headache, dizziness, tinnitus, diplopia, trembling

CV: ↓ HR, ↓ BP, syncope, angina, tachyarrhythmias

GI: Nausea, ↑ LFTs

Pulmonary: Dyspnea, coughing

Other: ↑ Glucose, myalgias, muscle cramps, rash

Dosage:
25 mg PO tid (max. 50 mg tid)

Contraindications:
Cardiogenic shock, advanced heart block, ↑ QT interval, recent MI

Drug Interactions:
Cimetidine ↑ effect

Key Points:
Use with diuretics, β-blocker, Ca-channel blockers, epinephrine, volatile anesthetics can ↑ CV depressant effects

ESMOLOL

Trade Name:
Brevibloc

See Chapter 16, "Beta-Blockers"

FLECAINIDE

Trade Name:
Tambocor

Indications:
Ventricular tachycardia, paroxysmal SVT, atrial fibrillation/flutter

FLECAINIDE *continued*

Pharmacokinetics:	Onset: <1 h; bioavailability: 87%; peak: 1–6 h; protein binding: 40%; Vd: 4.9 L/kg; Cl: 5.6 mL/min/kg; $T_{1/2}$ β: 14–20 h; therapeutic level: 0.2–11 μg/mL; extensively metabolized by liver, excreted in urine
Pharmacodynamics:	Class IC antiarrhythmic analog of procainamide, ↓ SA node, automaticity, ↑ conduction times in His-Purkinje system, ↑ ERP, ↑ APD
CNS:	Dizziness, diplopia, headache, tremor, tinnitus, fatigue, anxiety
CV:	↓ HR, ↓ BP, arrhythmias, angina, flushing, edema, palpitation, (−) inotrope
GI:	Nausea, vomiting, constipation, cramps, dyspepsia, anorexia
Pulmonary:	Dyspnea, wheezing
Dosage:	100 mg PO bid (max. 400–600 mg/d)
Contraindications:	Advanced heart block (without pacemaker), cardiogenic shock, recent MI
Drug Interactions:	Amiodarone, quinidine, cimetidine ↑ effect; ↑ CV depression with disopyramide, verapamil, β-blockers; smoking ↓ effect
Key Points:	Long-acting drug with potent CV depressant effects can enhance anesthesia-induced hypotension

LIDOCAINE

Trade Name:	**Xylocaine**
Indications:	Ventricular arrhythmias, status epilepticus, local anesthesia
Pharmacokinetics:	Onset: <2 min; bioavailability: 20%; peak: <10 min; protein binding: 60%; duration: 0.5–2 h; Vd: 1 L/kg; Cl: 9.2 mL/min/kg; therapeutic level: 1–5 μg/mL; $T_{1/2}$ β: 1–2 h; extensively metabolized in liver to active metabolites, excreted in urine
Pharmacodynamics:	Class IB antiarrhythmic, ↓ automaticity, ↓ ERP, ↓ APD, inhibits reentry mechanisms
CNS:	Drowsiness, perioral paresthesias, agitation, tinnitus, diplopia, slurred speech, disorientation, tremors, convulsions, dizziness
CV:	↓ HR, ↓ BP, arrhythmias, asystole
GI:	Nausea, vomiting
Pulmonary:	Respiratory arrest, status asthmaticus
Dosage:	300 mg (4–5 mg/kg) IM, 0.5–1 mg/kg as IV bolus (max. 3–5 mg/kg), 10–50 μg/kg/min infusion (ventricular arrhythmias 2° to MI); 1 mg/kg IV, then 0.5 mg/kg after 2 min (status epilepticus)

LIDOCAINE *continued*

Contraindications:
: Stokes-Adams syndrome, Wolff-Parkinson-White syndrome, heart block (in absence of pacemaker); allergic to amide-type local anesthetics

Drug Interactions:
: β-blockers and cimetidine ↑ effect

Key Points:
: ↑ Neuromuscular blocking effect of succinylcholine; small doses (1–2 mL 1% lidocaine) are useful in ↓ pain on injection of anesthetic drugs

MAGNESIUM

Other Name:
: **Mag Sulfate**

See Chapter 7, "Anticonvulsants"

MEXILETINE

Trade Name:
: **Mexitil**

Indications:
: Ventricular arrhythmias, diabetic neuropathic pain

Pharmacokinetics:
: Onset: 0.5–2 h; bioavailability: 90%; peak: 2–3 h; protein binding: 55%; duration: 6–8 h; Vd: 4.9 L/kg; Cl: 6.3 mL/min/kg; $T_{1/2}$ β: 10 h; therapeutic level: 0.5–2 μg/mL; metabolized in liver, excreted in urine

Pharmacodynamics:
: Class IB antiarrhythmic, lidocaine analog, Na^+ channel antagonist

CNS:
: Dizziness, headache, diplopia, confusion, tremor, ataxia, tinnitus, paresthesias, insomnia

CV:
: Palpitations, angina, ↑ HR, ↓ CO, ↑ SVR, arrhythmias, edema

GI:
: Nausea, vomiting, anorexia, ↑ LFTs, heartburn, dry mouth

Other:
: Bone marrow suppression, dyspnea

Dosage:
: 150–300 mg PO q 8 h (max. 400 mg q 8 h)

Contraindications:
: Cardiogenic shock, advanced heart block (without pacemaker), recent MI, breast-feeding

Drug Interactions:
: Pentobarbitol, phenytoin, rifampin ↓ effects; antacids, atropine, opioids ↓ absorption; metoclopramide ↑ absorption; carbonic amylase inhibitors ↓ excretion

Key Points:
: High doses can cause CNS stimulation (e.g., seizures) and may ↑ anesthetic requirement

MORICIZINE

Trade Name:	**Ethmozine**
Indications:	Ventricular tachycardia
Pharmacokinetics:	Onset: 1 h; bioavailability: 38%; peak: 0.5–2 h; protein binding: 95%; duration: 10–24 h; $T_{1/2}$ β: 6–14 h; 1st-pass metabolism, excreted in urine (39%) and feces (56%)
Pharmacodynamics:	Class IB antiarrhythmic, phenothiazine derivative, ↓ inward sodium current, ↓ AV antiaccessory pathway conduction ↑ PR, ↑ QRS
CNS:	Headache, dizziness, paresthesias, fatigue, diplopia, insomnia, asthenia
CV:	Arrhythmias, CHF, palpitations, angina, ↓ PVR, thrombophlebitis
GI:	Dry mouth, nausea, vomiting, diarrhea, dyspepsia, ↑ LFTs
Pulmonary:	Dyspnea
Other:	Urinary frequency/retention, dysuria, myalgia, diaphoresis, rash
Dosages:	200–300 mg PO q 8 h
Contraindications:	Cardiogenic shock, advanced heart block (without pacemaker)
Drug Interactions:	Digoxin and β-blockers ↑ PR interval; cimetidine ↓ clearance; ↑ theophylline clearance
Key Points:	In presence of electrolyte abnormalities, ↑ arrhythmias during general (volatile) anesthesia

PHENYTOIN

Trade Name:	**Dilantin**
Indications:	Ventricular arrhythmias, SVT, QT prolongation, tonic-clonic seizures, status epilepticus, neuropathic pain
Pharmacokinetics:	Onset: <2 min; bioavailability: 90%; peak: 1–3 h; protein binding: 90%; duration: 4–12 h; Vd: 0.64 L/kg; Cl: 5.9 mL/min/kg; $T_{1/2}$ β: 18–30 h; therapeutic level: 10–20 μg/mL; metabolized via hydroxylation to inactive metabolites, excreted in urine
Pharmacodynamics:	Class IB antiarrhythmic, ↓ sodium ion influx, stabilizes neural membranes, ↓ APD, ↓ ERP, ↓ QT interval, ↑ AV nodal conduction
CNS:	Drowsiness, nystagmus, vertigo, ataxia, blurred vision, insomnia, confusion, slurred speech, headache, nervousness
CV:	Periarteritis nodosa, ↓ BP

PHENYTOIN *continued*

GI:	Nausea, vomiting, constipation, gingival hyperplasia, ↑ LFTs
Other:	Bone marrow depression, hyperglycemia, osteomalacia, Stevens-Johnson syndrome, toxic epidermal necrolysis, rash
Dosage:	100 mg IV q 5 min until arrhythmia is controlled (max. 700 mg/d); 15 mg/kg PO, then 7.5 mg/kg followed by 4–6 mg/kg/d
Contraindications:	Sinus bradycardia, advanced heart block, Adams-Stokes syndrome
Drug Interactions:	Allopurinol, amiodarone, benzodiazepines, chloramphenicol, dicumarol, disulfiram, isoniazid, cimetidine, sulfonamides ↑ effect; ↑ hepatic drug metabolism via cytochrome P_{450}; theophylline ↑ clearance; ↑ CNS toxicity of local anesthetics; lithium and antipsychotics ↓ seizure threshold; ↑ warfarin-induced anticoagulation
Key Points:	Chronic use ↑ fentanyl and nondepolarizing muscle relaxant requirements during surgery

PROCAINAMIDE

Trade Names:	**Procanbid SR, Pronestyl**
Indications:	Atrial flutter, PAT, ventricular tachycardia and fibrillation
Pharmacokinetics:	Onset: <30 min (IV/IM), 1–2 h (oral); bioavailability: 85%; peak: 15–60 min (IV/IM); 0.5–1.5 h (oral); protein binding: 20%; therapeutic level: 3–10 µg/mL; duration: 3–6 h; $T_{1/2}$ β: 2–5 h; metabolized to *N*-acetyl-procainamide (active), excreted in urine
Pharmacodynamics:	Class IA arrhythmic, ↓ myocardial excitability, ↓ automaticity, ↓ CV, ↑ ERP, ↑ APD, anticholinergic activity, ↑ AV nodal conduction
CNS:	Psychosis, confusion, seizures, dizziness, depression
CV:	Ventricular asystole, ↑ HR, ↓ PVR, ↓ BP, AV block
GI:	Anorexia, nausea, vomiting, diarrhea, bitter taste, ↑ LFTs
Other:	Drug fever, pancytopenia, pruritus, lupus-like vasculitis, Raynaud's, Coombs' (+) hemolytic anemia, myalgias, angioedema
Dosage:	0.5–1 g PO q 4–6 h; 1 g IV (give in 100 mg boluses over 2–4 min)
Contraindications:	Prolonged QT interval, advanced heart block (without pacemaker), myasthenia gravis, SLE-like reaction, allergic to procaine

PROCAINAMIDE *continued*

Drug Interactions:	Atropine, diphenhydramine, TCAs ↑ anticholinergic effects; cimetidine ↑ effect
Key Points:	Vagolytic effects on AV node may accelerate ventricular response to AF; use with muscle relaxants may prolong neuromuscular blockade

PROPAFENONE

Trade Name:	**Rythmol**
Indications:	Ventricular arrhythmias
Pharmacokinetics:	Onset: <1 h; bioavailability: 95%; peak: 3–4 h; protein binding: 95%; $T_{1/2}$ β: 6–13 h (10–32 h in slow metabolizers); metabolized in liver to two active metabolites, excreted in urine
Pharmacodynamics:	Class IC antiarrhythmic; ↑ PR, QRS, QT; ↑ ERF; ↓ AV conduction; weak β-adrenergic, Ca-channel blockade
CNS:	Dizziness, somnolence, fatigue, tinnitus, anxiety, insomnia, syncope, tremor, diplopia, headache
GI:	Nausea, vomiting, cramps, dyspepsia, anorexia, flatulence, dry mouth, metallic taste
CV:	↓ HR, ↓ BP, angina, edema, CHF, atrial flutter/fibrilation
Pulmonary:	Dyspnea, wheezing
Other:	Diaphoresis, rash, arthralgias, agranulocytosis
Dosage:	150 mg PO tid (max. 900 mg/d)
Contraindications:	Cardiogenic shock, CHF, advanced heart block, active bronchospasm, electrolyte imbalances
Drug Interactions:	Quinidine and cimetidine ↑ effect, ↑ levels of digoxin, metoprolol, propranolol
Key Points:	Use of large amounts of epinephrine-containing local anesthetics ↑ risks of CNS toxicity

PROPRANOLOL

Trade Name:	**Inderal**
	See Chapter 16, "Beta-Blockers"

QUINIDINE

Trade Names:	**Quinora, Quinalan**
Indications:	Atrial flutter and fibrillation, paroxysmal SVT, frequent PACs/PCVs, ventricular tachycardia

QUINIDINE *continued*

Pharmacokinetics:	Onset: 0.5–2 h; bioavailability: 80%; peak: 2–4 h; protein binding: 90%; duration: 6–8 h; Vd: 2–3 L/kg; therapeutic level: 1.5–4 µg/mL; Cl: 4.7 mL/min/kg; $T_{1/2} \beta$: 5–12 h; hepatic metabolism to active metabolites, excreted in urine
Pharmacodynamics:	Class IA, antiarrhythmic, ↓ automaticity, ↑ EPR, ↑ APD, ↓ AV nodal refractioness (↑ conductance), anticholinergic effect
CNS:	Dizziness, headache, fatigue, ataxia, tinnitus, diplopia, "cinchonism"
CV:	↑ HR, ↓ BP, syncope
GI:	Nausea, vomiting, diarrhea, ↑ LFTs, anorexia, abdominal pain, ↑ salivation
Pulmonary:	Wheezing, respiratory arrest
Other:	Drug fever, photosensitivity, myalgias, SLE-like angioedema, blood dyscrasias, unusual taste
Dosage:	200–400 mg PO qid; 600 mg q 8–12 h; 200 mg IM
Contraindications:	Prolonged QT syndrome, advanced heart block, allergic to cinchona
Drug Interactions:	Amiodarone and cimetidine ↑ effect; verapamil and antihypertensives ↑ CV depression; nifedipine, phenytoin, rifampin ↓ effect; ↑ coumarin effect
Key Points:	↑ Anticholinergic effects of muscle relaxants and enhances residual muscle weakness

SOTALOL

Trade Name:	**Betapace**
	See Chapter 16, "Beta-Blockers"

TOCAINIDE

Trade Name:	**Tonocard**
Indications:	Ventricular arrhythmias, myotonic dystrophy
Pharmacokinetics:	Onset: <30 min; bioavailability: 95%; peak: 0.5–2 h; protein binding: 50%; duration: 8 h; Vd: 3.0 L/kg; therapeutic level: 6–12 µg/mL; Cl: 2.6 mL/min/kg; $T_{1/2} \beta$: 11–23 h; hepatic metabolism to inactive metabolites, excreted in urine
Pharmacodynamics:	Class IB antiarrhythmic, ↓ automaticity, ↓ ERP, ↓ APD of His-Purkinje fibers, inhibits reentry mechanisms

TOCAINIDE *continued*

CNS:	Dizziness, tremor, confusion, tinnitus, diplopia, fatigue, headache, paresthesias
CV:	↓ HR, ↓ BP, palpitations
GI:	Nausea, vomiting, anorexia, diarrhea, ↑ LFTs
Pulmonary:	Fibrotic changes, interstitial pneumonitis, edema
Other:	Blood dyscrasias, rash, diaphoresis, Stevens-Johnson syndrome
Dosage:	400–600 mg PO q 8 h (max. 2400 mg/d); ↓ dose with hepatorenal impairment
Contraindications:	Allergic to amide-type local anesthetics, advanced AV block (without pacemaker), CHF
Drug Interactions:	Lidocaine ↑ CNS toxicity; cimetidine and rifampin ↓ effect; metoprolol ↓ CV depression
Key Points:	Less CV depression than lidocaine; use β-blockers sparingly during anesthesia to avoid ↑ CV depression

VERAPAMIL

Trade Names:	**Calan, Isoptin, Verelan**
	See Chapter 19, "Calcium Channel Blockers"

5

Anticholinergics

ATROPINE

Trade Name:	**Same**
Indications:	Reversal of neuromuscular blockade (in combination with anticholinesterase drug), antisialagogue, brady-arrhythmias, bronchoconstriction, visceral spasm, peptic ulcer disease, organophosphate poisoning, biliary and renal colic
Pharmacokinetics:	Onset: <2 min; peak: 3–5 min; protein binding: 50%; duration: 2–4 h; Vd: 210 L; $T_{1/2}$ β: 2–3 h; hepatic metabolism, excretion unchanged in urine
Pharmacodynamics:	Competitive acetylcholine antagonist at central and peripheral muscarinic receptors
CNS:	Sedation, excitement, confusion, antiemetic, ↓ tremor, dizziness, mydriasis, cycloplegia, insomnia
CV:	↑ HR (usual effect), ↓ HR (low dose), palpitations
GI:	↓ Secretions, ↓ lower esophageal sphincter tone, ↑ gastroesophageal reflux, ↓ biliary spincter tone, dysphagia, altered taste
Pulmonary:	Mucous plug formation, bronchodilator effect (relaxation of bronchial smooth muscle), nasal congestion, ↑ airway dead space
Other:	↓ Lacrimal secretions, abolishes HR variability in fetus, neuromuscular and ganglionic blockage (at high dose), ↑ intraocular pressure, ↑ body temperature, ↓ sweating
Dosage:	0.5–1.0 mg IV q 5–10 min (max. 2 mg) (bradyarrhythmias/asystole); 0.2–0.6 mg IM 20–40 min before surgery (antisialagogue); 0.01 mg/kg IV (in combination with cholinesterase inhibitor for reversal of neuromuscular blockade); 0.025–0.05 mg/kg inhaled q 4–6 h (max. 2.5 mg) (bronchodilators); 1–2 mg IV/IM q 20–30 min (organophosphate poisoning); 10–20 μg/kg IV/IM, 30 μg/kg PO (children)
Contraindications:	Narrow-angle glaucoma, obstructive uropathy (e.g., BPH), paralytic ileus, pyloric stenosis, toxic megacolon, acute hemorrhage, asthma, myasthenia gravis, allergic to sodium metabisulfites
Drug Interactions:	Sedative/hypnotics ↑ CNS depression; haloperidol ↑ IOP; urinary alkalinizers ↓ elimination; MAOIs ↑ anticholinergic effects and ↓ metabolism; opioids ↑ constipation and urinary retention
Key Points:	For reversal, use with edrophonium (vs neostigmine); more potent vagolytic (vs antisialagogue) effects than glycopyrrolate; avoid anesthetic drugs that ↑ HR (e.g., ketamine)

GLYCOPYRROLATE

Trade Name:	**Robinul**
Indications:	Reversal of neuromuscular blockade (in combination with anticholinesterase drug), antisialagogue, bradyarrhythmias, peptic ulcer disease, and organophosphate poisoning
Pharmacokinetics:	Onset: 1–2 min (IV), 15–30 min (IM); bioavailability: 20%; peak: 30–60 min; duration: 3–7 h; $T_{1/2}$ β: 1.25 h; quaternary amine does not cross blood-brain barrier; hepatic metabolism (80%), excreted in feces and urine
Pharmacodynamics:	Competitive acetylcholine antagonist at peripheral muscarinic receptors
CNS:	Peripheral neuropathy, blurred vision, mydriasis
CV:	↑ HR, ↓ HR (small dose), atrial arrhythmias, palpitations
GI:	↓ Secretions, ↓ lower esophageal sphincter tone, dyspepsia ↓ motility/gastric emptying, nausea, vomiting, constipation, bloating
GU:	Urinary retention/hesitancy, impotence
Pulmonary:	Mucous plug formation, bronchodilator effect (2° to relaxation of bronchial smooth muscle), ↑ airway dead space
Other:	↓ Lacrimal secretions, urticaria; anhidrosis (heat stroke)
Dosage:	0.005 mg/kg IV q 2–3 min (bradyarrhythmias); 0.005 mg/kg IM/IV (0.2–0.3 mg) (antisialagogue) IM before induction of anesthesia; 0.2 mg IV per 1 mg of neostigmine, or 5 mg of pyridostigmine (reversal of neuromuscular blockade); 1–2 mg PO tid, or 0.1–0.2 mg IV/IM tid (peptic ulcer disease)
Contraindications:	Obstructive uropathy, obstructive/ileus, pyloric stenosis, myasthenia gravis, glaucoma, Down syndrome, ulcerative colitis/toxic megacolon
Drug Interactions:	Antacids, ketoconazole, levodopa ↓ absorption; urinary alkalinizers delay elimination; ↑ anticholinergic effects of antihistamines, disopyramide, meperidine, phenothiazine, procainaimide, quinidine, TCAs, and MAOIs; opioids ↑ risk of constipation and urinary retention
Key Points:	For use with neostigmine (vs edrophonium) in reversal of neuromuscular blockade; more prominent antisecretogogue (vs vagolytic) effect compared with atropine

HYOSCYAMINE

Trade Name:	**Cystospaz**
Indications:	Visceral spasms, adjunctive therapy for endoscopy
Pharmacokinetics:	Onset: 2 min (IV), 20–30 min (oral); peak: 15–30 min (IM/IV), 30–60 min (oral); protein binding: 50%; duration: 4–12 h; $T_{1/2}$ β: 7 h; crosses blood-brain barrier; metabolized in liver, excreted in urine
Pharmacodynamics:	Competitively blocks acetylcholine at central and peripheral muscarinic receptors
CNS:	Headache, insomnia, drowsiness, dizziness, blurred vision, cycloplegia, mydriasis, photophobia, ↑ IOP, nervousness
CV:	↑ HR, palpitations
GI:	Dry mouth, dysphagia, ↓ GI motility and ↓ gastric acid secretion, constipation, dyspepsia, paralytic ileus
GU:	Urinary hesitancy/retention, impotence
Other:	Urticaria, ↓ sweating (anhidrosis), drug fever
Dosage:	0.125–0.25 mg PO qid; 0.25–0.5 mg IM/IV tid
Contraindications:	Glaucoma, obstructive uropathy, ulcerative colitis, toxic megacolon, intestinal obstruction or atony, myasthenia gravis, acute hemorrhage
Drug Interactions:	Antacids ↓ absorption; amantadine, antihistamines, phenothiazines, and TCAs ↓ effects; ↓ haloperidol effect
Key Points:	Potential for ↑ risk of regurgitation during induction of anesthesia; may induce heat stroke

IPRATROPIUM

Trade Name:	**Atrovent**
Indications:	Bronchospasm associated with chronic bronchitis, emphysema, COPD, asthma, rhinorrhea
Pharmacokinetics:	Onset: <5 min; peak: <15 min; duration: 3–4 h; hepatic metabolism, excreted 1° in feces
Pharmacodynamics:	Inhibits vagally mediated reflexes, ↓ acetylcholine at bronchial muscarinic receptors, ↓ intracellular cyclic GMP
CNS:	Headache, blurred vision, dizziness, insomnia, tremor, anxiety
CV:	↑ HR, palpitations, angina
GI:	Dry mouth, nausea
Pulmonary:	↓ Airway secretions, bronchodilation, bronchitis, cough, dyspnea
Other:	Myalgias, arthralgias, rash

IPRATROPIUM *continued*

Dosage:	0.03% and 0.06% (18 µg/metered spray); 2–4 puffs q 3–4 h (max. 2 mg)
Contraindications:	Narrow-angle glaucoma, bladder neck obstruction, prostatic hypertrophy, sensitivity to soya lecithin (soybeans, peanuts)
Drug Interactions:	β-agonist and antimuscarinics ↑ efficacy; ↓ miotics
Key Points:	Enhanced sensitivity with atropine; delayed onset of bronchodilation; use with ketamine and desflurane may ↑ tachycardia

OXITROPIUM

Trade Name:	**Oxivent**
Indications:	Asthma, COPD
Pharmacokinetics:	Onset: 60–90 min; duration: 6–8 h; minimal systemic absorption, no tolerance with prolonged use
Pharmacodynamics:	Competitive muscarinic acetylcholine receptor antagonist in bronchial smooth muscle
Pulmonary:	Paradoxical bronchoconstriction (due to hypotonic solution)
Other:	Dry mouth, glaucoma, urinary retention
Dosage:	200 µg metered dose inhaler q 6–12 h
Contraindications:	Sensitivity to preservatives (benzalkonium, EDTA)
Drug Interactions:	↑ Efficacy with theophylline
Key Points:	Long-acting ipratropium that is synergistic with theophylline

OXYBUTYNIN

Trade Name:	**Ditropan**
Indications:	Neurogenic bladder disorders
Pharmacokinetics:	Onset: 0.5–1 h; peak: 3–4 h; duration: 6–10 h; metabolized in liver, excreted in urine
Pharmacodynamics:	Direct spasmolytic and antimuscarinic (↓ urge to void), ↓ detrusor muscle contractions (↑ bladder capacity)
CNS:	Dizziness, insomnia, restlessness, hallucinations, cycloplegia, ↓ lacrimation, mydriasis, amblyopia, somnolence, headache
CV:	↑ HR, palpitations, vasodilation
GI:	Nausea, vomiting, dry mouth, constipation

OXYBUTYNIN *continued*

GU:	Urine retention/hesitancy, UTI
Other:	Rash, ↓ sweating (heat stroke), ↓ lactation
Dosage:	5 mg PO q 6–12 h (max. 20 mg/d); 36 mg TTS
Contraindications:	Myasthenia gravis, glaucoma, GI obstruction, paralytic ileus, toxic megacolon, intestinal atony (elderly), obstructive uropathy
Drug Interactions:	↓ Acetaminophen absorption; ↑ level of digoxin and atenolol; ↓ level of haloperidol, levodopa; phenothiazine ↑ anticholinergic effects
Key Points:	↑ Sedative effects of CNS depressants during perioperative period

SCOPOLAMINE

Trade Names:	**Scopace, Isopto Hyoscine, Transdermal Scop**
Indications:	Antisialagogue, antiemetic, motion sickness/vertigo, iritis luveitis
Pharmacokinetics:	Onset: <30 min; 4–6 h (TTS); peak: 1 h (24 h TTS); duration: 6–8 h (72 h TTS); $T_{1/2}$ β: 1.6–3.3 hr; crosses both blood-brain and placental barriers; hepatic metabolism, urinary excretion
Pharmacodynamics:	Competitive antagonist of acetylcholine at muscarinic receptors, blocking vagal inhibition at SA node, ↓ secretion and GI motility
CNS:	Sedation, confusion, amnesia, agitation, dizziness, blurred vision, headache, ↑ IOP, antiemetic effect, ↓ parkinsonism tremor; mydriasis, cycloplegia
CV:	↑ HR (large dose), ↓ HR (small dose), palpitations
GI:	Dry mouth, ↓ lower esophageal sphincter tone, ↓ GI gastric emptying (↑ residual gastric volume), constipation
Pulmonary:	↓ Secretions (mucus plugging), bronchodilation, ↑ airway dead space
Other:	↓ Lacrimal secretions, ↓ sweating, rash, flushing
Dosage:	0.2–0.6 mg IM/IV before surgery; apply 1.5 mg TTS patch evening prior to surgery; 0.006 mg/kg IM (max. 0.3 mg in children)
Contraindications:	Narrow-angle glaucoma, dementia, BPH, paralytic ileus, pyloric stenosis, asthma/COPD, myasthenia gravis, toxic megacolon, sensitivity to belladonna alkaloids
Drug Interactions:	Haloperidol ↓ IOP; urinary alkalinizers ↓ elimination; MAOIs ↑ effects and ↓ metabolism; opioids ↑ risk of constipation and urinary retention

SCOPOLAMINE *continued*

Key Points:	↑ Sedative effects of CNS depressants; more potent than atropine in ↓ salivation and ocular dysfunction but less potent with respect to cardiac and smooth muscle effects

TIOTROPIUM

Trade Name:	**Spiriva**
Indications:	Bronchial asthma (acute), COPD
Pharmacokinetics:	Bioavailability: low (<20%); protein binding: 72%; Cl: 10–15 mL/kg/min; $T_{1/2}$ β: 5–6 d; excreted 1° unchanged in urine
Pharmacodynamics:	Long-acting muscarinic receptor antagonist
CNS:	Blurry vision
GI:	Dry mouth
Pulmonary:	Wheezing (on inhalation)
Dosage:	10–20 μg/d (10 μg/puff)
Contraindications:	Sensitivity to atropine, ipratropium, or oxitropium; narrow-angle glaucoma, BPH, pregnancy
Drug Interactions:	Avoid coadministration of other anticholinergic drugs
Key Points:	↓ Doses of anticholinergics during perioperative period

6

Anticoagulants and Procoagulants

ABCIXIMAB

Trade Name:	**ReoPro**
Indications:	Maintain patency of coronary vessels after PTCA, unstable angina
Pharmacokinetics:	Onset: <5 min; peak: 5–10 min; duration: 10–60 min; $T_{1/2}$ β: 30 min, remains platelet-bound for up to 15 d
Pharmacodynamics:	Blocks binding of fibrinogen to glycoprotein receptors, ↓ platelet aggregation
CNS:	Dizziness, anxiety, hypesthesia, confusion, blurred vision
CV:	Arrhythmias, ↓ BP, peripheral edema
GI:	Dyspepsia, nausea, vomiting, diarrhea
Pulmonary:	Pleural effusion, pleurisy, pneumonia
Other:	Bleeding, thrombocytopenia, leukocytosis
Dosage:	0.25 mg/kg IV over 30 min, then 0.125 µg/mL/min for 12 h (10 µg/min)
Contraindications:	Active bleeding, history of CVA (<2 yr), thrombocytopenia, AV malformation, severe hypertension
Drug Interactions:	Anticoagulants and antiplatelet agents ↑ risk of bleeding
Key Points:	Platelet count, prothrombin, and activated prothrombin times should be evaluated before surgery

ACETYLSALICYLIC ACID (ASA)

Other Name:	**Aspirin**
Indications:	Thrombosis prophylaxis (with ASCVD, atrial fibrillation, aortocoronary graft, and TIAs), pericarditis after MI, analgesic, antipyretic, anti-inflammatory (Kawasaki syndrome, rheumatic fever, arthritis)
Pharmacokinetics:	Onset: 5–15 min (↑ by food); peak: 0.5–4 h; duration: 1–3 hr; Vd: 170 mL/kg; $T_{1/2}$ β: 15–30 min; irreversibly acetylates platelets, highly metabolized in liver, excreted in urine
Pharmacodynamics:	Inhibits prostaglandin synthesis (↓ cyclooxygenase activity), ↓ thromboxane A_2, ↓ platelet aggregation, peripheral vasodilation
CNS:	Tinnitus
GI:	Dyspepsia, nausea, vomiting, gastric/duodenal ulcers, ↑ GI bleeding
Other:	Reye's syndrome (in children); hepatotoxicity (with high doses), ↓ uric acid excretion, ↑ bleeding time, hematomas

ACETYLSALICYLIC ACID (ASA) *continued*

Dosage:	81–325 mg/d (antithrombotic); 0.325–1.2 g/d (arthritis); 60–130 mg/kg/d (children); 60–100 mg/kg (anti-inflammatory)
Contraindications:	Active peptic ulcer disease, G6PD deficiency, hemophilia, von Willebrand's disease, telangiectasia, flulike symptoms in children
Drug Interactions:	↑ Bleeding with anticoagulants and thrombolytics; alcohol, corticosteroids, and NSAIDs ↑ risk of GI bleeding; ↓ spironolactone diuretic effect; aminoglycoside, loop diuretics, cisplatin, vancomycin ↑ ototoxicity; ↑ lithium level
Key Points:	Avoid aspirin in children with viral infection and exacerbations of asthma; hemostasis during surgery potentiated by anticoagulants and thrombolytics; ↓ gastric secretion and dyspepsia; use of H_2 antagonist or PPI

ALTEPLASE (TISSUE PLASMINOGEN ACTIVATOR [TPA])

Trade Name:	**Activase**
Indications:	Coronary thrombolysis in acute MI, pulmonary embolism, acute ischemic stroke, peripheral arterial occlusion
Pharmacokinetics:	Onset: <2 min; peak: 45 min; duration: 4 h; Cl: 480 mL/min; $T_{1/2}$ β: <10 min; metabolized in liver, excreted in urine
Pharmacodynamics:	Synthetic plasminogen activator, converts tissue plasminogen to plasmin, produces local fibrinolysis
CNS:	Intracranial hemorrhage
CV:	Arrhythmias, ↓ BP, edema
GI:	Nausea, vomiting
Other:	Bleeding, fever
Dosage:	60 mg IV (initially), then 10–20 mg or 20 mg/h (max. 100 mg)
Contraindications:	Active bleeding, CVA with seizure, severe hypertension, bleeding diathesis, intracranial hemorrhage/neoplasm, AVM, aneurysm
Drug Interactions:	Heparin, vitamin K antagonists, and antiplatelet drugs (abciximab, aspirin, dipyridamole) ↑ risk of bleeding
Key Points:	Coagulation panel should be checked prior to surgery

AMINOCAPROIC ACID

Trade Name:	**Amicar**
Indications:	Acute bleeding (2° to hyperfibrinolysis), antidote for streptokinase and urokinase, prophylaxis against recurrent subarachnoid hemorrhage
Pharmacokinetics:	Onset: <1 h; peak: 2 h; duration: 3–5 h; Vd: 30 L; Cl: 169 mL/min; no metabolism, excreted 1° unchanged in urine
Pharmacodynamics:	Inhibits plasminogen activators, blocks antiplasmin by ↓ fibrinolysis
CNS:	Confusion, seizures, dizziness, malaise, headache, tinnitus
CV:	↓ BP, ↓ HR, arrhythmias, thrombosis, edema
GI:	Cramps, diarrhea, nausea, vomiting, ↑ LFTs, abdominal pain
Other:	Acute renal failure, myopathy, ↑ K^+, lacrimation, pruritus, rash, bone marrow suppression
Dosage:	4–5 g IV initially, then 1 g/h × 8 h (max. 30 g/d); 5–30 g/d in divided doses; 100 mg/kg initially, then 33 mg/kg/h (max. 18 g/m^2/d) (children)
Contraindications:	Active intravascular clotting, presence of DIC (without heparin)
Drug Interactions:	Estrogens ↑ risk of bleeding; do not mix with Factor IX Complex or anti-inhibitor coagulant concentrates
Key Points:	Avoid rapid IV infusion to minimize risk of CV depression (e.g., administer loading dose over 1 h)

ANAGRELIDE

Trade Name:	**Agrylin**
Indications:	Essential thrombocythemia
Pharmacokinetics:	Onset: <10 min; peak: 1 h; duration: 6–12 h; $T_{1/2}$ β: 1.3 h; extensively metabolized, excreted in urine
Pharmacodynamics:	Inhibits cAMP diphosphate and collagen-induced platelet aggregation, platelet-reducing effect
CNS:	Malaise, dizziness, headache, insomnia, CVA, nervousness, paresthesias, syncope, tinnitus, asthenia
CV:	Arrhythmias, angina, edema, ↑ HR, CHF, vasodilation
GI:	Anorexia, flatulence, dyspepsia, melena, gastritis, diarrhea, nausea
GU:	Dysuria, hematuria
Pulmonary:	Dyspnea, asthma, pneumonia, bronchitis
Other:	Myalgias, arthralgia, dehydration, pruritus, rash, urticaria, photosensitivity, anemia, fever, rhinitis, epistaxis; ecchymoses, alopecia

ANAGRELIDE *continued*

Dosages: 0.5–1 mg PO q 6–12 h (max. 10 mg/d)

Contraindications: Severe cardiovascular disease

Drug Interactions: Sucralfate ↓ absorption

Key Points: ↑ CV depressant effects of general anesthetics

ANTIHEMOPHILIC FACTOR

Trade Names: **Advate, Alphanate, Bioclate, Helixate, Hemofil M, Recombinate**

Indications: Hemophilla A (Factor VIII deficiency)

Pharmacokinetics: Onset: <2 min; peak: <10 min; duration: 12 h; $T_{1/2}$ β: 4–24 h; eliminated rapidly from plasma, consumed during blood clotting; does not cross placental or blood-brain barrier

Pharmacodynamics: Replaces deficient clotting factor that converts prothrombin to thrombin
CV: Chest tightness
GI: Nausea
Pulmonary: Bronchospasm
Other: Fever, urticaria, ↓ PT/PTT, ↑ risk of hepatitis B and HIV

Dosage: Highly individualized

Contraindications: Sensitivity to murine protein

Drug Interactions: None known

Key Points: Check coagulation profile prior to surgery; Advate and Recombinate are recombinants (rAHF)

ANTISTREPTASE (ANISOYLATED PLASMINOGEN-STREPTOKINASE ACTIVATOR COMPLEX [APSAC])

Trade Name: **Eminase**

Indications: Coronary thrombolysis (after acute MI)

Pharmacokinetics: Onset: <2 min; peak: <10 min; duration: 4–6 h; $T_{1/2}$ β: 88–112 min; rapidly deacylated to active streptokinase-plasminogen complex

Pharmacodynamics: Covalently modified complex of streptokinase and Lys-plasminogen, activates endogenous fibrinolysis to produce plasmin
CNS: Cerebral and retinal hemorrhage
CV: ↓ BP, arrhythmias
GI: Hemorrhage

ANTISTREPTASE
(APSAC) *continued*

Pulmonary:	Bronchospasm, dyspnea, hemoptysis
Other:	Hematuria, arthralgias, hematoma, urticaria, pruritus, rash
Dosage:	30-unit vial, infuse over 2–5 min
Contraindications:	Active bleeding, aneurysm, AVM, severe hypertension
Drug Interactions:	Anticoagulants or antiplatelet drugs ↑ risk of bleeding; steroids, cephalosporins, ethacrinic acid, and valproic acid ↑ risk of hemorrhage
Key Points:	Drugs that alter platelet function (e.g., NSAIDs, dipyridamole, ASA, heparin) ↑ risk of intraoperative bleeding

ANTITHROMBIN III

Trade Name:	**Thrombate**
Indications:	Hereditary antithrombin III deficiency (prophylaxis and adjunct treatment of thromboembolism)
Pharmacokinetics:	Binds to epithelium, removes antithrombin III clotting factor complexes from circulation; metabolism and excretion not known
Pharmacodynamics:	Normalizes coagulation-inhibiting capability, inhibits formation of thromboemboli, inactivates plasmin
CV:	Vasodilation, ↓ BP
GU:	Diuresis, dehydration
Dosage:	100–500 IU/min loading infusion, then maintenance infusion (60% of loading dose) for 2–8 d
Contraindications:	NK
Drug Interactions:	Heparin ↑ anticoagulant effect
Key Points:	Check coagulation profile before surgery

ARGATROBAN

Trade Name:	**Acova**
Indications:	Prevention or treatment of thrombosis with heparin-induced thrombocytopenia (HIT)
Pharmacokinetics:	Onset: <2 min; peak: 5 min; protein binding: 54%; duration: <10 min (after infusion); $T_{1/2} \beta$: 39–51 min; metabolized in liver (P_{450}); excreted 1° in feces
Pharmacodynamics:	Reversibly binds to the thrombin active site, inhibits thrombin-catalyzed reactions (direct thrombin inhibitor)
CNS:	Dysesthesias, fever

ARGATROBAN *continued*

CV:	Arrhythmias (AF, VT), ↓ BP, cardiac arrest
GI:	Abdominal pain, diarrhea, bleeding, nausea, vomiting
GU:	Hematuria, UTI, ↑ BUN/Cr
Pulmonary:	Dyspnea, hemoptysis, coughing, pneumonia
Other:	Anemia, sepsis, ↑ bleeding time

Dosages: 150–350 μg/kg over 3–5 min, then 2–20 μg/kg/min (max. 30 μg/kg/min)

Contraindications: Major bleeding, severe hypertension, intracranial hemorrhage

Drug Interactions: Thrombolytics and oral anticoagulants ↑ risk of bleeding

Key Points: Check coagulation profile before regional anesthetic technique, and avoid perioperative hypertension

CLOPIDOGREL

Trade Name: **Plavix**

Indications: Recent CVA, MI, peripheral arterial occlusion, acute coronary syndrome (i.e., unstable angina and non–Q wave MI)

Pharmacokinetics: Onset: 2 h; bioavailability: 50%; peak: 4–6 h; protein binding: 94%; duration: 5–7 d; $T_{1/2}$ β: 8 h; extensively metabolized in liver, excreted in urine and feces

Pharmacodynamics: Inhibits binding of ADP to its platelet receptor, modifying ADP receptors, and inhibiting platelet aggregation

CNS:	Depression, paresthesia, fatigue, headache, dizziness
CV:	Angina, edema, palpitations, ↑ BP, syncope
GI:	Diarrhea, gastritis, dyspepsia, nausea, vomiting
Pulmonary:	Dyspnea, URI, cough, epistaxis, rhinitis
Other:	Purpura, rash, pruritus, UTI, myalgias, arthralgia

Dosages: 75–300 mg PO qd

Contraindications: Intracranial hemorrhage, peptic ulcer, internal bleeding

Drug Interactions: ↑ Bleeding with aspirin, NSAIDs, heparin, and warfarin

Key Points: Coagulation profile should be checked before surgery

DALTEPARIN

Trade Name: **Fragmin**

Indications: Prophylaxis against DVT, unstable angina or non–Q wave MI

Pharmacokinetics: Onset: <1 h; bioavailability: 87%; peak: 4 h; duration: 6–12 h; Vd: 40–60 mL/kg; $T_{1/2}$ β: 2–3 h; metabolism/excretion is not known

DALTEPARIN *continued*

Pharmacodynamics:	Low–molecular weight heparin derivative, inhibits Factor Xa and thrombin by $\uparrow$ antithrombin levels
CNS:	Insomnia
CV:	$\downarrow$ BP (due to blood loss)
GI:	Nausea, vomiting, constipation, $\uparrow$ LFTs
Other:	Thrombocytopenia, hematoma, pruritus, rash, ecchymoses, fever
Dosage:	2500 IU SC; 1–2 h before surgery; repeat daily for 5–10 d (DVT prophylaxis); 120 IU/kg SC q 12 h (unstable angina)
Contraindications:	Sensitivity to heparin, pork products, active major bleeding, thrombocytopenia [(+) antiplatelet antibody]
Drug Interactions:	Anticoagulants and platelet inhibitors may $\uparrow$ risk of bleeding
Key Points:	Prophylaxis against DVT for "at-risk" surgical patients (>40 yr, obese, anesthesia >30 min, history DVT or PE) undergoing abdominal or major joint replacement surgery; hemorrhagic complications treated with protamine (1 mg/100 U)

DANAPAROID

Trade Name:	**Orgaran**
Indications:	Prophylaxis of postoperative DVT, treatment of thromboembolism
Pharmacokinetics:	Onset: <1 h; bioavailability: 100%; peak: 2–5 h; duration: 8–12 h; Cl: 0.36 L/h; $T_{1/2}$ β: 24 h: 1° eliminated in urine
Pharmacodynamics:	Glycosaminoglycuronan antithrombotic, which prevents fibrin formation via thrombin inhibition by anti-Xa and anti-IIa effects
CNS:	Headache, dizziness, insomnia
CV:	$\downarrow$ BP (due to bleeding)
GI:	Nausea, constipation
Other:	Fever, pain on injection, pruritus
Dosage:	750 anti-Xa units SQ bid for 7–10 d
Contraindications:	Sensitivity to pork products, severe hemorrhage diathesis (e.g., hemorrhagic state, hemophilia, ITP)
Drug Interactions:	Oral anticoagulants and/or platelet inhibitors $\uparrow$ effect
Key Points:	Monitoring anticoagulants using PT or thrombotest is unreliable <5 h after drug injection

DESIRUDIN

Trade Name:	**Iprivask**
Indications:	DVT prophylaxis
Pharmacokinetics:	Onset: rapid; peak: 10–15 min; $T_{1/2}$ β: 2–3 h
Pharmacodynamics:	Recombinant hirudin, selective thrombin inhibitor
CV:	Leg edema
GI:	Nausea, tarry stools
Pulmonary:	Emboli (due to DVT), epistaxis
Other:	Hematomas, anemia, anaphylactic reactions, ↑ aPTT/TT
Dosage:	15 mg SC q 12 h (10 min before surgery), then 9–12 d postoperatively
Contraindications:	Sensitivity to hirudins, use of heparin or dextran, ↑ BP, bleeding/coagulation disorders, hepatorenal insufficiency
Drug Interactions:	Anticoagulants, abciximab, clopidogrel, dipyridamole, IIb/IIIa antagonists, glycoprotein, NSAIDs, ASA ↑ effects
Key Points:	Risk of neuraxial hematoma with continuous epidural anesthesia; ↓ risk of thrombocytopenia (vs heparins)

DIPYRIDAMOLE

Trade Names:	**Aggrenox, Persantine**
	See Chapter 39, "Vasodilators"

ENOXAPARIN

Trade Name:	**Lovenox**
Indications:	Prevention and treatment of DVT, unstable angina, and non–Q wave MI
Pharmacokinetics:	Onset: <2 min; bioavailability: 90%; peak: 3–5 h; duration: 24 h; Vd: 6 L; $T_{1/2}$ β: 4–5 h; metabolized in liver, excreted in urine
Pharmacodynamics:	Low–molecular weight heparin binds to antithrombin III, inhibits Factor Xa and thrombin, blocks conversion of fibrinogen to fibrin
CV:	Edema, angina, arrhythmias
GI:	Nausea, ↑ LFTs
Other:	Thrombocytopenia, bleeding complications, local irritation, rash, angioedema, anemia

ENOXAPARIN *continued*

Dosage:	30–40 mg SC q 12 h for 7–10 d (DVT prophylaxis); 1 mg/kg SC q/2 h for 2–8 d (ischemia); 1 mg/kg SC q 12 h for 5–7 d (acute DVT)
Contraindications:	Active bleeding, thrombocytopenia, sensitivity to heparin or pork products, diabetic retinopathy, severe hypertension
Drug Interactions:	↑ Risk of hemorrhage with anticoagulants, NSAIDs, salicylates, aspirin, and dipyridamole; valproic acid and plicamycin ↓ platelet aggregation
Key Points:	Potential for neurologic injury (e.g., spinal/epidural hematomas) when used with major regional anesthetic technique (e.g., indwelling epidural catheters); patients with heparin-induced thrombocytopenia at ↑ risk of hemorrhage

FONDAPARINUX

Trade Name:	**Arixtra**
Indications:	Prophylaxis against blood clots after major orthopedic surgery
Pharmacokinetics:	Onset: <2 min; bioavailability: 100%; peak: 2–3 h; protein binding: 94%; duration: 12–24 h; Cl: 34 mg/h; $T_{1/2} \beta$: 17–21 h; no metabolism, eliminated unchanged in urine
Pharmacodynamics:	Inhibits Factor Xa by binding to antithrombin III, ↓ formation of thrombin and blood clots
CNS:	Headache, dizziness, confusion, insomnia
CV:	↓ BP, edema
GI:	Nausea, vomiting, dyspepsia, constipation, ↑ LFTs
GU:	UTI, urinary retention
Other:	Hemorrhage, anemia, thrombocytopenia, hypokalemia, purpura, fever
Dosage:	2.5 mg/d SC for 5–9 d
Contraindications:	Severe renal impairment (CrCl <30 mL/min), major active bleeding, bacterial endocarditis, thrombocytopenia/antiplatelet antibody
Drug Interactions:	NSAIDs, platelet inhibitors, and anticoagulants ↑ risk of bleeding
Key Points:	Use with continuous spinal/epidural anesthesia ↑ risk of developing hematoma; anticoagulant effect lasts 2–4 d

HEPARIN

Trade Name:	**Same**
Indications:	DVT, pulmonary embolism, acute MI, unstable angina, cardiopulmonary bypass, DIC, adjunct to thrombolytic regimen
Pharmacokinetics:	Onset: <2 min (IV), 20–60 min (SC); peak: 2–4 h; duration: 4–6 h; Vd: 40–60 mL/kg; Cl: 10 min; $T_{1/2}$ β: 1–2 h; removed by reticuloendothelial system; does not cross placental barrier or into breast milk
Pharmacodynamics:	Accelerates formation of antithrombin III-thrombin complex, inactivates thrombin, prevents conversion of fibrinogen to fibrin
CNS:	Headache
CV:	↓ BP (due to hemorrhage), ↑ clotting time (↑ PTT), vasospasm
Other:	Hypoaldosteronism, thrombocytopenia, thrombosis ("white clot syndrome"), skin necrosis, hematoma, anaphylactoid reactions
Dosages:	5000–10,000 U IV, then 4000–5000 U q 4 h or 20,000–40,000 U/24 h (DVT/PE); 50 U/kg, then 50–100 U/kg q 4 h (children); 25–100 U/kg IV q 4 h (DIC); 5000 U SC q 8–12 h (prophylaxis)
Contraindications:	Active bleeding, blood dyscrasias, intracranial hemorrhage
Drug Interactions:	Digitalis, tetracyclines, antihistamines, and nicotine ↓ effect; platelet inhibitors, warfarin, cephalosporins, and penicillin ↑ effect
Key Points:	Major regional anesthetic techniques should be performed with caution immediately after discontinuation of heparin

PENTOXIFYLLINE

Trade Name:	**Trental**
Indications:	Intermittent claudication, improve blood flow to extremities, high-altitude sickness, sickle cell disease, diabetic neuropathy
Pharmacokinetics:	Onset: <1 h; bioavailability: >90%; peak: 2–4 h; duration: 6–8 h; $T_{1/2}$ β: 0.5–1.5 h; 1st-pass metabolism by liver (and erythrocytes), eliminated in urine
Pharmacodynamics:	Hemorrheologic action, ↓ blood viscosity, ↑ erythrocyte flexibility
CNS:	Headache, anxiety, confusion, tremor, blurred vision, anorexia

PENTOXIFYLLINE *continued*

CV:	↓ BP, angina, pedal edema
GI:	Dyspepsia, nausea, vomiting, flatus, constipation, dry mouth
Other:	Epistaxis, nasal congestion, pruritis, bone marrow suppression, laryngitis
Dosage:	400 mg PO tid (with meals)
Contraindications:	Sensitivity to methylxanthines (e.g., caffeine, theophylline, theobromine), recent cerebral or retinal hemorrhage
Drug Interactions:	↑ Theophylline levels; antiplatelet drugs and anticoagulants ↑ bleeding; antihypertensives ↑ hypotensive effect
Key Points:	↑ Hypotensive effect of regional and general anesthetic technique (especially in the elderly), ↑ risk of bleeding

PROTAMINE

Trade Name:	**Same**
Indications:	Heparin antidote
Pharmacokinetics:	Onset: <1 min; peak: <5 min; duration: 2 h; $T_{1/2}$ β: 1–3 h; heparin-protamine complex degraded, excreted in urine
Pharmacodynamics:	Forms complex with heparin, anticoagulant effect
CNS:	Lassitude, fatigue
CV:	↓ HR, pulmonary hypotension, ↓ BP, ↓ CO
GI:	Nausea, vomiting
Pulmonary:	Pulmonary edema, dyspnea
Other:	Cutaneous flushing, ↓ heparin-prolonged PTT
Dosage:	1 mg IV per 90–115 U heparin over 1–3 min (max. 50 mg/10 min)
Contraindications:	Sensitivity to antidote (e.g., fish allergy)
Drug Interactions:	Incompatible with antibiotics (e.g., cephalosporins, penicillins)
Key Points:	After cardiac surgery, reversal of heparin should be monitored by PTT

RETEPLASE

Trade Name:	**Retavase**
Indications:	Acute MI
Pharmacokinetics:	Onset: <2 min; peak: <10 min; duration: 30–60 min; Cl: 250–450 mL/min; $T_{1/2}$ β: 13–16 min; metabolized in liver and kidney

RETEPLASE *continued*

Pharmacodynamics:	Catalyzes cleavage of plasminogen to generate plasmin, leading to fibrinolysis
CNS:	Intracranial hemorrhage, fever
CV:	Arrhythmias, cholesterol embolization
GI:	Nausea, vomiting, GI bleeding
Other:	Anemia, bleeding tendency (e.g., hematuria, IV sites)
Dosage:	10.8 U IV over 2 min, repeat in 30 min
Contraindications:	Active bleeding, history of CVA, recent intracranial or spine surgery, uncontrolled hypertension, AVM, ruptured aneurysm
Drug Interactions:	Heparin, oral anticoagulants, platelet inhibitors, and vitamin K antagonists ↑ risk of bleeding
Key Points:	↑ Risk of hemorrhage in elderly and parturients and after recent surgery

STREPTOKINASE

Trade Name:	**Streptase**
Indications:	Lysis of thrombi with acute MI, pulmonary embolism, acute venous and arterial thrombosis
Pharmacokinetics:	Onset: <1 min; peak: 0.5–2 h; duration: 12–24 h; $T_{1/2}$ β: 18–83 min; eliminated by circulating antibodies and reticuloendothelial system
Pharmacodynamics:	Stimulates conversion of plasminogen to plasmin
CNS:	Headache, cerebral hemorrhage, polyneuropathy
CV:	Arrhythmias, ↓ BP, vasculitis
Pulmonary:	Difficulty breathing, bronchospasm, apnea
Other:	Major bleeding, periorbital edema, nausea, myalgias, interstitial nephritis, angioedema
Dosage:	1.5 million U IV, or 20,000 U directly into coronary artery followed by 2000 U/min for 1 h (acute MI); 250,000 U over 30 min, followed by 100,000 U/h (thromboembolism)
Contraindications:	Hemorrhagic stroke, embolic or thrombotic stroke (<6 mo), intracranial surgery or trauma (<2 mo), uncontrolled hypertension, active internal bleeding, recent surgery (<10 d), bleeding diathesis, acute pancreatitis, SBE, diabetic retinopathy
Drug Interactions:	Anticoagulant or antiplatelet drugs ↑ risk of bleeding; aminocaproic acid inhibits activating effect; streptokinase is antigenic
Key Points:	Regional anesthetic techniques should be utilized only after normal fibrinolysis has been established; ↑ risk of bleeding in all surgical patients for up to 6 mo

TENECTEPLASE

Trade Name:	**TNKase**
Indications:	Acute MI
Pharmacokinetics:	Onset: <1 min; peak: <2 min; duration: 20–24 min; Cl: 99–119 mL/min; $T_{1/2}$ β: 90–130 min; hepatic metabolism, urinary excretion
Pharmacodynamics:	Human tissue plasminogen activator, binds to fibrin and converts plasminogen to plasmin
CNS:	Intracranial hemorrhage, CVA
GI/GU:	Hematuria, GI bleeding
Other:	Epistaxis, IV site bleeding, hematoma, cholesterol embolism
Dosage:	25–50 mg IV over 5 sec
Contraindications:	Active bleeding, CVA, intracranial or spine surgery (in <2 mo), aneurysm, uncontrolled hypertension, AVM
Drug Interactions:	Anticoagulant and antiplatelet drugs ↑ risk of bleeding
Key Points:	Coagulation profile should be checked before regional anesthetic block is performed (especially in pregnant and elderly patients)

THROMBIN

Trade Names:	**Thrombogen, Thrombostat**
Indications:	Operative site bleeding
Pharmacokinetics:	Not available
Pharmacodynamics:	Catalyzes conversion of fibrogen to fibrin
CV:	Intravascular clotting
Other:	Fever
Dosage:	100 U/mL to area where clotting is needed (max. 2000 U/mL); use dry powder for bone bleeding
Contraindications:	Sensitivity to bovine products
Drug Interactions:	None known
Key Points:	Do *not* inject into large blood vessels (may result in severe intravascular clotting)

TICLOPIDINE

Trade Name:	**Ticlid**
Indications:	Reduce risk of thrombotic CVA, thrombosis after coronary stents cerebral infarction (if aspirin intolerant)

TICLOPIDINE *continued*

Pharmacokinetics:	Onset: <1 h; bioavailability: >80%; peak: 2 h; protein binding: 98%; duration: 8–12 h; $T_{1/2}$ β: 0–15 h (with repeat dose ↑ 4–5 d); metabolized by liver, excreted 1° in urine
Pharmacodynamics:	Blocks ADP-induced platelet aggregation, prolongs bleeding time
CNS:	Headache, dizziness, peripheral neuropathy, tinnitus
GI:	Diarrhea, nausea, anorexia, dyspepsia, vomiting, flatulence, GI bleeding, cholestatic jaundice, ↑ LFTs
Other:	Urticaria, asthenia, epistaxis, nephrotic syndrome, hematuria, rash, pancytopenia, hypoextremia, arthralgias, myositis, serum sickness
Dosage:	250 mg PO bid (with food)
Contraindications:	TTP, aplastic anemia, hemostatic disorders, severe liver impairment, intracranial or GI bleeding
Drug Interactions:	↑ Antiplatelet effect of aspirin and NSAIDs; antacids ↓ level; cimetidine ↓ metabolism; ↑ levels of digoxin, theophylline, phenytoin
Key Points:	Operative site bleeding can be treated with methylprednisolone

TINZAPARIN

Trade Name:	**Innohep**
Indications:	DVT (with or without pulmonary embolism)
Pharmacokinetics:	Onset: 2–3 h; peak: 4–5 h; duration: 18–24 h; $T_{1/2}$ β: 3–4 h; partially metabolized in liver, excreted in urine
Pharmacodynamics:	Low–molecular weight heparin, inhibits Factor Xa and thrombin (II_2) by binding plasma protease inhibitor (antithrombin)
CNS:	Headache, confusion, insomnia, dizziness, intracranial bleeding
CV:	Arrhythmias, angina, thromboembolism, pedal edema
GI:	Anorectal bleeding, constipation, flatulence, melena, nausea, vomiting, dyspepsia, ↑ LFTs
GU:	Dysuria, urinary retention, hematuria, vaginal hemorrhage, UTI
Pulmonary:	Dyspnea, pulmonary embolus, pneumonia
Other:	Epistaxis, hemarthrosis, pancytopenia, myalgias, rash, purpura
Dosage:	175 anti-Xa III U/kg/d SC for 6 d
Contraindications:	Sensitivity to heparin, sulfites, benzyl alcohol, pork products, major bleeding, and heparin-induced thrombocytopenia

TINZAPARIN *continued*

Drug Interactions: Oral anticoagulants, antiplatelets, and thrombolytics ↑ risk of bleeding; antacids ↓ absorption

Key Points: Coagulation profile should be checked before major surgery; may be ↑ risk of bleeding with major regional nerve block techniques

UROKINASE

Trade Name: **Abbokinase**

Indications: Lysis of acute pulmonary emboli, venous thrombi, coronary artery thrombosis, lysis of arterial thrombus, catheter occlusion

Pharmacokinetics: Onset: <10 min; peak: 0.5–4 h; duration: 4 h; $T_{1/2}$ β: 10–20 min; rapidly metabolized in liver, eliminated in urine and bile

Pharmacodynamics: Thrombolytic, activates conversion of plasminogen to plasmin
CNS: Cerebral hemorrhage
CV: Arrhythmias, phlebitis, ↑ HR
GI: Nausea, vomiting
Other: Bleeding at IV and surgical sites, hematoma formation, dyspnea, epistaxis, rash, ecchymoses, fever, chills

Dosage: 5000 U into IV line (catheter occlusion); 6000 U/min for up to 2 h (coronary thrombolysis); 4400 U/kg over 10 min, followed by 4400 U/kg/h for 12 h (pulmonary embolus)

Contraindications: Hemorrhagic stroke, embolic or thrombotic stroke (<6 mo), intracranial surgery or trauma (<2 mo), severe hypertension, AVM, active bleeding (<2 wk), surgical trauma (<10 d), postpartum bleeding diathesis, acute pancreatitis, diabetic retinopathy

Drug Interactions: ↑ Risk of bleeding with concomitant use of antiplatelet drugs or anticoagulants; aminocaproic acid ↓ effect

Key Points: Coagulation profile should be checked before administering major regional anesthetic techniques; discontinue heparin and reverse oral anticoagulants; avoid in pregnant and postpartum patients

WARFARIN

Trade Name:	**Coumadin**
Indications:	Atrial fibrillation, rheumatic valvular disease, prosthetic heart valves, DVT, post-MI, peripheral vascular disease (PVD)
Pharmacokinetics:	Onset: 0.5–3 d; peak: 3–4 d; protein binding: 99%; duration: 2–5 d; Vd: 0.14 L/kg; Cl: 0.045 mL/min/kg; $T_{1/2}$ β: 1–3 d; metabolized by liver, excreted in urine
Pharmacodynamics:	Inhibition of vitamin K–dependent activation of clotting factors (II, VII, IX, X, and prothrombin)
GI:	Anorexia, nausea, cramps, stomatitis, diarrhea, oral ulcers, ↑ LFT, jaundice, vomiting, diarrhea
Other:	Hemorrhage, gangrene, urticaria, hematuria, fever, dermatitis, alopecia, "purple toe" syndrome, paresthesia
Dosage:	2–5 mg/d IV/IM, then 2–10 mg/d PO (based on PT/INR)
Contraindications:	Pregnancy, bleeding dyasthesis, severe hepatorenal disease, severe hypertension, SBE, aneurysm, ascorbic acid deficiency, polycythemia vera, vitamin K deficiency, psychosis, recent surgery
Drug Interactions:	Trimethoprim-sulfamethoxazole and cimetidine ↓ elimination; cholestyramine ↓ absorption; aspirin, acetaminophen, and NSAIDs ↑ effect; cephalosporins inhibit interconversion of vitamin K; ↑ risk of bleeding
Key Points:	Prothrombin time should be checked before surgery; if regional anesthetic technique is indicated, recommend spinal (vs epidural) for central neuraxis blockade (avoid catheters); many drugs and herbal medications can alter the response to warfarin

7

Anticonvulsants

CARBAMAZEPINE

Trade Names:	**Tegretol, Epitol**
Indications:	Tonic-clonic and partial seizures, bipolar affective disorders, trigeminal and glossopharyngeal neuralgia, restless leg syndrome, chorea
Pharmacokinetics:	Onset: 1–2 h; peak: 2–12 h; protein binding: 75%; duration: 8–12 h; Vd: 1–3 L/kg; Cl: 0.05 L/kg/h; $T_{1/2}$ β: 25–65 h (↓ 12–17 h with chronic administration); metabolized by liver to active metabolite, excreted 1° in urine
Pharmacodynamics:	Antineuralgic action, ↓ seizure propagation
CNS:	Dizziness, blurred vision, ataxia, nystagmus, dysarthria, drowsiness, headache, syncope, fatigue
CV:	Arrhythmias, CHF, angina, pedal edema
GI:	Diarrhea, nausea, vomiting, jaundice, ↑ LFTs, anorexia, stomatitis
GU:	Urinary frequency/retention, impotence, glycoseuria/albuminuria
Pulmonary:	Dyspnea, pneumonitis, respiratory depression
Other:	Bone marrow depression, SIADH, chills, fever, rash, urticaria, Stevens-Johnson syndrome, muscle twitching, pancreatitis
Dosage:	50–100 mg PO qid, 100–200 mg bid (max. 1.6 g/d); 10–20 mg/kg/d (max. 1 g/d) (children)
Contraindications:	Bone marrow depression, sensitivity to TCAs, use of MAOIs
Drug Interactions:	Acetaminophen, theophylline, phenytoin, warfarin, haloperidol ↓ effect; TCAs, MAOIs, phenothiazines ↑ CNS depression; cimetidine, macrolides, isoniazide, valproic acid, diltiazem, verapamil ↑ effect
Key Points:	↑ Risk of arrhythmias with sympathomimetic drugs; ↑ hepatotoxicity of volatile anesthetics (?)

CLONAZEPAM

Trade Name:	**Klonopin**
Indications:	Absence, myoclonic and tonic-clonic seizures, panic disorders, infantile spasms
Pharmacokinetics:	Onset: 20–60 min; bioavailability: 90%; peak: 1–2 h; protein binding: 85%; duration: 6–12 h; Vd: 2.0–4.8 L/kg; Cl: 0.04–0.07 L/kg/h; $T_{1/2}$ β: 18–40 h; hepatic metabolism, renal elimination
Pharmacodynamics:	Benzodiazepine, which inhibits GABA receptors in limbic system, thalamus, hypothalamus

CLONAZEPAM *continued*

CNS:	Drowsiness, ataxia, tremor, nystagmus, dysarthria confusion; withdrawal symptoms (e.g., restlessness, insomnia, psychosis, seizures)
CV:	Palpitations, $\downarrow$ BP ($\downarrow$ PVR)
GI:	Nausea, vomiting, constipation, gastritis, anorexia
GU:	Dysuria, enuresis, nocturia, urinary retention
Pulmonary:	Respiratory depression, $\uparrow$ oral secretions, dyspnea
Other:	Muscle weakness, myalgias, rash, bone marrow suppression

Dosage:	0.5–1 mg PO tid (max. 20 mg/d); 0.01–0.03 mg/kg/d (children)
Contraindications:	Severe hepatic disease, acute narrow angle glaucoma
Drug Interactions:	$\uparrow$ CNS depressants (e.g., anticonvulsants, alcohol); $\uparrow$ elimination of cimetidine, contraceptives, disulfiram, erythromycin; valproic acid $\uparrow$ seizures
Key Points:	$\uparrow$ CNS depressant effects of general anesthetics and opioid analgesics; glycopyrrolate is useful in $\downarrow$ oral secretions

ETHOSUXIMIDE

Trade Name:	**Zarontin**
Indications:	Absence (petit mal) seizures
Pharmacokinetics:	Onset: <2 h; peak: 3–7 h; protein binding: negligible; duration: 12–24 h; Vd: 0.6–0.7 L/kg; Cl: 0.012–0.016 L/kg/h; $T_{1/2}$ β: 30–60 h; extensively metabolized and excreted in urine
Pharmacodynamics:	Suppresses spike and wave activity by depressing neuronal transmission in motor cortex and basal ganglia
CNS:	Confusion, coma, drowsiness, headache, irritability, myopia
GI:	Nausea, vomiting, cramps, dyspepsia, anorexia, diarrhea
GU:	Vaginal bleeding, hematuria, urinary frequency
Pulmonary:	Respiratory depression, hiccups
Other:	Pancytopenia, gingival hyperplasia, tongue swelling, trismus, $\downarrow$ muscle tone, urticaria

Dosage:	250 mg PO bid (max. 1.5 g/d); 20 mg/kg/d (children)
Contraindications:	Severe hepatorenal disease, intermittent porphyria, succinimide allergic
Drug Interactions:	Carbamazepine, phenobarbital and hydantoins $\downarrow$ levels, $\uparrow$ phenytoin levels
Key Points:	Additive CNS depression with anesthetic drugs, $\downarrow$ anesthetic requirement

FELBAMATE

Trade Name:	**Felbatol**
Indications:	Partial seizures
Pharmacokinetics:	Onset: <1 h; peak: 2–3 h; protein binding: 25%; duration: 12–24 h; Vd: 756 mL/g; Cl: 26 mL/h/kg; $T_{1/2}$ β: 22 h; excreted in urine
Pharmacodynamics:	Anticonvulsant activity (due to generalized CNS depression)
CNS:	Somnolence, dizziness, insomnia, headache, fatigue
CV:	Arrhythmias
GI:	Anorexia, nausea, vomiting, dyspepsia, constipation, ↑ SGPT
Pulmonary:	URI, rhinitis
Dosage:	1–2 g/d PO (adult); 15 mg/kg/d (children)
Contraindications:	Blood dyscrasias, severe hepatic dysfunction
Drug Interactions:	↓ Level of carbamazepine, ↑ level of phenytoin and valproic acid
Key Points:	↑ Sedative effects of general anesthetic drugs

FOSPHENYTOIN

Trade Name:	**Cerebyx**
Indications:	Status epilepticus, seizures during neurosurgery
Pharmacokinetics:	Onset: 15–30 min (conversion to active metabolite); peak: 30–60 min; protein binding: 95%; Vd: 4.3–10.8 L; excretion unknown
Pharmacodynamics:	Prodrug of phenytoin, stabilizes neuronal membranes by inhibiting calcium channels
CNS:	Dysarthria, ↑ ICP, ataxia, drowsiness, nystagmus, tinnitus, agitation, asthenia, paresthesia, diplopia
CV:	↓ HR, ↑ BP, vasodilation, QT prolongation
GI:	Dry mouth, nausea/vomiting, constipation, tongue edema, bad taste
Other:	Hypokalemia, myalgias, rash, pruritus, ecchymosis, pneumonia
Dosage:	15–20 mg/kg IV initially, then 4–6 mg/kg/d
Contraindications:	Sinus bradycardia, advanced heart block, Adams-Stokes syndrome, sensitivity to hydantoins
Drug Interactions:	Benzodiazepines, chloramphenicol, cimetidine, disulfiram, isoniazid, phenothiazines, succinimides, sulfonamides, valproic acid ↓ metabolism; phenothiazines,

FOSPHENYTOIN *continued*

	barbiturates, carbamazepine, diazoxide, ethanol, rifampin, theophylline ↑ metabolism; antacids, charcoal ↓ absorption; ↓ effects of dopamine, furosemide, levodopa, nondepolarizing muscle relaxants, coumarin, digoxin, furosemide, theophylline, quinidine; TCAs ↓ seizure threshold
Key Points:	Can ↑ central effects of inhalational anesthetics and local anesthetics; ↓ effects of muscle relaxants and fentanyl opioids

GABAPENTIN

Trade Name:	**Neurontin**
Indications:	Partial seizures, after herpetic neuralgia, chronic pain
Pharmacokinetics:	Onset: <1 h; bioavailability: 60%; minimal protein binding; duration: 6–12 h; Vd: 58 L; elimination $T_{1/2}$ β: 5–7 h; not metabolized, excreted unchanged in urine
Pharmacodynamics:	Anticonvulsant with analgesic-like activity
CNS:	Somnolence, dizziness, ataxia, tremor, diplopia, amnesia
CV:	Peripheral edema, vasodilation
GI:	Nausea, vomiting, dyspepsia, flatulence, constipation, ↑ appetite
Other:	Impotence, myalgias, pruritis, hyperlipidemia, hypoestrogenia
Dosage:	300–600 mg tid (max. 3.6 g/d); 10–40 mg/kg/d (children)
Contraindications:	Severe renal dysfunction
Drug Interactions:	↓ Absorption with antacids
Key Points:	Opioid-sparing effects when administered during the perioperative period

LAMOTRIGINE

Trade Name:	**Lamictal**
Indications:	Partial seizures, Lennox-Gastaut syndrome
Pharmacokinetics:	Peak plasma concentration: 1.4–4.8 h; protein binding: 55%; Vd: 0.9–1.3 L/kg; metabolized by glucuronide conjugation, excreted in urine
Pharmacodynamics:	Anticonvulsant, ↓ release of glutamate and aspartate in the brain
CNS:	Dizziness, somnolence, blurred vision, amnesia, confusion, nystagmus, vertigo, headache, ataxia, seizures, dysarthria

LAMOTRIGINE *continued*

CV:	Postural hypotension, palpitations, ↑ HR, vasodilation, edema
GI:	Dry mouth, dysphagia, stomatitis, nausea, dyspepsia, rectal hemorrhage, peptic ulcer, anorexia, ↑ LFTs
Other:	Acne, alopecia, urticara, rash (Stevens-Johnson syndrome or toxic epidermal necrolysis), dysmenorrhea, vaginitis, hyperglycemia, rhinitis, epistaxis, myalgias, tooth pain, pharyngitis, photosensitivity
Dosage:	25 mg/d PO; 0.15 mg/g/d (children)
Contraindications:	Severe hepatorenal and cardiac impairment
Drug Interactions:	Phenytoin, carbamazepine, phenobarbital ↓ effect; inhibits folate synthesis, valproic acid ↑ effect
Key Points:	Abrupt drug withdrawal lowers seizure threshold

MAGNESIUM

Other Name:	**Mag Sulfate, Epsom Salt**
Indications:	Seizure prevention, pre-eclampsia or eclampsia, acute nephritis, acute hypomagnesemia, atypical ventricular tachycardia, "torsades de pointes"
Pharmacokinetics:	Onset: 1 h; peak: <30 min; duration: 0.5–4 h; no metabolism, excreted in urine
Pharmacodynamics:	CNS and respiratory depressant, causes vasodilation and ↓ neuromuscular transmission
CNS:	Drowsiness, flaccid paralysis (↓ reflexes)
CV:	↓ BP; CV collapse; prolongs PR, QRS, QT interval
Pulmonary:	Respiratory paralysis, dyspnea
Other:	Hypothermia, hypocalcemia, diaphoresis, flushing
Dosage:	4–5 g IV/IM q 4 h (max. 30–40 g/d) (seizures); 100–200 mg/kg IV/IM q 4–6 h (max. 8–15 g/d); 1–6 g IV, then 3–20 mg/min (ventricular arrhythmias); 4–6 g IV over 20 min, then 2–4 g/h for 12–24 h (preterm labor)
Contraindications:	Heart block, MI, renal failure, toxemia of pregnancy
Drug Interactions:	Cardiotoxicity with digoxin; alcohol ↑ CNS depression; IV calcium neutralizes side effects
Key Points:	↑ Neuromuscular relaxants; ↑ CNS depressant effects of anesthetics

PENTOBARBITAL

Trade Name:	**Nembutal**
Indications:	Seizures, insomnia, premedication
Pharmacokinetics:	Onset: 10–25 min; bioavailability: high; peak: 0.5–1 h; protein binding: 40%; duration: 3–4 h; $T_{1/2}$ β: 35–50 h; metabolized in liver, eliminated in urine
Pharmacodynamics:	Nonselective depressant of both pre- and postsynaptic membrane excitability by facilitating the action of GABA in the CNS
CNS:	Somnolence, paradoxical excitement, hallucinations
CV:	↓ HR, ↓ BP, syncope
GI:	Nausea, vomiting
Pulmonary:	Respiratory depression
Other:	Porphyria, rash, Stevens-Johnson syndrome, angioedema
Dosage:	100 mg IV (max. 500 mg) (seizures); 20–40 mg q 6–12 h (sedation/insomnia); 2–6 mg/kg (children)
Contraindications:	Porphyria, severe respiratory disease
Drug Interactions:	Antidepressants, sedative-hypnotics, alcohol, antihistamines, opioids ↑ CNS and respiratory depression; corticosteroids, digitoxin, doxycycline, theophylline, estrogens, rifampin ↑ metabolism; disulfiram, MAOIs, valproic acid ↓ metabolism (↑ level)
Key Points:	Use with other barbiturates, benzodiazepines, IV anesthetics ↑ CNS, respiratory, cardiovascular depressive effects

PHENOBARBITAL

Trade Names:	**Luminal, Solfoton**
Indications:	Partial seizures, generalized clonic-tonic seizures, status epilepticus, sedation, insomnia, drug withdrawal
Pharmacokinetics:	Onset: 5–30 min; peak: 0.5–2 h; protein binding: 50%; duration: 4–12 h; Vd: 0.6 L/kg; Cl: 0.008 L/kg/h; $T_{1/2}$ β: 5–7 h; hepatic metabolism, renal elimination
Pharmacodynamics:	CNS depressant, which ↓ spread of epileptogenic foci by enhancing GABA at both pre- and postsynaptic membranes
CNS:	Drowsiness, paradoxical excitement, withdrawal symptoms, seizures, tolerance/dependence, nystagmus, ataxia
CV:	Arrhythmia, ↓ HR, ↓ BP, thrombophlebitis
GI:	Nausea, vomiting, constipation, porphyria

PHENOBARBITAL *continued*

Pulmonary:	Respiratory depression, apnea
Other:	Megaloblastic anemia, erythema multiforma, Stevens-Johnson syndrome
Dosage:	60–100 mg PO; 200–300 mg IM/IV (seizures); 1–6 mg/kg PO; 4–6 mg/kg/d IM/IV (children); 100–200 mg PO; 100–320 mg IM (sedation/insomnia)
Contraindications:	Severe respiratory disease, porphyria, hepatic failure
Drug Interactions:	↑ Metabolism of warfarin, phenytoin, phenylbutazone, prednisone, hydrocortisone, digoxin; valproic acid, and chloramphenicol ↓ effect; ↑ sedation with CNS depressants
Key Points:	Use with other barbiturates, benzodiazepines, IV anesthetics ↑ CNS, respiratory, cardiac depression

PHENYTOIN

Trade Name:	**Dilantin**
	See Chapter 4, "Antiarrhythmics"

PRIMIDONE

Trade Name:	**Mysoline**
Indications:	Partial (psychomotor) seizures, generalized tonic-clonic seizures, benign familial (essential) tremor
Pharmacokinetics:	Onset: <30 min; peak: 3–4 h; protein binding: <20%; duration: 8–24 h; Vd: 0.6 L/kg; Cl: 0.013–0.041 L/kg/h; $T_{1/2} \beta$: 4–12 h; metabolized in liver to isphenobarbital, excreted in urine
Pharmacodynamics:	Nonspecific CNS depressant with anticonvulsant activity
CNS:	Drowsiness, nystagmus, ataxia, fatigue, dizziness, diplopia, restlessness, paranoia, headache
GI:	Nausea, vomiting, anorexia
Other:	Blood dyscrasias, impotence, polyuria, rash
Dosage:	100–750 mg/d PO (<2 g/d) in divided doses (adults); 10–20 mg/kg/d (children)
Contraindications:	Porphyria, sensitivity to phenobarbital, breast-feeding
Drug Interactions:	Acetazolamide, carbamazepine, succinimides ↓ level; hydantoins, isoniazid, nicotinamide ↑ level
Key Points:	↑ CNS depressant effects of inhalational and IV anesthetics ↑ sedation, as well as respiratory and cardiovascular depression

TIAGABINE

Trade Name:	**Gabitril**
Indications:	Partial seizures
Pharmacokinetics:	Onset: <30 min; bioavailability: 90%; peak: 30–60 min; protein binding: 90%; duration: 7–9 h; $T_{1/2}$ β: 7–9 h; metabolized in liver by P_{450} enzymes, excreted 1° in feces
Pharmacodynamics:	Anticonvulsant, ↑ activity of GABA at postsynaptic membranes
CNS:	Dizziness, asthenia, somnolence, tremor, ataxia, speech disorder, agitation, confusion, paresthesia, nystagmus, amnesia
CV:	Vasodilation, postural hypotension
GI:	Abdominal pain, nausea/vomiting, diarrhea, ↑ appetite, mouth ulcer
Other:	Cough, rash, pruritus, myasthenia, myalgia, UTI
Dosage:	4 mg/d PO in divided doses (max. 56 mg/d)
Contraindications:	Breast-feeding
Drug Interactions:	↓ Valproic level; carbamazepine, phenobarbital, phenytoin ↑ metabolism
Key Points:	When administered prior to general anesthesia, ↑ CNS depressive effects can prolong early recovery

TOPIRAMATE

Trade Name:	**Topamax**
Indications:	Partial, generalized tonic-clonic seizures, Lennox-Gastaut syndrome
Pharmacokinetics:	Onset: <30 min; bioavailability: 80%; peak: 2 h; protein binding: 15%; duration: 24 h; $T_{1/2}$ β: 21 hr; minimal metabolism, excreted 1° unchanged in urine
Pharmacodynamics:	↑ Activity of GABA and glutamate activity receptor, Na-channel blocking action
CNS:	Somnolence, ataxia, inattention, amnesia, suicidal thoughts, dizziness, tremor, hallucinations, nystagmus, tinnitus, insomnia, anxiety, anorexia
CV:	Peripheral edema, palpitations, angina
GI:	Gingivitis, dyspepsia, nausea, vomiting, flatulence, dry mouth
GU:	Dysmenorrhea (hot flashes, bleeding), dysuria, impotence, UTI, urinary incontinence, hematuria, vaginitis, renal calculus
Pulmonary:	Cough, dyspnea, bronchitis, pharyngitis, sinusitis, epistaxis
Other:	Anemia, leukopenia, myalgia, acne, alopecia, diaphoresis

TOPIRAMATE *continued*

Dosage:	25–50 mg/d PO (max. 40 mg/d); 5–9 mg/kg/d (children)
Contraindications:	Acute myopia with angle-closure glaucoma
Drug Interactions:	Carbamazepine and phenytoin ↓ level; carbonic anhydrase inhibitors ↑ renal stone formation; ↓ effect of hormonal contraceptives; phenobarbital and valproic acid ↑ level
Key Points:	Potential ↑ CNS depression and prolonged recovery from general anesthesia if administered before surgery

VALPROIC ACID

Trade Names:	**Depakene, Depakote**
Indications:	Simple (petit mal) and complex absence seizures
Pharmacokinetics:	Onset: <15 min; bioavailability: >90%; peak: 0.5–5 h; protein binding: 90%; duration: 12–24 h; Vd: 0.17 L/kg; Cl: 0.016 L/kg/h; $T_{1/2}$ β: 11–20 h; metabolized extensively, eliminated in urine
Pharmacodynamics:	Anticonvulsant activity due to ↑ GABA in the brain
CNS:	Drowsiness, tremor, ataxia, nystagmus, diplopia, dysarthria, incoordination, confusion, dizziness, asthenia, restlessness, irritability, headache
GI:	Nausea, vomiting, abdominal cramps, dyspepsia, ↑ LFTs, diarrhea
Other:	↓ Platelet aggregation, ↑ bleeding time, hematomas, bone marrow suppression, myalgias, rash, alopecia, pruritus, photosensitivity, pancreatitis
Dosage:	10–15 mg/kg/d PO (max. 60 mg/kg/d); 15–45 mg/kg/d (children)
Contraindications:	Severe hepatic dysfunction, pregnancy
Drug Interactions:	Chlorpromazine, cimetidine, salicylates ↑ levels; ↑ bleeding with anticoagulants and NSAIDs; carbamazepine, phenytoin, primidone, phenobarbital ↑ metabolism
Key Points:	↑ Fentanyl and nondepolarizing relaxant requirements due to ↑ hepatic clearance; use with halogenated anesthetics ↑ hepatoxicity; naloxone partially reverses CNS depression

ZONISAMIDE

Trade Name:
: **Zonegran**

Indications:
: Partial seizures

Pharmacokinetics:
: Onset: 1–2 h; peak: 3–5 h; protein binding: 40%; duration: 24–48 h; $T_{1/2}$ β: 63 h; extensively binds to erythrocytes; metabolized by cytochrome P_{450} and excreted in urine

Pharmacodynamics:
: Antiseizure activity 2° to blockade of sodium and calcium channels, stabilizing neuronal membranes, and ↓ hypersynchronization

CNS:
: Headache, dizziness, ataxia, tremor, asthenia, nystagmus, confusion, tinnitus, nervousness, paresthesias, diplopia, anorexia, somnolence

GI:
: Nausea, vomiting, bad taste, diarrhea, dyspepsia, dry mouth

Other:
: Cough, ecchymoses, rash, pruritus

Dosage:
: 100 mg PO qd (max. 400 mg/d)

Contraindications:
: Sensitivity to sulfonamides, CRF (CrCl <50 mL/min)

Drug Interactions:
: Hepatic cytochrome P_{450} metabolized drugs ↑ metabolism

Key Points:
: Abrupt withdrawal may precipitate seizure (i.e., status epilepticus)

8

Antiemetics and Antinauseants

APREPITANT

Trade Name:	**Emend**
Indications:	Chemotherapy-induced emesis, PONV
Pharmacokinetics:	Onset: 1–2 h; bioavailability: 65%; peak: 4 h; protein binding: 95%; Vd: 70 L; Cl: 60–90 mL/min; $T_{1/2}$ β: 9–13 h; crosses blood-brain barrier; extensively metabolized in liver, excreted 1° in feces
Pharmacodynamics:	Highly selective substance P/neurokinin-1 (NK-1) receptor antagonist
CNS:	Dizziness, hiccups, fatigue, headache
CV:	Postural hypotension (reflex ↑ HR)
GI:	Diarrhea, ↓ appetite, dehydration, abdominal pain, LFTs
Other:	Hiccups, dehydration
Dosage:	80–125 mg/d PO (prophylaxis), then 80 mg/d
Contraindications:	Pimozide, terfenadine, and astemizole ↑ side effects
Drug Interactions:	↓ Effect of OCPs; cytochrome P_{450} inhibitors ↑ effect; P_{450} inducers ↓ effect; 5-HT$_3$ antagonists and dexamethasone ↑ antiemetic effect
Key Points:	↑ Effects of other antiemetics (as part of a multimodal regimen for antiemetic prophylaxis), may ↑ postoperative sedation due to ↓ hepatic metabolism of benzodiazepines and IV anesthetics

CHLORPROMAZINE

Trade Name:	**Thorazine**
	See Chapter 9, "Antipsychotics"

CYCLIZINE

Trade Name:	**Marezine**
Indications:	Prevention and treatment of PONV, motion sickness
Pharmacokinetics:	Onset: 30–60 min; peak: 2–3 h; duration: 4–24 h; metabolized in the liver, excreted in the urine
Pharmacodynamics:	↓ Labyrinth excitability, ↓ CTZ stimulation
CNS:	Drowsiness, blurred vision, hallucinations, tinnitus, restlessness
CV:	↑ HR, ↓ BP, palpitations
GI:	Dry mouth, anorexia, cholestatic jaundice, constipation
GU:	Urinary retention and frequency
Other:	Rash, urticaria

CYCLIZINE *continued*

Dosage:	50 mg PO (prophylaxis); 50 mg IM (treatment); 1 mg/kg (children)
Contraindications:	GI tract or bladder neck obstruction, BPH, asthma
Drug Interactions:	Aminoglycosides, cisplatin, loop diuretics, ASA, vancomycin can mask ototoxicity
Key Points:	↑ CNS depressant effects of analgesics, anxiolytics, anesthetics

DIMENHYDRINATE

Trade Name:	**Dramamine**
Indications:	Prevention and treatment of PONV, dizziness/vertigo
Pharmacokinetics:	Onset: <1 h; peak: 1–2 h; protein binding: 98%; duration: 3–6 h; metabolized in liver, excreted in urine
Pharmacodynamics:	Antihistaminic (H_1 receptor antagonist); antiemetic, antivertigo, and anticholinergic activity
CNS:	Drowsiness, ↓ labyrinthine function, diplopia
Other:	Dry mouth, chest tightness (wheezing), dysuria
Dosage:	0.25–7.75 mg/kg PO/IV q 4–6 h (max. 400 mg/d); 25–50 mg (0.5–1.25 mg/kg) q 6–8 h, max.; 300 mg/d (children)
Contraindications:	Neonates, BPH, sensitivity to benzyl alcohol
Drug Interactions:	↑ Ototoxicity of antibiotics; ↓ effect of apomorphine; ↑ CNS depression produced by anesthetic drugs and alcohol
Key Points:	Consists of diphenhydramine (Benadryl) and dimenhydrinate, possesses greater anticholinergic activity than other H_1-antagonists

DEXAMETHASONE

Trade Name:	**Decadron**
	See Chapter 37, "Steroids"

DRONABINOL

Trade Name:	**Marinol**
Indications:	Chemotherapy-induced nausea and vomiting, appetite stimulation

DRONABINOL *continued*

Pharmacokinetics:	Onset: 30–60 min; bioavailability: 90%; peak: 2–4 h; protein binding: 99%; duration: 24–48 h; metabolized in liver, excreted 1° in feces
Pharmacodynamics:	Synthetic cannabinoid with sympathomimetic activity; inhibits CTZ
CNS:	Dizziness, euphoria, ataxia, hallucinations, amnesia, paranoia, speech difficulties, visual disturbances, asthenia
CV:	↑ HR, orthostatic hypotension, vasodilation, palpitations, flushing
GI:	Dry mouth, ↑ appetite, diarrhea, nausea, vomiting
Dosage:	2.5–5 mg PO bid (max. 20 mg/d)
Contraindications:	Active drug abuse, pregnancy, breast-feeding
Drug Interactions:	Anticholinergics and antihistamines ↑ drowsiness; TCAs, amphetamines, and sympathomimetics ↑ BP and HR; alcohol, opioids, and benzodiazepines ↑ CNS depression
Key Points:	↑ Sedative effects of benzodiazepines and general anesthetics; causes dysphoric reactions in the elderly

DROPERIDOL

Trade Name:	**Inapsine**
Indications:	Prophylaxis and treatment of PONV, delirium
Pharmacokinetics:	Onset: <10 min; peak: 30 min; duration: 2–4 h; Vd: 2.4 L/kg; Cl: 14.1 mL/kg/min; $T_{1/2}$ β: 1.73 h; crosses blood-brain and placental barriers; metabolized in liver, excreted in urine and feces
Pharmacodynamics:	α-Adrenergic and dopaminergic receptor blockade at the CTZ
CNS:	Tranquilization, dysphoria, extrapyramidal reactions, hallucinations, apprehension, restlessness, drowsiness, dizziness
CV:	↓ BP, ↑ HR, QT prolongation (torsades de pointes)
Pulmonary:	Respiratory depression
Dosage:	0.625–1.25 mg IV; 25–50 μg/kg (children)
Contraindications:	Congenital long QT syndrome, severe dysphoric reaction
Drug Interactions:	Alcohol ↑ CNS depression; ↓ pressor effect of epinephrine
Key Points:	↑ Sedative, respiratory, cardiovascular depressant effects of opioid analgesics and general anesthetics; used for antiemetic prophylaxis after induction of anesthesia

GRANISETRON

Trade Name:	**Kytril**
Indications:	Chemotherapy-induced emesis, PONV
Pharmacokinetics:	Onset: 1–2 h; peak: 3–4 h; protein binding: 65%; duration: 24–36 h; Vd: 2.2 L/kg;
	Cl: 3.5 mL/min/kg; $T_{1/2}$ β: 11 h; metabolized by liver, excreted in urine
Pharmacodynamics:	Long-acting $5\text{-}HT_3$ antagonist, stimulates serotonin receptors in CTZ
CNS:	Headache, dizziness, asthenia, somnolence
CV:	↓ HR, flushing
GI:	Flatulence, dyspepsia, ↑ LFT
GU:	UTI, oliguria
Other:	Alopecia, rash, leukopenia
Dosage:	0.2–1 mg PO/IV; 40 μg/kg (children)
Contraindications:	Sensitivity to other $5\text{-}HT_3$ antagonists
Drug Interactions:	None known
Key Points:	Long-acting $5\text{-}HT_3$ antagonist that is effective in postdischarge period; use in combination with dexamethasone ↑ antiemetic activity

HYDROXYZINE

Trade Names:	**Atarax, Vistaril**
	See Chapter 10, "Antihistamines"

MECLIZINE

Trade Name:	**Antivert**
Indications:	Dizziness, motion sickness, PONV
Pharmacokinetics:	Onset: 1 h; peak: 2–4 h; duration: 8–24 h; $T_{1/2}$ β: 6 h; metabolized in liver, excreted unchanged in feces
Pharmacodynamics:	↓ Labyrinth excitability, ↓ CTZ stimulation
CNS:	Drowsiness, restlessness, hallucinations, blurred vision, tinnitus
CV:	↓ BP, ↑ HR
GI:	Dry mouth, constipation
GU:	Urinary retention and frequency
Other:	Urticaria, rash
Dosage:	25–100 mg/d PO

MECLIZINE *continued*

Contraindications:	Severe asthma, BPH, glaucoma
Drug Interactions:	Masks ototoxicity due to aminoglycosides, cisplatin, loop diuretics, ASA
Key Points:	↑ CNS depressant effects of anesthetic drugs

METOCLOPRAMIDE

Trade Name:	**Reglan**
Indications:	Gastroesophageal reflux, PONV, chemotherapy-induced emesis, diabetic gastroparesis, facilitates gastric emptying
Pharmacokinetics:	Onset: <30 min; bioavailability: >75%; peak: 1–2 h; duration: 1–2 h; Vd: 2.8 L/kg; $T_{1/2}$ β: 3–6 h; excretion 1° via kidney
Pharmacodynamics:	Dopamine receptor antagonist, gastrokinetic agent
CNS:	Drowsiness, dizziness, ↑ extrapyramidal reactions, ↑ parkinsonian symptoms, ↓ seizure threshold, restlessness, fatigue
GI:	↑ Lower esophageal sphincter tone, ↓ gastric volume, ↓ intestinal transit time, diarrhea, nausea
GU:	Urinary frequency, amenorrhea
Other:	Galactorrhea, ↑ prolactin, porphyria, gynecomastia, impotence
Dosage:	10–20 mg PO/IV; 0.1–0.25 mg/kg (children)
Contraindications:	Bowel obstruction, perforation, or hemorrhage, pheochromocytoma, epilepsy, use other antiemetics with extrapyramidal side effects
Drug Interactions:	↑ Absorption of acetaminophen, ASA, diazepam, lithium; anticholinergics and opioids ↓ effects on GI motility; MAOIs ↑ BP
Key Points:	For antiemetic prophylaxis, administer at end of surgery in combination with a 5-HT₃ antagonist; ↓ residual gastric volume prior to induction of general anesthesia (e.g., diabetics, morbid obesity, "full stomach")

ONDANSETRON

Trade Name:	**Zofran**
Indications:	Chemotherapy-induced emesis (CIE), PONV
Pharmacokinetics:	Onset: <1 h; bioavailability: 60%; peak: 1–2 h; duration: 6–12 h; Vd: 2.3 L/kg; Cl: 6–8 mL/kg/min; $T_{1/2}$ β: 4–6 h

ONDANSETRON *continued*

Pharmacodynamics:	Selective 5-HT$_3$ receptor antagonist
CNS:	Headache, dizziness, extrapyramidal reactions
GI:	↑ LFTs
Other:	Warm sensation (in epigastrium), fever, flushing
Dosage:	4–8 mg IV or 8–16 mg PO (PONV); 50–100 µg/kg IV (children); 16–32 mg PO (CIE); 150 µg/kg PO (children)
Contraindications:	Sensitivity to other 5-HT$_3$ antagonists; orally disintegrating tablet (ODT) contains aspartane (PKU)
Drug Interactions:	NK
Key Points:	Optimal timing of IV administration for antiemetic prophylaxis is end of surgery; ↑ efficacy when combined with droperidol, metoclopramide, dexamethasone, and/or acupoint stimulation

PALONOSETRON

Trade Name:	**Aloxi**
Indications:	Chemotherapy-induced nausea and vomiting, PONV
Pharmacokinetics:	Onset: <15 min; peak: 30 min; protein binding: 62%; Vd: 8.3 L/kg; Cl: 160 mL/kg/h; T$_{1/2}$ β: 40 h; hepatic metabolism, excreted in bile and urine
Pharmacodynamics:	Selective 5-HT$_3$ receptor antagonist
CNS:	Headache, dizziness, fatigue, insomnia
CV:	Arrhythmia, QT prolongation
GI:	Constipation, diarrhea, abdominal pain
Dosage:	0.25 mg IV (3 µg/kg)
Contraindications:	Prolonged QT interval, sensitivity to 5-HT$_3$ antagonists
Drug Interactions:	Low potential for drug interactions
Key Points:	Can ↑ QT prolongation of anesthetic drugs

PERPHENAZINE

Trade Name:	**Trilafon**
Indications:	Psychosis, PONV, hiccups
Pharmacokinetics:	Onset: 0.5–1 h; peak: 1–3 h; protein binding: 90%; Vd: 20.2 L/kg; Cl: 1.8 mL/kg/min; T$_{1/2}$ β: 9–10 h; extensive hepatic metabolism, excreted 1° in urine
Pharmacodynamics:	Phenothiazine, which blocks dopamine receptors in CTZ

PERPHENAZINE *continued*

CNS:	Tranquilizing, ↓ seizure threshold, extrapyramidal reactions, tardive dyskinesia, drowsiness, pseudo-parkinsonism
CV:	Postural hypotension, vasodilation (↓ PVR), ↑ HR, (−) inotrope, ↑ QT_c interval
GI:	Dry mouth, jaundice, constipation, ↓ gastric secretion and motility
Other:	Galactorrhea (↑ prolactin), agranulocytosis, Δ blood glucose

Dosage:	5 mg IM q 6 h (PONV); 4–16 mg PO tid (max. 48 mg/d) (psychosis)
Contraindications:	Bladder neck obstruction, BPH, pyloroduodenal obstruction
Drug Interactions:	Antacids ↓ absorption; ↓ sympathomimetic effects; ↑ lithium toxicity; ↑ BP response to antihypotensive drugs
Key Points:	↑ Postoperative sedation and orthostatic hypotensive effects of CNS depressant drugs

PROCHLORPERAZINE

Trade Name:	**Compazine**
Indications:	Prevention and treatment of nausea and vomiting, psychosis
Pharmacokinetics:	Onset: <30 min; bioavailability: 25%; peak: 2–4 h; protein binding: 90%; duration: 6–12 h; Vd: 20 L/kg; Cl: 33 mL/kg/min; $T_{1/2}$ β: 7 h; extensive hepatic metabolism, excreted in urine
Pharmacodynamics:	Phenothiazine-like, which blocks dopamine receptor in CTZ
CNS:	Tranquilization, dizziness, drowsiness, blurred vision, ↓ seizure threshold, ↑ extrapyramidal reactions
CV:	Orthostatic hypotension, ↑ HR, (−) inotropic action
GI:	Dry mouth, jaundice, constipation, ↓ gastric secretion/motility, ileus
GU:	Urinary retention, dark urine, ↓ ejaculation, menstrual irregularities
Other:	Galactorrhea (↑ prolactin), ↑ appetite
Dosage:	5–10 mg PO/IM q 3–4 h; 10–25 mg supp; 0.4 mg/kg (children)
Contraindications:	Severe liver or cardiac disease, central neuroaxis block (children)
Drug Interactions:	Antacids ↓ absorption; ↓ sympathetic response to ephedrine; ↑ postural hypotension, pimozide ↑ QT interval, β-blockers, phenytoin ↑ levels

PROCHLORPERAZINE *continued*

Key Points: ↑ Anesthesia-induced CNS depression, contributing to postoperative sedation, hypotension, respiratory depression

PROMETHAZINE

Trade Name: **Phenergan**

Indications: Prevention and treatment of PONV, motion sickness, drug allergic reactions (e.g., pruritus, urticaria, and dermatitis), anxiety

Pharmacokinetics: Onset: 3–5 (IV), 20 min (IM), 15–60 min (oral); duration: 4–6 h; extensive hepatic metabolism, excreted in urine and feces

Pharmacodynamics: Phenothiazine-type H_1-blocker, with antimuscarinic action at CTZ

CNS: Drowsiness, disorientation, tremor, extrapyramidal symptoms, blurred vision, dizziness, tinnitus, fatigue

CV: Hemodynamic instability, cardiac arrest

GI: Dry mouth, obstructive jaundice, nausea, vomiting

Other: Blood dyscrasias, urinary retention, hyperglycemia, rash

Dosage: 12.5–25 mg IM or 25 mg PO bid; 0.25–0.5 mg/kg q 6 h (children)

Contraindications: Intestinal obstruction, BPH, bladder neck obstruction, seizure disorders, CNS depression, neonates, breast-feeding

Drug Interactions: ↑ Sedative effects of benzodiazepines, opioids, alcohol; avoid use with MAOIs; antithyroid drugs ↑ risk of agranulocytosis; ↓ α-adrenergic effects of epinephrine; ↓ effects of L-dopa in parkinsonism

Key Points: ↑ CNS depressant effects of general anesthetics (e.g., sedation)

TRANSDERMAL SCOPOLAMINE

Trade Name: **Transderm Scōp**

Indications: Motion sickness, PONV

Pharmacokinetics: Onset: 4–6 h; peak: 12–24 h; duration: 72 h; metabolized via enzymatic hydrolysis to scopine and tropic acid, <10% excreted in urine

TRANSDERMAL SCOPOLAMINE *continued*

Pharmacodynamics:	Competitive antagonist of acetylcholine at muscarinic receptors
CNS:	Drowsiness, dizziness, amnesia, hallucinations, restlessness, confusion, blurred vision, mydriasis, cycloplegia
CV:	↓ HR (low dose); ↑ HR (high dose), flushing
GI:	↓ Alivation, ↓ gastric secretions and motility, dyspepsia
GU:	Urinary hesitancy and retention
Other:	Bronchial mucous plugs, rash
Dosage:	1.5 mg TTS (patch)
Contraindications:	Belladonna alkaloids, narrow-angle glaucoma, bladder neck obstruction, ↑ digoxin levels, alcohol intoxication
Drug Interactions:	Additive effects with other anticholinergic drugs
Key Points:	Apply patch the evening prior or morning of surgery for prophylaxis against PONV; possesses more profound effects than atropine on salivation and ocular function, less effect on HR and smooth muscle

TRIMETHOBENZAMIDE

Trade Name:	**Tigan**
Indications:	PONV
Pharmacokinetics:	Onset: <30 min; bioavailability: 68%; peak: 1–2 h; duration: 2–4 h; metabolized in liver, excreted in urine and feces
Pharmacodynamics:	Centrally acting nonphenothiazine antiemetic, weak antihistamine
CNS:	Drowsiness, Parkinson-like symptoms, dizziness, disorientation, headaches, blurred vision, dystonic reactions, seizures
CV:	↓ BP, ↑ HR
GI:	↓ GI motility, diarrhea, jaundice
Other:	Reye's syndrome, pain at injection site, muscle cramps, blood dyscrasias
Dosage:	200–250 mg PO tid; 100 mg IM; 100–200 mg tid (children)
Contraindications:	Sensitivity to benzocaine; children with acute febrile illness
Drug Interactions:	CNS depressants ↑ toxicity; masks symptoms of ototoxicity
Key Points:	↑ CNS depressant effect of anesthetics and opioid analgesics

9

Antipsychotics

CHLORPROMAZINE

Trade Name:	**Thorazine**
Indications:	Psychosis, treatment of nausea and vomiting, intractable hiccups, Tourette's syndrome, behavioral disorders
Pharmacokinetics:	Onset: 0.5–1 h; bioavailability: 20; peak: 2 h; protein binding: 90%; duration: 4–6 h; Vd: 21 L/kg; Cl: 9.1 mL/kg/min; $T_{1/2}$ β: 30 h; extensively metabolized, excreted in urine
Pharmacodynamics:	Phenothiazine with antiadrenergic, peripheral anticholinergic, ganglionic blocking, antihistaminic, antiserotonin activity
CNS:	Drowsiness, ↓ seizure threshold, retinopathy, restlessness, ↑ extrapyramidal symptoms, ataxia, photosensitivity
CV:	↓ BP, ↓ PVR (α-adrenergic blockade), ↑ HR, (−) inotropic action, palpitations, ECG changes
GI:	Nausea, constipation, ↓ gastric secretion and motility, jaundice
Other:	Thick secretions, dry mouth, ↓ ejaculation, gynecomastia, bone marrow suppression, ↑ prolactin, dystonic reactions
Dosage:	25–50 mg q 4–6 h (antipsychotic effect); 3–6 mg/kg/d (children); 12.5–50 mg IM q 3–4 h (PONV); 1 mg/kg (children)
Contraindications:	Reye's syndrome, CNS depression, severe cardiovascular disease
Drug Interactions:	↑ Sedative and anticholinergic effects of centrally active drugs; ↓ seizure threshold with metrizamide; false-positive test for urine bilirubin and pregnancy; lithium ↑ toxicity; ↑ valproic acid levels
Key Points:	↑ CNS depressant effects of anesthetic drugs; consider giving folinic acid or vitamin B_{12} at the end of anesthesia in patients with blood disorders if N_2O is used; may precipitate if given with thiopental, atropine, solutions with a pH <5

CLOZAPINE

Trade Names:	**Clozaril, Fazaclo (ODT)**
Indications:	Schizophrenia
Pharmacokinetics:	Onset: <1 h; peak: 2–3 h; protein binding: 97%; duration: 4–12 h; $T_{1/2}$ β: 4–66 h; highly metabolized, excreted in urine and feces
Pharmacodynamics:	Antipsychotic that binds to dopamine receptors in limbic system

CLOZAPINE *continued*

CNS:	Dizziness, drowsiness, tremor, hypokinesia, ataxia, slurred speech, depression, myoclonus, seizures, headache, fever
CV:	Cardiomyopathy, ↓ BP, ↑ HR, orthostatic hypotension
GI:	Constipation, nausea, vomiting, dry mouth, ↑ salivation, dyspepsia
GU:	Abnormal ejaculation, urinary frequency/retention
Other:	Bone marrow suppression, rash, diaphoresis, weight gain
Dosage:	12.5–50 mg, then 50–100 mg/d (max. 450 mg/d)
Contraindications:	Epilepsy, severe CNS depression, myleosuppressive disorders
Drug Interactions:	↑ Anticholinergic drugs; ↑ levels of drugs metabolized by cytochrome P_{450} (e.g., antidepressants, carbamazepine); antihypertensives and benzodiazepines ↑ hypotensive effect; ↑ digoxin and warfarin levels, ↓ phenytoin level
Key Points:	Use with general anesthesia may delay recovery and ↑ risk of postoperative sedation, hypotension, respiratory depression

FLUPHENAZINE

Trade Name:	**Prolixin**
Indications:	Psychotic disorders
Pharmacokinetics:	Onset: <1 h; peak: 1–2 h; protein binding: 90%; duration: 7.5 h; Vd: 8–10 L/kg; $T_{1/2}$ α: 1.5 h, β: 14 h; hepatic metabolism, excreted 1° in urine
Pharmacodynamics:	Phenothiazine that blocks postsynaptic CNS dopamine receptors
CNS:	↓ Seizure threshold, dizziness, dystonia, extrapyramidal symptoms, NMS, poikilothermic effect, blurred vision
CV:	Prolonged QT interval, quinidine-like effect, ↑ HR, vasodilation, orthostatic hypotension
GI:	Dry mouth, nausea, ↑ LFTs, jaundice, constipation
GU:	Urine retention, dark urine, ↓ ejaculation, amenorrhea
Other:	↓ Vasopressin, ↑ prolactin secretion, bone marrow suppression, photosensitization, gynecomastia, weight changes
Dosage:	0.5–10 mg PO q 6–8 h (max. <20 mg/d); 1.25 mg IM q 6–8 h
Contraindications:	Coma, Parkinson's disease, bone marrow suppression, hepatic encephalopathy; sulfite allergic (parenteral formulation)

FLUPHENAZINE *continued*

Drug Interactions: ↑ Effects of alcohol, barbiturates, organophosphate insecticides, anticholinergics; ↑ risk of arrhythmia with antiarrhythmics; antacids ↓ absorption; TCAs and phenytoin ↓ metabolism; caffeine ↑ metabolism; β-blocker ↑ levels

Key Points: ↑ CNS effects of anesthetic and analgesic drugs; carefully titrate centrally active antihypertensive (e.g., clonidine) to avoid profound hypotension; intraoperative hypotension should *not* be treated with epinephrine (use phenylephrine)

HALOPERIDOL

Trade Name: **Haldol**

Indications: Psychosis, alcohol dependence, delirium, Tourette's syndrome

Pharmacokinetics: Onset: <1 h; bioavailability: 60%; peak: 3–6 h; protein binding: 90%; duration: 6–12 h; metabolized extensively in liver, excreted 1° in urine

Pharmacodynamics: Antipsychotic that blocks postsynaptic CNS dopamine and peripheral anticholinergic receptors, possesses antiemetic and ganglionic blocking activity

CNS: NMS, seizures, extrapyramidal reactions, tardive dyskinesia, drowsiness, confusion, vertigo, blurred vision, headaches, anorexia

CV: ↑ HR, arrhythmias (due to QT prolongation)

GI: Dyspepsia, nausea, vomiting, jaundice, ↑ LFTs, constipation

GU: Urinary retention, priapism, menstrual irregularities

Other: Dry mouth, leukopenia, rash, diaphoresis, gynecomastia

Dosage: 0.5–10 mg PO bid (max. 100 mg/d); 2–5 mg IM q 6–8 h (max. 0.15 mg/kg/d)

Contraindications: Parkinsonism, severe depression (or coma)

Drug Interactions: Antacids ↓ absorption; antiarrhythmics ↑ risk of arrhythmias; anticholinergics ↑ side effects; ephedrine ↓ BP response; centrally acting drugs ↑ sedation, ↑ toxicity of levodopa; β-blocker and phenytoin ↑ toxicity; smoking metabolism (↓ levels)

Key Points: ↑ Sedative and hypotensive effects and prolongs recovery after anesthesia; impairs tolerance to hemorrhage and hypotension (due to absence of compensatory reflexes)

MESORIDAZINE

Trade Name:	Serentil
Indications:	Schizophrenia, psychoneurotic anxiety, alcoholism
Pharmacokinetics:	Onset: <1 h; peak: 2–4 h; protein binding: 90%; duration: 4–6 h; metabolized extensively in liver, excreted 1° in urine
Pharmacodynamics:	Phenothiazine that blocks postsynaptic blockade of CNS dopamine receptors, peripheral α- and ganglionic blocker with antihistaminic and antiserotonin activity
CNS:	Extrapyramidal reactions, tardive dyskinesia, drowsiness, NMS, blurred vision, retinitis pigmentosa, dizziness
CV:	↓ BP, ↑ HR, arrhythmias, ↑ QT interval
GI:	Dry mouth, nausea, vomiting, constipation, ↑ LFTs
GU:	Urinary incontinence, ↓ ejaculation, menstrual irregularity, enuresis
Other:	Leukopenia, aplastic anemia, thrombocytopenia, gynecomastia, lactation, weight gain, photosensitivity, muscle weakness
Dosage:	50–100 mg PO tid or 25 mg q 6–8 h IM (max. 200 mg/d) (schizophrenia); 25 mg bid (max. 200 mg/d) (alcoholism)
Contraindications:	Coma, arrhythmias, prolonged QT interval
Drug Interactions:	Sedative-hypnotics, MAOIs, opioids, phenothiazines, β-blockers, anticholinergic cytochrome P_{450} inhibitors ↑ effects; $α_2$-agonists ↓ BP response; antacids ↓ absorption
Key Points:	↑ CNS effects of general anesthetics and opioid analgesics, potentially delaying recovery from anesthesia; avoid use of adjunctive drugs that prolong QT interval

OLANZAPINE

Trade Name:	Zyprexa
Indications:	Schizophrenia, bipolar disorder, manic episodes
Pharmacokinetics:	Onset: 1–2 h; peak: 6 h; protein binding: 93%; Vd: 1 L/kg; $T_{1/2}$ β: 21–54 h; 1st-pass hepatic metabolism via glucoronidation and cytochrome P_{450} oxidation, excreted 1° in urine
Pharmacodynamics:	Antipsychotic that antagonizes CNS dopamine and serotonin receptors and peripheral adrenergic, cholinergic, histaminergic receptors

OLANZAPINE *continued*

CNS:	Somnolence, agitation, insomnia, akathisia, tardive dyskinesia, hypertonia, suicidal tendencies, NMS, parkinsonism, amblyopia, corneal lesion, dizziness, personality disorders, tremor
CV:	Orthostatic hypotension, angina, ↑ HR, pedal edema
GI:	Dry mouth, thirst, ↑ appetite, ↑ salivation, nausea, vomiting, constipation, dyspepsia
GU:	Hematuria, metrorrhagia, UTI, urinary incontinence
Pulmonary:	Cough, dyspnea, pharyngitis
Other:	Eosinophilia, neck rigidity, vesiculobullous rash, asthenia
Dosage:	5–15 mg/d PO, then ↑ 5 mg/d (max. 20 mg/d)
Contraindications:	Severe cardiac or cerebrovascular disease
Drug Interactions:	Antihypertensives, diazepam, alcohol ↑ hypotension; fluvoxamine ↓ clearance; carbamazepine, omeprazole, rifampin ↑ clearance
Key Points:	↑ Hypotension associated with general anesthesia

PIMOZIDE

Trade Name:	**Orap**
Indications:	Tourette's syndrome (suppression of tics)
Pharmacokinetics:	Onset: 2–3 h; bioavailability: 50%; peak: 4–12 h; metabolized in liver (1st-pass effect), excreted 1° in urine
Pharmacodynamics:	Antipsychotic that blocks CNS dopamine receptors, anticholinergic, antiemetic, α-blockade, anxiolytic effects
CNS:	Drowsiness, headache, insomnia, NMS, extrapyramidal symptoms, tardive dyskinesia, blurred vision, asthenia
CV:	Prolonged QT interval, ↑ HR
GI:	Dry mouth, constipation
GU:	Impotence, urinary frequency
Other:	Muscle rigidity, rash, diaphoresis, fever
Dosage:	1–2 mg/d PO (max. 20 mg/d); 0.5 mg/kg/d (children)
Contraindications:	Simple tics, cardiac arrhythmias, congenital QT prolongation
Drug Interactions:	Amphetamine, ↑ tics; ↑ anticonvulsant dosages; ↑ risk of arrhythmias with epinephrine, antidepressants, antipsychotics, antiarrhythmics
Key Points:	Use with general anesthetics and opioid analgesics prolongs recovery from anesthesia, ↑ risk of respiratory depression and oversedation

PROCHLOPERAZINE

Trade Name: **Compazine**

                      See Chapter 8, "Antiemetics and Antinauseants"

QUETIAPINE

Trade Name: **Seroquel**

Indications: Psychotic disorders

Pharmacokinetics: Onset: <30 min; peak: 1–2 h; protein binding: 83%;
                      Vd: 10 L/kg; $T_{1/2}$ β: 6 h; extensively metabolized in
                      liver, excreted 1° in urine

Pharmacodynamics: Antipsychotic that antagonizes dopamine (D_2) and
                      serotonin type-2 (5-HT_2) receptors
  CNS: Dizziness, headache, somnolence, dysarthria, ear pain
  CV: Orthostatic hypotension, ↑ HR, pedal edema
  GI: Dry mouth, dyspepsia, constipation, pharyngitis
  Other: Leukopenia, cough, dyspnea, rash, sweating

Dosage: 25 mg PO bid, ↑ to 300–400 mg/d

Contraindications: Severe cerebrovascular disease, seizure disorders

Drug Interactions: Anticholinergics ↑ side effects; ↑ sedation; erythromycin,
                      fluconazole, cimetidine, ketoconazole ↓ clearance;
                      antagonizes effects of dopamine agonists; ↑ lorazepam
                      effects; barbiturates, carbamazepine, glucocorticoids,
                      rifampin ↑ metabolism

Key Points: ↑ CNS depression prolongs recovery from anesthesia;
                      orthostatic hypotension can occur in the early
                      postoperative period

RISPERIDONE

Trade Name: **Risperdal**

Indications: Psychotic disorders, schizophrenia

Pharmacokinetics: Onset: <0.5 h; bioavailability: 70%; peak: 1 h;
                      protein binding: 90%; $T_{1/2}$ β: 20 h; duration: 12 h;
                      metabolized extensively in liver by cytochrome P_{450},
                      excreted 1° in urine

Pharmacodynamics: Antipsychotic that antagonizes dopamine (D_2) and
                      serotonin (5-HT_2) receptors
  CNS: Extrapyramidal symptoms, NMS, insomnia, agitation,
                      blurred vision, dizziness, headache, somnolence
  CV: Orthostatic hypotension, ↑ HR, QT prolongation
  GI: Constipation, nausea, dyspepsia, anorexia

RISPERIDONE *continued*

Other:	Rhinitis, cough, rash, arthralgias
Dosage:	1 mg PO bid (max. 8 mg/d)
Contraindications:	Breast-feeding, congenital QT prolongation
Drug Interactions:	↑ Effects of antihypertensives; antagonizes dopamine agonists; carbamazepine ↑ clearance; clozapine ↓ clearance
Key Points:	Droperidol ↑ extrapyramidal symptoms and QT prolongation, additive CNS depression with general anesthetics may prolong recovery and ↑ postural hypotension after surgery

THIORIDAZINE

Trade Name:	**Mellaril**
Indications:	Psychotic disorders, dementia, dysthymic disorders
Pharmacokinetics:	Onset: 0.5–1 h; peak: 2–4 h; protein binding: 90%; duration: 4–6 h; metabolized in liver, excreted in urine
Pharmacodynamics:	Antipsychotic that blocks postsynaptic blockade of CNS dopamine receptors, peripheral α- and ganglionic blocking activity
CNS:	NMS, extrapyramidal reactions, tardive dyskinesia, drowsiness, blurred vision, ↑ appetite
CV:	Orthostatic hypotension, ↑ HR, ↑ QT interval (torsades de pointes)
GI:	Dry mouth, nausea, vomiting, diarrhea, jaundice
GU:	↓ Ejaculation, urine retention, menstrual irregularities
Other:	Leukopenia, agranulocytosis, weight gain, photosensitivity, hyperprolactinemia, dermatitis
Dosage:	25–100 mg PO tid (to 800 mg/d); 0.5–3 mg/kg/d (children)
Contraindications:	Coma, CHF
Drug Interactions:	Sedative-hypnotics, MAOIs, opioids, phenothiazines, antidepressants, anticholinergics inhibit cytochrome P_{450} and ↑ effects; α_2-agonists ↓ BP response; ↑ arrhythmias with drugs that ↑ QT interval; ↓ effects of dopamine agonists
Key Points:	↑ CNS depressant effects of general anesthetics, barbiturates, opioids; ↑ risk of hypotension and respiratory depression; avoid adjuncts that prolong the QT interval

THIOTHIXENE

Trade Name:	**Navane**
Indications:	Psychosis, acute agitation
Pharmacokinetics:	Onset: 10–30 min; peak: 1–6 h; protein binding: >90%; duration: 8–12 h; metabolized in liver, excreted 1° in feces
Pharmacodynamics:	Antipsychotic that blocks postsynaptic CNS dopamine receptor, α-blockade
CNS:	NMS, extrapyramidal reactions, tardive dyskinesia, drowsiness, dizziness, blurred vision
CV:	↓ BP, ↑ HR
GI:	Dry mouth, nasal congestion, nausea, vomiting, constipation, ↑ LFTs
GU:	Urine retention, ↓ ejaculation, gynecomastia, amenorrhea
Other:	Leukopenia/agranulocytosis, photosensitivity, weight gain, rash
Dosage:	4 mg IM tid (max. 30 mg/d) (agitation); 2–5 mg PO bid (max. 60 mg/d) (psychosis)
Contraindications:	Coma, blood dyscrasias
Drug Interactions:	Caffeine, smoking ↑ metabolism; sun exposure ↑ photosensitivity
Key Points:	Inhalation and IV anesthetics ↑ CNS depressive effects and prolong recovery from anesthesia

TRIFLUOPERAZINE

Trade Name:	**Stelazine**
Indications:	Schizophrenia, psychotic disorders, anxiety states
Pharmacokinetics:	Onset: 0.5–1 h; peak: 24 h; protein binding: >90%; duration: 4–6 h; metabolized in liver, excreted in urine
Pharmacodynamics:	Phenothiazine that blocks postsynaptic CNS dopamine receptors in CTZ, peripheral α- and ganglionic blockade
CNS:	NMS, extrapyramidal reactions, tardive dyskinesia, dystonias, restlessness, dizziness, drowsiness, blurred vision, headache
CV:	Orthostatic hypotension, ↑ HR, arrhythmias
GI:	Dry mouth, constipation, nausea, jaundice, ↑ LFTs
GU:	Urinary retention, menstrual irregularity
Other:	Leukopenia/agranulocytosis, photosensitivity, rash, gynecomastia
Dosage:	1–2 mg PO bid (max. 6 mg/d) (anxiety); 1–5 mg bid (max. 40 mg/d) or 1–2 mg IM q 4–6 h; 1 mg bid (max. 15 mg/d) or 1 mg IM bid (children) (schizophrenia)

TRIFLUOPERAZINE *continued*

Contraindications:	Coma, bone marrow suppression
Drug Interactions:	Barbiturates, lithium, caffeine, smoking ↓ effects; propylthiouracil ↑ agranulocytosis; ↓ pressor effects of sympathomimetics; centrally acting antihypertensives (e.g., clonidine, guanabenz, guanadrel, methyldopa, reserpine) block ↓ BP; β-blockers ↑ CV toxicity
Key Points:	Prolongs recovery from general anesthesia and ↑ perioperative hypotension

ZIPRASIDONE

Trade Name:	**Geodon**
Indications:	Schizophrenia
Pharmacokinetics:	Onset: 1–3 h; peak: 6–8 h; duration: 12 h; $T_{1/2}$ β: 7 h; metabolized in liver via cytochrome P_{450}, excreted in urine
Pharmacodynamics:	Antipsychotic that antagonizes CNS dopamine and serotonin receptors
CNS:	Somnolence, extrapyramidal symptoms, cogwheel rigidity, paresthesia, blurred vision, dizziness
CV:	Orthostatic hypotension, ↓ HR, QT prolongation
GI:	Nausea, vomiting, dyspepsia, rectal hemorrhage
Other:	Cough, tooth pain, rash, diaphoresis, rhinitis
Dosage:	20 mg PO bid (max. 200 mg/d); 10 mg IM q 2 h
Contraindications:	Congenital QT syndrome, recent MI, acute heart failure
Drug Interactions:	Carbamazepine ↓ level; diuretics ↑ arrhythmias; ketoconazole ↑ level
Key Points:	Check electrolytes before surgery to ↓ risk of arrhythmias; avoid adjunctive drugs that prolong QT interval

10

Antihistamines

ACRIVASTINE

Trade Name:	**Semprex (with pseudoephedrine)**
Indications:	Rhinitis (due to seasonal allergies and chronic urticaria), dermographism
Pharmacokinetics:	Onset: rapid; peak: 70 min; protein binding: 50%; duration: 4–8 h; Vd: 0.8 L/kg; Cl: 3 mL/kg/min; $T_{1/2}\ \beta$: 2 h; minimal metabolism, 1° excreted unchanged in urine
Pharmacodynamics:	Competitive histamine (H_1) antagonist
CNS:	Headache, drowsiness, dizziness
CV:	↑ HR, ↑ BP (due to psuedoephedrine)
GI:	Dry mouth
Dosage:	8 mg PO qid (pseudoephedrine 60 mg)
Contraindications:	Renal impairment, sensitivity to triprolidine
Drug Interactions:	↑ Sedative effect of other antihistamines, TCAs, sedative-hypnotics; ↑ antimuscarinic effect of TCAs and MAOIs (↑ pseudoephedrine CV effects)
Key Points:	↑ Anesthetic-induced sedation and anticholinergic activity

AZATADINE

Trade Name:	**Optimine**
Indications:	Allergic rhinitis
Pharmacokinetics:	Onset/peak/duration: NK; metabolized by liver, excreted in urine
Pharmacodynamics:	Phenothiazepine-type H_1 blocker with antiserotonergic and anticholinergic activity
CNS:	Drowsiness, diplopia, tinnitus, tremor, seizures, dizziness, ataxia
CV:	↓ BP, ↑ BP (with ↑ HR), arrhythmias
Pulmonary:	Wheezing, dry (thick) secretions
Other:	Agranulocytosis, anemia, diaphoresis, urinary retention, nausea, vomiting, dyspepsia
Dosage:	1 mg PO bid
Contraindications:	Sensitivity to cyproheptadine and use of MAOIs
Drug Interactions:	MAOIs prolong anticholinergic activity
Key Points:	Possesses prolonged anticholinergic action; ↓ vasopressor response to epinephrine

AZELASTINE

Trade Name:	**Astelin**
Indications:	Allergic conjunctivitis, seasonal allergic rhinitis, vasomotor rhinitis
Pharmacokinetics:	Onset: <3 min; peak: 2–3 h; duration: 8–12 h
Pharmacodynamics:	Selective H_1-histamine antagonist, inhibits release of histamine
CNS:	Fatigue, headaches, dizziness, drowsiness, blurred vision
GI:	Bitter taste, dry mouth, sinusitis, nausea
Pulmonary:	Wheezing, dyspnea, paroxysmal sneezing
Other:	↑ Weight, pruritus, flulike symptoms
Dosage:	1–2 puffs (137 µg/puff) bid; 1 gtt 0.05% bid
Contraindications:	Sensitivity to H_1-receptor antagonist
Drug Interactions:	↑ Sedative effects of alcohol and other CNS depressants
Key Points:	May reduce the IV anesthetic requirement

BROMPHENIRAMINE, CARBETAPENTANE, PYRILAMINE

Trade Names:	**Ryna, Rynatuss, Tussi**
Indications:	Common cold, nasal congestion, URI, asthma, bronchitis, menstrual cramping
Pharmacokinetics:	NK
Pharmacodynamics:	H-1 receptor antagonist, antitussive (carbetapentane), inhibits histamine at H-1 receptors, anticholinergic effects
CNS:	Drowsiness, dizziness, insomnia, nervousness, dry eyes
CV:	↓BP
GI:	Dry mouth
GU:	Urinary retention
Dosages:	*Brompheniramine:* 0.0875–1.25 mg/kg SC q 6 h *Carbetapentane:* 60–120 mg PO q 12 h *Pyrilamine:* 30–60 mg PO q 12 h; 15–30 mg q 12 h (children)
Contraindications:	Uncontrolled hypertension, MAO inhibitors
Drug Interactions:	Tranquilizers, alcohol, other antihistamines ↑ sedation; MAOIs ↑ anticholinergic and sedative effects
Key Points:	↑ CNS depressant effects of anesthetic drugs

CETIRIZINE

Trade Name:	**Zyrtec**
Indications:	Seasonal allergy, chronic urticaria
Pharmacokinetics:	Onset: <30 min; peak: 0.5–1.5 h; protein binding: 93%; duration: 24 h; excreted 1° unchanged in urine
Pharmacodynamics:	Selective inhibition of peripheral H_1 receptors
CNS:	Drowsiness, fatigue
GI:	Dry mouth
Dosage:	5–10 mg/d PO; 2.5 mg/d (children)
Contraindications:	Sensitivity to hydroxyzine
Drug Interactions:	↑ Sedation with CNS depressants, alcohol, anticholinergics; theophylline ↓ clearance
Key Points:	Enhanced CNS depression with anesthetic drugs, ↑ postoperative sedation

CHLORPHENIRAMINE

Trade Name:	**Chlor-Trimeton**
Indications:	Nasal congestion, rhinitis, urticaria, conjunctivitis, allergic reactions (with pruritus, urticaria, angioedema)
Pharmacokinetics:	Onset: 15–30 min; peak: 2–3 h; protein binding: 72%; duration: 4–8 h; $T_{1/2}$ β: 8 h; excreted in urine as inactive metabolites
Pharmacodynamics:	Peripheral-acting H_1 receptor antagonist
CNS:	Drowsiness
CV:	↓ BP, vasodilation
GI:	↓ Appetite, nausea, vomiting, dyspepsia
Pulmonary:	Bronchodilation, thick secretions
Other:	Dry mouth, cough, urinary retention
Dosage:	2–8 mg PO q 4–6 h
Contraindications:	Acute asthmatic attack, breast-feeding, narrow-angle glaucoma, BPH, pyloroduodenal obstruction, bladder neck obstruction
Drug Interactions:	MAOI and β-blockers ↑ effect
Key Points:	↑ CNS depressant effects of general anesthetics and anticholinergic activity; sedation is less than with most other antihistamines

CIMETIDINE

Trade Name:	**Tagamet**
	See Chapter 3, "Antacids and Antisecretories"

CLEMASTINE

Trade Name:	**Tavist**
Indications:	Nasal congestion, rhinitis, urticaria, allergic reactions
Pharmacokinetics:	Onset: 15–60 min; peak: 2–5 h; duration: 10–12 h; hepatic metabolism, excreted in the urine
Pharmacodynamics:	Peripheral acting H_1-receptor antagonist
CNS:	Drowsiness, headache, dizziness, incoordination, restlessness
CV:	↓ BP, ↑ HR
GI:	Dyspepsia, nausea, vomiting
Pulmonary:	Bronchodilation, dry mucous membranes, thick bronchial secretions
Other:	Bone marrow suppression, dry mouth, cough, urinary retention
Dosage:	1.34–2.68 mg PO bid
Contraindications:	Acute asthmatic attack, severe hypertension, ↑ IOP, breast-feeding
Drug Interactions:	↑ Sedation with CNS depressants and alcohol; MAOIs prolong anticholinergic effect
Key Points:	↑ CNS depressants, anticholinergics, seizure-inducing anesthetic drugs

CYPROHEPTADINE

Trade Name:	**Periactin**
Indications:	Rhinitis, urticaria, conjunctivitis; allergic reactions; appetite stimulant, cluster headaches, Cushing's syndrome
Pharmacokinetics:	Onset: <30 min; peak: 6–9 h; duration: 8–12 h; hepatic metabolism, excreted in urine and feces
Pharmacodynamics:	Peripheral-acting H_1-receptor antagonist
CNS:	Drowsiness, headaches, dizziness, ataxia, confusion, restlessness
CV:	↓ BP, ↑ HR, palpitations
GI:	Dyspepsia, nausea, vomiting, dry mouth
Pulmonary:	Bronchodilatation, dry mucous membranes, thick secretions

CYPROHEPTADINE *continued*

Other:	Blood dyscrasias, cough, urinary retention/frequency, weight gain
Dosage:	4 mg PO tid
Contraindications:	Acute asthmatic attack, severe hypertension, ↑ IOP
Drug Interactions:	↑ CNS depression with hypnotics-sedatives, tranquilizers, alcohol; MAOIs prolong anticholinergic effect
Key Points:	Preoperative use with general anesthetics may prolong recovery and ↑ anticholinergic symptoms

DESLORATADINE

Trade Name:	**Clarinex**
Indications:	Seasonal allergy, pruritis, urticaria
Pharmacokinetics:	Onset: <1 h; peak: 2–4 h; protein binding: 85%; $T_{1/2} \beta$: 27 h; does not cross blood-brain barrier; extensive hepatic metabolism, excreted in urine and feces
Pharmacodynamics:	Long-acting, tricyclic H_1-receptor histamine antagonist
CNS:	Somnolence, fatigue, headache
GI:	Dry mouth, nausea
Other:	Myalgia, pharyngitis
Dosage:	5 mg/d PO
Contraindications:	Sensitivity to loratadine, breast-feeding
Drug Interactions:	None reported
Key Points:	Use with general anesthetics ↑ sedation and may prolong recovery

DIMENHYDRINATE

Trade Name:	**Dramamine**
	See Chapter 8, "Antiemetics and Antinauseants."

DIPHENHYDRAMINE

Trade Names:	**Benadryl, Dytan-D**
Indications:	Nasal congestion, rhinitis, urticaria, conjunctivitis, allergic reactions; anaphylaxis, pruritus, motion sickness, Parkinson's disease

DIPHENHYDRAMINE *continued*

Pharmacokinetics:	Onset: <30 min; peak: 1–4 h; protein binding: 82%; duration: 4–8 h; $T_{1/2}$ β: 2–4 h; excreted as inactive metabolites in urine
Pharmacodynamics:	Central antimuscarinic action and H_1 receptor antagonist at smooth muscle
CNS:	Drowsiness, excitement, dizziness, insomnia, headache
CV:	Palpitations, ↓ BP
GI:	Dyspepsia, nausea, vomiting, diarrhea
Pulmonary:	Bronchodilatation, nasal congestion, thick secretions
Other:	Dry mouth, cough, urinary retention
Dosage:	25–50 mg PO/IM q 4–6 h, 6.25–12.5 mg IM (children)
Contraindications:	Acute asthma, narrow-angle glaucoma, use of MAOIs
Drug Interactions:	↑ Sedative effects of CNS depressants and alcohol; MAOIs ↑ anticholinergic effects
Key Points:	Vasopressor effects of epinephrine may be blunted, and residual sedation can delay recovery from general anesthesia; Dytan-D contains the antihistamine (25 mg) and phenylephrine (7.5–10 mg)

EPINASTINE

Trade Name:	**Elastat**
Indications:	Allergic conjunctivitis (antipruritic)
Pharmacokinetics:	NK
Pharmacodynamics:	H_1-receptor antagonist, inhibits histamine release from mast cell
CNS:	Sedation, drowsiness
Pulmonary:	URI, pharyngitis
Other:	Burning in eye, folliculosis, hyperemia, pruritus
Dosage:	0.05% topical solution, 1 gtt bid
Contraindications:	Not for IV or PO use, sensitivity to benzalkonium
Drug Interactions:	NK
Key Points:	Excessive use could produce sedation

FAMOTIDINE

Trade Name:	**Pepcid**
	See Chapter 3, "Antacids and Antisecretories"

HYDROXYZINE

Trade Names:	**Atarax, Vistaril**
Indications:	Anxiety, hyperkinesia, allergic reactions emesis, pruritus
Pharmacokinetics:	Onset: 15–30 min; peak: 2–4 h; Cl: 32.1 mL/kg/min; duration: 4–6 h; Vd: 18.5 L/kg; $T_{1/2}$ β: 20–25 h; hepatic metabolism to active metabolite, excreted in urine
Pharmacodynamics:	CNS depression, peripheral H_1 receptor antagonist
CNS:	Somnolence, tremor
Other:	Dry mouth, pain at injection site
Dosage:	50–100 mg PO qid; 25 mg PO tid (pruritus); 25–100 mg IM q 4–8 h; 1.1 mg/kg IM q 4–6 h (children)
Contraindications:	Narrow-angle glaucoma, prostatic hypertrophy, pregnancy
Drug Interactions:	↑ Sedative effects of anesthetics, opioids, alcohol; ↓ sympathomimetic effects of epinephrine
Key Points:	↑ CNS depressant effects of anesthetics and ↓ volatile anesthetic requirement

LORATADINE

Trade Name:	**Claritin**
Indications:	Nasal congestion, allergic rhinitis, urticaria, conjunctivitis
Pharmacokinetics:	Onset: 1–3 h; peak: 8–10 h; protein binding: 97%; duration: 24 h; $T_{1/2}$ β: 8–11 h; metabolized by cytochrome P_{450} to active metabolite, excreted 1° in urine
Pharmacodynamics:	Peripheral-acting tricyclic H_1 receptor antagonist
CNS:	Headache, somnolence, fatigue
Other:	Dry mouth
Dosage:	10 mg/d PO
Contraindications:	Breast-feeding
Drug Interactions:	↓ Erythromycin; licorice prolongs QT interval
Key Points:	Less CNS depressant effects on anesthetic and analgesic drugs than other antihistaminic compounds

NIZATIDINE

Trade Name: **Axid**

See Chapter 3, "Antacids and Antisecretories"

RANITIDINE

Trade Name: **Zantac**

See Chapter 3, "Antacids and Antisecretories"

11

Anti-inflammatory Analgesics

ACETAMINOPHEN

Trade Name:	**Tylenol**
Indications:	Acute (and chronic) pain, inflammation, and fever; osteoarthritis
Pharmacokinetics:	Onset: <1 h; peak: 1–3 h; protein binding: 25%; duration: 3–4 h; Vd: 0.94 L/kg; Cl: 19.3 L/h; $T_{1/2}$ β: 1–4 h; extensively metabolized in liver, excreted in urine
Pharmacodynamics:	Inhibition of prostaglandin synthesis, blocks endogenous pyrogen
CNS:	Analgesia, somnolence, asthenia, insomnia, nervousness
GI:	Nausea, vomiting, ↑ LFTs, jaundice, constipation
Other:	Bone marrow suppression, hypoglycemia, rash, antipyretic
Dosage:	500–1500 mg q 4–6 h (max. 4 g/d); or 1–2 g IV; 20–40 mg/kg, then 10–15 mg/kg q 4–6 h (children)
Contraindications:	Viral hepatitis, phenylketonuria, hepatorenal impairment, alcoholism
Drug Interactions:	↑ Hepatotoxicity with alcohol, ↑ anticoagulant effect, ↑ nephropathy with NSAIDs; caffeine ↑ effect; antacids ↓ absorption
Key Points:	Useful adjuvant as part of a multimodal analgesic regimen; produces dose-dependent opioid-sparing effects; IV formulation under investigation

ASPIRIN (ACETYLSALICYLIC ACID [ASA])

See Chapter 6, "Anticoagulants and Procoagulants," and Appendix I, "Oral Analgesic Drug Combinations"

CELECOXIB

Trade Name:	**Celebrex**
Indications:	Osteo- and rheumatoid arthritis, familial adenomatous polyposis, dysmenorrhea, acute postoperative pain
Pharmacokinetics:	Onset: <1 hr; peak: 2–3 hr; highly protein bound; duration: 6–12 h; $T_{1/2}$ β: 11 h; metabolized by cytochrome P_{450}, excreted 1° in urine
Pharmacodynamics:	NSAID with selective inhibition of COX-2 isoenzyme
CNS:	Dizziness, insomnia, headache, anxiety
GI:	Abdominal pain, flatulence, dyspepsia, ↑ LFTs, bleeding, diarrhea

CELECOXIB *continued*

Pulmonary:	URI, dyspnea
Other:	Rash, edema, hypophosphatemia, ↑ creatinine level
Dosage:	200–400 mg PO initially, then 100–200 mg PO bid
Contraindications:	Late pregnancy, severe hepatic impairment, sensitivity to sulfonamides, ASA, NSAIDs, Stevens-Johnson syndrome
Drug Interactions:	↓ Effect of ACE inhibitors; aspirin and alcohol ↑ risk of gastric ulceration; ↑ lithium level; fluconazole ↑ level
Key Points:	Postoperative opioid-sparing effect when administered for premedication and pre-emptive analgesia

DICLOFENAC

Trade Name:	**Voltaren**
Indications:	Acute and chronic pain, inflammation, osteo- and rheumatoid arthritis, ankylosing spondylitis
Pharmacokinetics:	Onset: 10 min; peak: 30 min; protein binding: 100%; duration: 8 h; Vd: 0.15 L/kg; Cl: 15.6 L/h; $T_{1/2}$ β: 1.5 h; extensive 1st-pass hepatic metabolism, excreted in urine and bile
Pharmacodynamics:	Inhibition of prostaglandin synthesis
CNS:	Dizziness, blurred vision, tinnitus, hallucinations
CV:	↑ BP, pedal edema, CHF, arrhythmias, palpitations
GI:	Mucosal ulceration/bleeding, jaundice, ↑ LFTs
GU:	Proteinuria, nephrotic syndrome, interstitial nephritis
Pulmonary:	Bronchospasm (asthmatics)
Other:	↓ Platelet aggregation (reversible), Δ glucose level, blood dyscrasias
Dosage:	50–100 mg PO/IM q 8–12 h (max. 200 mg/d)
Contraindications:	Peptic ulceration, GI bleeding, asthma, porphyria, late pregnancy, allergic reactions to ASA or NSAIDs, porphyria
Drug Interactions:	↓ Levels of methotrexate, lithium, digoxin; sodium and water retention ↓ effect of diuretics and antihypertensives; NSAIDs and acetaminophen ↑ nephropathy and GI ulceration; ↑ lithium and aminoglycoside level; colestipol and sucralfate ↓ absorption; sun exposure ↑ photosensitivity
Key Points:	↓ Postoperative inflammation when administered systematically (or topically); ↑ operative bleeding and hematoma formation (?)

DIFLUNISAL

Trade Name:	**Dolobid**
Indications:	Acute and chronic pain, inflammation, rheumatoid arthritis
Pharmacokinetics:	Onset: 1 h; peak: 2–3 h; duration: 8–12 h; Vd: 0.11 L/kg; Cl: 0.35–0.49 L/h; $T_{1/2}$ β: 8–12 h; metabolized in liver, excreted in urine
Pharmacodynamics:	Salicylic acid derivative that inhibits prostaglandin synthesis
CNS:	Dizziness, insomnia, fatigue, tinnitus, headache, somnolence
GI:	Nausea, vomiting, dyspepsia, flatulence
Other:	↓ Platelet aggregation (reversible), ↑ bleeding time, hyperkalemia, hypouricemia, Stevens-Johnson syndrome, rash
Dosage:	250–500 mg PO q 8–12 h (max. 1.5 g/d)
Contraindications:	Peptic ulceration, GI bleeding, asthma
Drug Interactions:	↑ Levels of methotrexate, verapamil, nifedipine, lithium, digoxin; ↓ effect of diuretics and antihypertensives; NSAIDs or acetaminophen ↑ nephropathy; ↑ bleeding with anticoagulants; ↑ risk of Reye's syndrome
Key Points:	When administered preoperatively, potential for ↑ operative site bleeding analogous to other nonselective NSAIDs

ETODOLAC

Trade Name:	**Lodine**
Indications:	Osteo- and rheumatoid arthritis, acute and chronic pain
Pharmacokinetics:	Onset: 30 min; peak: 1–2 h; duration: 4–12 h; protein binding: 99%; extensively metabolized in liver, excreted 1° in urine
Pharmacodynamics:	Inhibition of prostaglandin biosynthesis
CNS:	Asthenia, depression, drowsiness, dizziness
GI:	Dyspepsia, nausea, vomiting, flatulence, ulceration/bleeding, ↑ LFTs
Other:	Leukopenia, thrombocytopenia, pruritus, rash, Stevens-Johnson syndrome, asthma, dysuria, urinary frequency
Dosage:	200–400 mg PO q 6–8 h
Contraindications:	Aspirin and NSAID-induced asthma

ETODOLAC *continued*

Drug Interactions:	Antacids ↓ level; aspirin and warfarin ↑ GI bleeding; ↑ level of phenytoin, digoxin, lithium, methotrexate; cyclosporin ↑ nephrotoxicity; β-blocker and diuretics ↑ effect
Key Points:	Potential for operative site bleeding when administered for premedication

ETORICOXIB

Trade Name:	**Arcoxia**
Indications:	Gouty, osteo-, and rheumatoid arthritis; dysmenorrhea, ankylosing spondylitis; acute and chronic pain
Pharmacokinetics:	Onset: <1 h; bioavailability: 85%; peak: 2–3 h; duration: 24 h; $T_{1/2}$ β: 20–30 h; metabolized extensively in liver, excreted 1° in urine
Pharmacodynamics:	Highly-selective COX-2 inhibitor
CV:	Fluid retention, pedal edema, hypertension
GI:	Dry mouth, ↑ LFTs
Dosage:	60–120 mg/d PO
Contraindications:	CHF, inflammatory bowel disease, severe hepatic impairment
Drug Interactions:	ACE inhibitors ↓ hypotensive effects; tacrolimus and cyclosporin ↑ nephrotoxicity
Key Points:	Potential usefulness as a pre-emptive analgesic before and after surgery due to long duration of action

FLURBIPROFEN

Trade Names:	**Ansaid, Ocufen**
Indications:	Acute and chronic pain, inflammation, rheumatic conditions
Pharmacokinetics:	Onset: <30 min; peak: 1–2 h; protein binding: 99%; duration: 6–12 h; Vd: 0.1 L/kg; Cl: 1.3 L/h; $T_{1/2}$ β: 6–10 h; metabolized in liver, excreted in urine
Pharmacodynamics:	Nonselective inhibition of prostaglandin synthesis
CNS:	Anxiety, insomnia, dizziness
CV:	Pedal edema
GI:	Mucosal; ulceration and bleeding, ↑ LFTs
GU:	UTI, hematuria
Dosage:	50–100 mg q 6–12 h (max. 300 mg/d); 9 gtt 0.03% solution before surgery

FLURBIPROFEN *continued*

Contraindications:	Peptic ulceration, GI bleeding, asthma, breast-feeding
Drug Interactions:	↑ Levels of methotrexate, lithium, digoxin; ↓ effect of diuretics and antihypertensive medication; other NSAIDs or acetaminophen ↑ nephropathy or GI ulceration; ↑ bleeding tendency with anticoagulants
Key Points:	Use for pre-emptive analgesia prior to surgery; may ↑ operative site bleeding

IBUPROFEN

Trade Names:	**Advil, Motrin, Nuprin**
Indications:	Acute and chronic pain, inflammation, fever, arthritis
Pharmacokinetics:	Onset: <1 h; bioavailability: 80%; peak: 1–2 h; Vd: 0.14 L/kg; Cl: 3.5 L/h; $T_{1/2}$ β: 2.5 h; metabolized in liver, excreted 1° in urine
Pharmacodynamics:	Nonselective inhibition of prostaglandin synthesis
CNS:	Dizziness, nervousness, aseptic meningitis, tinnitus
CV:	Peripheral edema, arrhythmia, ↓ BP, ↑ HR
GI:	Mucosal ulceration and bleeding
GU:	Azotemia, cystitis, hematuria, urinary retention
Pulmonary:	Bronchospasm (asthmatics), dyspnea
Other:	Reversible inhibition of platelet aggregation, ↑ bleeding time, Stevens-Johnson syndrome, rash, fever
Dosage:	300–800 mg q 4–6 h (max. 3.2 g/d); 30–40 mg/kg/d (children)
Contraindications:	Asthma, nasal polyps, peptic ulceration, renal impairment
Drug Interactions:	↑ Level of methotrexate, lithium, verapamil, digoxin; ↓ effects of diuretics and antihypertensives; NSAIDs, acetaminophen, gold ↑ nephropathy or GI bleeding; antacids ↓ absorption; ↑ bleeding with anticoagulants
Key Points:	Useful nonopioid analgesic as part of a multimodal regimen during the perioperative period, may ↑ operative site bleeding

INDOMETHACIN

Trade Name:	**Indocin**
Indications:	Pain, inflammation, rheumatoid and gouty arthritis, ankylosing spondylitis, dysmenorrhea, pericarditis, patent ductus arteriosus, cluster headache

INDOMETHACIN *continued*

Pharmacokinetics:	Onset: <1 h; peak: 1–2 h; duration: 6–8 h; highly protein bound; Vd: 0.2 L/kg; Cl: 6.3 L/h; $T_{1/2}$ β: 4–6 h; metabolized in liver, excreted in urine
Pharmacodynamics:	Inhibition of prostaglandin synthesis and phosphodiesterase
CNS:	Dizziness, depression, tinnitis, headache, fatigue
GI:	Nausea, dyspepsia
GU:	Hematuria, interstitial nephritis
Other:	↓ Platelet aggregation (reversible), bone marrow suppression, hypoglycemia
Dosage:	25–50 mg PO q 6–8 h (max. 200 mg/d); 50 mg PR; 0.25–0.6 mg/kg q 2 h (children)
Contraindications:	Asthma, GI bleeding, renal impairment, pregnancy, breast-feeding
Drug Interactions:	↑ Levels of methotrexate, lithium, verapamil, nifedipine, digoxin; ↓ effect of diuretics and antihypertensives; NSAIDs, acetaminophen, gold, alcohol ↑ risk of nephropathy and GI bleeding; ↑ bleeding with anticoagulants and thrombolytics
Key Points:	Produces opioid-sparing effect after surgery when administered preoperatively as rectal suppository; used in postoperative period

KETOPROFEN

Trade Names:	**Orudis, Oruvail**
Indications:	Acute and chronic pain, inflammation, osteo- and rheumatoid arthritis
Pharmacokinetics:	Onset: <30 min; peak: 1–2 h; highly protein bound; duration: 4–8 h; Vd: 0.11 L/kg; Cl: 5.2 L/h; $T_{1/2}$ β: 1.4 h; metabolized in liver, excreted in urine
Pharmacodynamics:	Nonselective inhibition of prostaglandin synthesis
CNS:	Dizziness, depression, tinnitus, headache
CV:	Peripheral edema
GI:	Dyspepsia, nausea, ↑ LFTs, flatulence
GU:	Nephrotoxicity
Other:	↓ Platelet aggregation (reversible), ↑ bleeding time, rash
Dosage:	50–75 mg PO q 6–8 h or 100–160 mg bid (max. 320 mg/d)
Contraindications:	Peptic ulceration, GI bleeding, asthma, sensitivity to ASA

KETOPROFEN *continued*

Drug Interactions: ↑ Levels of methotrexate, lithium, digoxin; ↓ effect of
                      diuretics and antihypertensives; NSAIDs,
                      acetaminophen, gold, alcohol ↑ nephropathy and GI
                      bleeding; ↑ bleeding with anticoagulants and
                      thrombolytics; sun exposure ↑ photosensitivity

Key Points: Nonselective NSAID with opioid-sparing properties
                      when administered during perioperative period

KETOROLAC

Trade Name: **Toradol**

Indications: Acute and postoperative pain

Pharmacokinetics: Onset: <10 min (IV/IM), <30 min (oral); peak: 1 h;
                      protein binding: 99%; duration: 6–8 h; Vd:
                      0.11–0.25 L/kg; Cl: 0.35–0.55 L/h; $T_{1/2}$ β: 4–8 h;
                      metabolized in liver, excreted in urine

Pharmacodynamics: Nonselective inhibition of prostaglandin synthesis
  CNS: Drowsiness, headache, dizziness
  CV: Pedal edema, ↑ BP, arrhythmia
  GI: Nausea, dyspepsia, mucosal ulceration/bleeding
  GU: Renal tubular dysfunction, ↑ creatine level
  Other: ↓ Platelet aggregation (reversible), thrombocytopenia,
                      purpura, diaphoresis, pruritus, rash

Dosage: 30–60 mg IV/IM initially, then 15–30 mg q 6 h
                      (max. 120 mg/d); 10 mg PO q 4–6 h

Contraindications: Peptic ulceration, GI bleeding, renal impairment,
                      renal artery stenosis, severe dehydration, asthma,
                      CHF, pregnancy, coagulopathy, abnormal platelet
                      function, concurrent use of nephrotoxic drugs

Drug Interactions: ↓ Levels of methotrexate, lithium, digoxin; ↓ effect of
                      diuretics and antihypertensives; NSAIDs,
                      acetaminophen, alcohol ↑ nephropathy or GI bleeding;
                      ↑ bleeding with anticoagulants and thrombolytics;
                      sun exposure ↑ photosensitivity

Key Points: Commonly used adjuvant during the perioperative period

LUMIRACOXIB

Trade Name: **Prexige**

Indications: Acute pain and inflammation, osteo- and rheumatoid
                      arthritis

Pharmacokinetics: NK (structural analog of diclofenac)

LUMIRACOXIB *continued*

Pharmacodynamics:	NSAID with selective inhibition of COX-2 isoenzyme
CNS:	Dizziness, insomnia, headache
GI:	Abdominal pain, flatulence, dyspepsia, ↑ LFTs (dose-dependent)
Dosage:	100–400 mg/d
Contraindications:	NK
Drug Interactions:	NK
Key Points:	Investigational drug that may prove useful as part of multimodal analgesic regimen in perioperative period

MAGNESIUM SALICYLATE

Trade Names:	**See Appendix I, "Oral Analgesic Drug Combinations"**

MEFENAMIC ACID

Trade Name:	**Ponstel**
Indications:	Acute pain, inflammation, rheumatoid arthritis, dysmenorrhea
Pharmacokinetics:	Onset: <1 h; peak: 2–3 h; highly protein bound; duration: 6–7 h; Vd: 1.3 L/kg; $T_{1/2}$ β: 3.5 h; metabolized in liver, excreted in urine
Pharmacodynamics:	Nonselective inhibition of prostaglandin synthesis
CNS:	Drowsiness, dizziness, headache
CV:	Edema
GI:	Mucosal ulceration and bleeding
GU:	Renal failure
Other:	Reversible inhibition of platelet aggregation
Dosage:	500 mg PO, then 250 mg q 6 h
Contraindications:	Peptic ulceration, GI bleeding, asthma
Drug Interactions:	↑ Levels of methotrexate, lithium, digoxin; ↓ effect of diuretics and antihypertensives; other NSAIDs, acetaminophen, alcohol ↑ nephropathy and GI bleeding; ↑ bleeding with anticoagulants and thrombolytics
Key Points:	Nonselective NSAID with nephrotoxicity and antiplatelet effects

MELOXICAM, OXAPROZIN

Trade Names:	**Mobic (meloxicam), Daypro (oxaprozin)**
Indications:	Osteoarthritis
Pharmacokinetics:	Onset: <1 h; bioavailability: 90%; peak: 3–5 h; protein binding: 99%; duration: 12–24 h; $T_{1/2}$ β: 15–30 h; extensively metabolized in liver, excreted in urine and feces
Pharmacodynamics:	Nonselective inhibition of prostaglandin synthetase
CNS:	Dizziness, headache
CV:	↑ HR, ↑ BP, pedal edema
GI:	Nausea, diarrhea, dyspepsia, flatulence, ↑ LTFs
Other:	Thrombocytopenia, rash, photosensitivity, angioedema
Dosages:	*Meloxicam:* 7.5–15 mg/d
	Oxaprozin: 1200–1800 mg/d
Contraindications:	Asthma, pregnancy, angioedema, sensitivity to ASA or NSAIDs
Drug Interactions:	↓ Effect of ACE inhibitors; aspirin and warfarin ↑ risk of bleeding; ↑ lithium level; sun exposure ↑ photosensitivity
Key Points:	May ↑ operative site and GI bleeding during the perioperative period

NABUMETONE

Trade Name:	**Relafen**
Indications:	Osteo- and rheumatoid arthritis
Pharmacokinetics:	Onset: 1–2 h; peak: 8–12 h; protein binding: 99%; duration: 12–24 h; $T_{1/2}$ β: 24 h; metabolized in liver, excreted 1° in urine
Pharmacodynamics:	Nonselective inhibitor of prostaglandin synthesis
CNS:	Dizziness, headache, fatigue, insomnia, nervousness, tinnitus
GI:	Diarrhea, dyspepsia, abdominal pain, nausea, vomiting, anorexia
Other:	Pruritus, rash, ↑ diaphoresis, pedal edema
Dosage:	0.5–1 g/d (max. 2 g/d)
Contraindications:	ASA- or NSAID-induced asthma, pregnancy
Drug Interactions:	Aspirin and alcohol ↑ risk of GI bleeding; ↑ cyclosporin, warfarin, and methotrexate toxicity
Key Points:	No known interaction with anesthetic drugs during perioperative period

NAPROXEN

Trade Name:	**Naprosyn**
Indications:	Acute and chronic pain, inflammation, acute gout, dysmenorrhea
Pharmacokinetics:	Onset: <1 h; peak: 2–4 h; highly protein bound; duration: 6–8 h; Vd: 0.1 L/kg; Cl: 0.3 L/h; $T_{1/2}$ β: 10–20 h; crosses placental barrier and in breast milk; metabolized in liver, excreted in urine
Pharmacodynamics:	Inhibition of prostaglandin synthesis
CNS:	Drowsiness, vertigo, confusion, tinnitus
CV:	Pedal edema, palpitations
GI:	Nausea, dyspepsia, constipation, ↑ LFTs
GU:	Nephrotoxicity
Pulmonary:	Bronchospasm, dyspnea
Other:	↓ Platelet aggregation (reversible), rash, urticaria, diaphoresis, pruritus
Dosage:	500 mg PO, then 250 mg q 6 h; 10 mg/kg/d in divided doses (children)
Contraindications:	GI ulceration/bleeding, nasal polyps, asthma, breast-feeding
Drug Interactions:	↑ Levels of methotrexate, lithium, digoxin; ↓ effect of diuretics and antihypertensives; NSAIDs, acetaminophen, alcohol ↑ nephropathy and GI bleeding; ↑ bleeding with anticoagulants and thrombolytics
Key Points:	Classical nonselective NSAID more commonly used for chronic pain and inflammation than acute postoperative pain

PARECOXIB

Trade Name:	**Dynastat**
Indications:	Acute pain
Pharmacokinetics:	Onset: <30 min; peak: 1–2 h; duration: 6–12 h; $T_{1/2}$ β: 8 h; converted to valdecoxib by enzymatic hydrolysis in the liver, excreted in urine
Pharmacodynamics:	Prodrug with active metabolite (valdecoxib) possessing selective COX-2–inhibiting activity
CNS:	Insomnia
CV:	Fluid retention, myocardial ischemia
GI:	Dyspepsia
GU:	Oliguria, ↓ renal tubular function
Other:	Toxic epidermal necrolysis (Stevens-Johnson syndrome), wound infections

PARECOXIB *continued*

Dosage:	20–40 mg IV/IM q 6–12 h (max. 80 mg/d)
Contraindications:	Sensitivity to sulfonamides/sulfur allergy, active GI bleeding, ulceration, severe hepatic impairment, CHF, colitis
Drug Interactions:	Fluconazole and ketoconazole ↓ metabolism; ↑ lithium level
Key Points:	Parenterally active COX-2–selective NSAID that produces opioid-sparing effects during the perioperative period; ↓ risk of perioperative bleeding (vs nonselective parenteral NSAIDs)

PIROXICAM

Trade Name:	**Feldene**
Indications:	Acute pain, inflammation, osteo- and rheumatoid arthritis
Pharmacokinetics:	Onset: 1 h; peak: 3–5 h; highly protein bound; duration: 48–72 h; Vd: 0.14 L/kg; Cl: 0.14 L/h; $T_{1/2}$ β: 45 h; metabolized in liver, excreted in urine
Pharmacodynamics:	Nonselective inhibition of prostaglandin synthesis
CNS:	Dizziness, drowsiness, tinnitus, headache
CV:	Pedal edema
GI:	Mucosal ulceration/bleeding, dyspepsia, nausea, constipation/diarrhea
GU:	Nephrotoxicity
Other:	Reversible inhibition of platelet aggregation, ↑ bleeding tendency, pancytopenia, ↑ BT, pruritus, rash, photosensitivity
Dosage:	20 mg/d PO or 10 mg PO q 12 h
Contraindications:	Peptic ulceration, GI bleeding, ASA- or NSAID-related asthma
Drug Interactions:	↑ Levels of methotrexate, lithium, digoxin ↓ effect of diuretics and antihypertensives; NSAIDs, acetaminophen, alcohol ↑ risk of nephropathy and GI bleeding; ginger, garlic, anticoagulants, thrombolytics ↑ risk of bleeding; sun exposure and St. John's Wort ↑ photosensitivity
Key Points:	More commonly used for chronic inflammatory-mediated pain than for acute perioperative pain

PROPACETAMOL

Trade Name:	**Pro-Dafalgan**
Indication:	Acute and postoperative pain
Pharmacokinetics:	Onset <30 min; prodrug that is rapidly metabolized to acetaminophen; duration 3–6 h; excreted in urine
Pharmacodynamics:	Inhibition of prostaglandin synthesis, blocks endogenous pyrogen
CNS:	Analgesia, antipyretic effects
GI:	Nausea, vomiting, ↑ LFTs, jaundice
Other:	Bone marrow suppression, hypoglycemia, rash, pain on injection
Dosage:	1–2 g IV/IM q 3–4 h
Contraindications:	Viral hepatitis, phenylketonuria, hepatorenal impairment, alcoholism
Drug Interactions:	↑ Hepatotoxicity with alcohol; ↑ nephropathy with NSAIDs; caffeine ↑ effect; antacids ↓ absorption
Key Points:	Parenterally active formulation of acetaminophen that can ↓ acute pain and need for opioid analgesics during perioperative period

ROFECOXIB

Trade Name:	**Vioxx**
Indications:	Acute and postoperative pain, osteo- and rheumatoid arthritis, dysmenorrhea
Pharmacokinetics:	Onset: <1 h; bioavailability: 93%; peak: 2–3 h; protein binding: 87%; $T_{1/2}$ β: 17 h; extensively metabolized in liver, excreted in urine
Pharmacodynamics:	Highly selective COX-2 inhibitor
CNS:	Headache, asthenia, aseptic meningitis, CVA
CV:	↑ BP, MI, ↓ HR, palpitations
GI:	Dyspepsia, nausea, abdominal pain, diarrhea/constipation, oral ulcers
Other:	Hyponatremia, muscle cramps, UTI/URI, pedal edema
Dosage:	12.5–50 mg/d PO; 50 mg (pre-emptive analgesia)
Contraindications:	Late pregnancy, CAD, severe hepatorenal disease, CHF
Drug Interactions:	↓ Effect of ACE inhibitors, furosemide, thiazides; ↑ GI bleeding with aspirin, smoking, alcohol; ↑ lithium, methotrexate, theophylline levels; ↑ warfarin effects; rifampin ↑ metabolism

ROFECOXIB *continued*

Key Points:	Long-acting nonopioid analgesic useful for premedication prior to elective surgery; opioid-sparing effect in postoperative period facilitates recovery process

TOLMETIN

Trade Name:	**Tolectin**
Indications:	Osteo- and rheumatoid arthritis
Pharmacokinetics:	Onset: <30 min; peak: 0.5–1.5 h; highly protein bound; duration: 24 h; $T_{1/2}$ β: 5 h; metabolized in liver, excreted in urine
Pharmacodynamics:	Nonselective inhibition of prostaglandin synthesis
CNS:	Headache, dizziness, drowsiness, asthenia, tinnitus
CV:	↑ BP, pedal edema, angina
GI:	Nausea, vomiting, abdominal pain, peptic ulceration, weight change, dyspepsia, diarrhea/constipation
GU:	↓ Renal function (with ↑ BUN/Cr), UTI
Dosage:	400 mg PO tid (max. 1800 mg/d); 4–8 mg/kg qid (children)
Contraindications:	ASA- or NSAID-related asthma, breast-feeding
Drug Interactions:	Anticoagulants and thrombolytics ↑ bleeding; ↑ toxicity of methotrexate; aspirin ↑ metabolism
Key Points:	Usefulness for perioperative analgesia has not been studied

VALDECOXIB

Trade Name:	**Bextra**
Indications:	Acute and postoperative pain, osteo- and rheumatoid arthritis, dysmenorrhea
Pharmacokinetics:	Onset: <1 h; bioavailability: 83%; peak: 2–3 h; protein binding: 98%; duration: 6–12 h; extensive hepatic metabolism, excreted in urine
Pharmacodynamics:	Selective inhibition of COX-2
CNS:	Dizziness, headache, neuropathy
CV:	↑ BP, angina, arrhythmia, CHF, pedal edema
GI:	Dyspepsia, nausea, vomiting, ↑ LFTs, constipation
Pulmonary:	URI, bronchospasm
Other:	Myalgia, rash (Stevens-Johnson syndrome), thrombocytopenia, leukopenia, menstrual irregularities, goiter, impotence

VALDECOXIB *continued*

Dosage:	40 mg initially, then 10–20 mg PO bid
Contraindications:	Asthma, severe renal or hepatic disease
Drug Interactions:	↓ Effect of ACE inhibitors; ↑ GI bleeding with aspirin; fluconazole and ketoconazole ↑ effects; ↑ lithium level; ↑ warfarin effect
Key Points:	Used as a premedication for pre-emptive analgesia after surgery; requires twice-daily dosing in postoperative period

12

Antimicrobials

AMIKACIN

Trade Name:	**Amikin**
Indications:	Infection with gram-(−) organisms resistant to kanamycin and gentamycin, tuberculosis
Pharmacokinetics:	Onset: <2 min; peak: <1 h; duration: 8–12 h; Vd: 0.35 L/kg; Cl: 94 mL/min; $T_{1/2}$ β: 2 h; excreted unchanged in urine
Pharmacodynamics:	Inhibition of ribosomal protein synthesis
CNS:	Otoxicity, encephalopathy
CV:	↓ BP, ↑ HR
Other:	Renal toxicity, bone marrow depression, ↑ LFTs, muscle weakness
Dosage:	5–7.5 mg/kg IV/IM q 8–12 h (max. 1.5 g/d); 10 mg/kg, then 7.5 mg/kg bid (children)
Contraindications:	Sensitivity to other aminoglycosides, renal impairment, neuromuscular disorders
Drug Interactions:	Diuretics, vancomycin, cyclosporin, amphotericin ↑ toxicity; synergism with bactericidal drugs; biphosphonates ↑ risk of hypocalcemia
Key Points:	↑ Muscle relaxant effects during surgery, ↑ requirement for neuromuscular reversal drugs

AMOXICILLIN

Trade Names:	**Amoxil, Wymox, Trimox, Augmentin (contains clavulanate)**
Indications:	UTI and URI (otitis media, sinusitis) with gram-(+) and gram-(−) organisms, *Haemophilus influenzae*, *Eikenella*, *Pasteurella* spp.
Pharmacokinetics:	Onset: <1 h; peak: 1–2 h; protein binding: minimal; duration: 6–8 h; $T_{1/2}$ β: 2 h; crosses placental barrier; partially metabolized, excreted in urine by renal tubular secretion
Pharmacodynamics:	Aminopenicillin and β-lactamase inhibitor
CNS:	Agitation, dizziness, insomnia, seizures
GI:	Nausea, vomiting, diarrhea, pseudomembranous colitis, ↑ LFTs, black "hairy" tongue, dyspepsia
Other:	Nephropathy, vaginitis, anemia, thrombocytopenia, leukopenia, anaphylaxis, rash
Dosage:	250–500 mg PO bid; 20–45 mg/kg/d (children)
Contraindications:	Sensitivity to β-lactam, cholestatic jaundice, mononucleosis

AMOXICILLIN *continued*

Drug Interactions:	↓ Elimination of methotrexate; probenecid ↓ renal elimination
Key Points:	Oral prophylaxis for bacterial endocarditis (2 g or 50 mg/kg) should be given 1 h prior to surgery

AMPHOTERICIN B

Trade Names:	**Amphocin, Fungizone**
Indications:	Fungal sepsis, pneumonia, meningitis
Pharmacokinetics:	Onset: <2 min; peak: 3 h; Vd: 0.08 L/kg; Cl: 0.46 mL/min/kg; $T_{1/2}$ β: 100–153 h; hepatic metabolism, excreted in urine
Pharmacodynamics:	Disruption of fungal cell membrane (polyene antibiotic)
CNS:	Headache, chills, fever, tremors
CV:	Arrhythmias, ↓ BP, asystole
GI:	Abdominal pain, hemorrhage, nausea, vomiting, diarrhea
Pulmonary:	Dyspnea, respiratory failure, wheezing
Renal:	Renal failure, hypokalemia
Other:	Fever, chills, sepsis, bone marrow suppression, rash, anemia
Dosage:	1 mg test dose infused over 20–30 min, ↑ dose to 0.5–1 mg/kg/d in divided doses, if no reaction occurs ↑ by 5–10 mg/d
Contraindications:	Renal failure
Drug Interactions:	↑ Nephrotoxicity of aminoglycosides; cisplatin and pentamidine ↓ effect; ↑ digoxin toxicity (due to hypokalemia)
Key Points:	Can ↑ neuromuscular blockade

AMPICILLIN

Trade Names:	**Omnipen, Principen, Amicill, Unasyn, Totacillin**
Indications:	Infections with gram-(+) and gram-(−) organisms (*H. influenzae*, *Escherichia coli*, *Proteus mirabilis*, *Salmonella* and *Shigella* spp.)
Pharmacokinetics:	Onset: <1 h; peak: 1–2 h; protein binding: 20%; duration: 6–8 h; Vd: 0.28 L/kg; Cl: 2 mL/min/kg; $T_{1/2}$ β: 1–2 h (10–24 h with ↓ CrCl; minimal metabolism, excreted 1° in urine
Pharmacodynamics:	Aminopenicillin bactericidal inhibition of cell wall synthesis

AMPICILLIN *continued*

CNS:	Myoclonic twitching, seizures
GI:	Nausea, vomiting, diarrhea, black "hairy" tongue, pseudomembranous colitis
Renal:	Interstitial nephritis
Other:	Bone marrow suppression, TTP, ↑ bleeding time, ↑ PTT, rash

Dosage: 2 g IV (plus gentamycin, 1.5 mg/kg IV, max. 80 mg), followed by 250–500 mg PO q 6 h regimen (endocarditis prophylaxis); 50 mg/kg IV followed by 25 mg/kg q 6 h (children); 1 to 2 g IM/IV q 3–4, 19–25 mg/kg q 3 h or 25–33 mg/kg q 4 h (max. 300 mg/kg) (meningitis, septicemia); 18–25 mg/kg IM/IV q 3 h or 25–33 mg/kg q 4 h (children)

Contraindications: β-lactam allergic (penicillins), mononucleosis, rash

Drug Interaction: Synergistic with aminoglycosides; sulbactam is a penicillinase (β-lactamase) inhibitor; allopurinol ↑ risk of rash; probenecid ↓ renal elimination

Key Points: May influence requirement for anticoagulants during CV surgery

AZITHROMYCIN

Trade Name: **Zithromax**

Indications: Infections with aerobic gram-(+) and gram-(−) microorganisms (except methicillin-resistant staph), chlamydias, mucoplasma

Pharmacokinetics: Onset: <1 h; peak: 2–5 h; duration: 12–24 h; Vd: 31 L/kg; Cl: 630 mL/min; $T_{1/2}$ β: 68 h; no metabolism; elimination: biliary (feces)

Pharmacodynamics:	Azalide, macrolide inhibitor of protein synthesis
GI:	Nausea/vomiting, abdominal pain, diarrhea
Other:	Rash, toxic epidermal necrolysis and Stevens-Johnson syndrome, cholestatic hepatitis, headache

Dosage: 500–1000 mg/d (slowly IV), followed by 250 mg/d for 4 d; 10 mg/kg IM/IV, followed by 5 mg/kg for 4 d (children)

Contraindications: Sensitivity to erythromycin, ergot toxicity

Drug Interactions: ↓ Metabolism by cytochrome P_{450} inhibitors, ↑ levels of erythromycin, theophylline, riazolam

Key Points: Can impair hepatic metabolism of anesthetic drugs, prolonging recovery

AZTREONAM

Trade Name:	**Azactam**
Indications:	Infections with gram-(−) bacteria
Pharmacokinetics:	Onset: <30 min; peak: 1 h; protein binding: 55%; duration: 6–8 h; Vd: 0.1–0.2 L/kg; $T_{1/2}$ β: 1.7 h; minimal metabolism, excreted 1° unchanged in urine
Pharmacodynamics:	Interaction with penicillin-binding proteins
CNS:	Seizure, paresthesias, confusion, insomnia
CV:	Arrhythmias, ↓ BP
GI:	Diarrhea, nausea/vomiting, ↑ LFTs, pseudomembranous colitis, cramps
Other:	Bone marrow suppression [(+) Coombs' reaction], ↑ PT, ↑ platelet aggregation, thrombophlebitis, ↓ renal function
Dosage:	2 g IV q 6–8 h (max. 8 g/d); ↓ dose by 50% with CrCl <30 mL/min; 2 g IV q 6–8 h (children)
Contraindications:	Elderly with impaired renal function
Drug Interactions:	Synergistic with aminoglycosides and β-lactam antibiotics; chloramphenicol ↓ effect; probenecid ↓ renal elimination
Key Points:	Vasodilators and IV anesthetics can ↑ depression

CEFAZOLIN, CEPHALEXIN, CEFADROXIL

Trade Names:	**Duricef (cefadroxil); Keflex (cephalexin); Ancef, Kefzol (cefazolin)**
Indications:	Prophylaxis and treatment of gram-(+) infections (1st-generation cephalosporins)
Pharmacokinetics:	Onset: <30 min; peak: 1–2 h; protein binding: 80%; duration: 8 h (↑ 12–24 h if CrCl <30 mL/min); Vd: 0.12 L/kg; CrCl: 0.95 mL/min/kg; $T_{1/2}$ β: 1–2 h (↑ 12–50 h with ↓ CrCl); no metabolism, urinary excretion
Pharmacodynamics:	Inhibits penicillin-binding proteins involved in cell wall synthesis
CNS:	Seizures (cefadroxil), dizziness, headache, confusion
GI:	Pseudomembranous colitis, nausea, vomiting, diarrhea, glossitis, ↑ LFTs
GU:	Genital pruritus, vaginitis, renal dysfunction

CEFAZOLIN, CEPHALEXIN, CEFADROXIL *continued*

Other:	Dyspnea, bone marrow suppression (pancytopenia), rash, oral candidiasis, serum sickness, angioedema, thrombophlebitis
Dosages:	*Cefadroxil/Cephalexin*: 1 g IV 0.5–1 h before surgery, then 0.5–1 g IV q 8 h for 24 h; 6.25–25 mg/kg IV q 6 h or 8–33 mg/kg q 8 h (children) *Cefazolin*: 0.25–1.5 g IV q 6–8 h
Contraindications:	β-lactam allergic (e.g., cephalosporine), breast-feeding
Drug Interactions:	Probenecid ↓ renal elimination; ↑ toxicity of nephrotoxic drugs (e.g., aminoglycosides, colistin, polymyxin B, vancomycin)
Key Points:	Dosages for perioperative prophylaxis should be reduced by 50% and dosing interval increased to q 12–24 h if CrCl <30 mL/min

CEFDINIR, CEFPODOXIME, CEFOPERAZONE

Trade Names:	**Omnicef (cefdinir), Vantin (cefpodoxime), Cefobid (cefoperazone)**
Indications:	Treatment of gram-(+) and gram-(−) aerobes (3rd-generation cephalosporins)
Pharmacokinetics:	Onset: <1 h; bioavailability: low (↑ with food); peak: 2–4 h; protein binding: 45%; duration: 12 h; Vd: 0.4 L/kg; $T_{1/2}$ β: 1.71 h; de-esterified to active metabolite (cefpodoxime), excreted 1° in urine
Pharmacodynamics: *CNS:* *GI:* *Other:*	Inhibits bacterial cell wall synthesis Headaches Diarrhea, nausea, vomiting, abdominal pain Vaginal candidiasis, rash
Dosage:	200–300 mg PO q 12 h (pneumonia, chronic bronchitis, gonorrhea); 100–250 mg PO q 12 h (max. 4 g/d) (pharyngitis or tonsillitis); 5–7 mg/kg q 12 (otitis media, [children])
Contraindications:	β-lactam allergic, breast-feeding, colitis
Drug Interactions:	Antacids ↓ absorption; probenecid ↓ renal elimination
Key Points:	Avoid alcohol for at least 72 h after dosing; adequate hydration during perioperative period ↓ risk of nephrotoxicity

CEFEPIME

Trade Name:	**Maxipime**
Indications:	Infections with aerobic gram-(+) and gram-(−) bacteria (4th-generation cephalosporins)
Pharmacokinetics:	Onset: 0.5 h; peak: 1–2 h; protein binding: 20%; Vd: 18 L; Cl: 120 mL/min; $T_{1/2} \alpha$: 2 h; minimally metabolized, excreted 1° in urine
Pharmacodynamics:	Inhibits bacterial cell wall synthesis
CNS:	Headache
GI:	Diarrhea, colitis, nausea, vomiting, oral candidiasis
Other:	Vaginitis, ↓ prothrombin activity, (+) Coombs' test, fever, rash
Dosage:	0.5–2 g IM q 12 h; 50 mg/kg q 12 h (children)
Contraindications:	Sensitivity to cephalosporins, penicillins, and β-lactams; severe colitis and renal insufficiency
Drug Interactions:	Aminoglycosides ↑ nephro- and ototoxicity; probenecid ↓ elimination; loop diuretics ↑ risk of nephrotoxicity
Key Points:	Adequate hydration during perioperative period minimizes nephrotoxicity

CEFOTETAN, CEFPROZIL, CEFOXITIN

Trade Names:	**Cefotan (cefotetan), Cefzil (cefprozil), Mefoxin (cefoxitin)**
Indications:	Prophylaxis and treatment of anaerobic infections (2nd-generation cephalosporins)
Pharmacokinetics:	Onset: <10 min; bioavailability: 95%; peak: <30 min; protein binding: 65%; duration: 8–12 h; Vd: 0.31 L/kg; Cl: 3.3 mL/min/kg; $T_{1/2} \beta$: 1 h; minimal metabolism, excreted 1° in urine
Pharmacodynamics:	Inhibits bacterial cell wall synthesis
CNS:	Dizziness
CV:	Thrombophlebitis, ↓ BP
GI:	Pseudomembranous colitis, nausea, diarrhea, ↑ LFTs
Renal:	Nephrotoxicity, ↑ BUN/Cr
Other:	Bone marrow suppression, dyspnea, rash, serum sickness
Dosage:	1 g IV q 6–8; 250 mg PO bid (mild infection); 1–2 g IV q 4 h or 2–3 g q 6–8 h; 500 mg PO bid (medium-severe infection); 2 g IV at 0.5–1 h before surgery, followed by 2 g at 4 h and 8 h after the first dose (perioperative prophylaxis); 13–27 mg/kg IV q 4 h or 20–40 mg/kg q 6 h; 15 mg/kg PO q 12 h (children)

CEFOTETAN, CEFPROZIL, CEFOXITIN *continued*

Contraindications:	β-lactam allergic (cephalosporins), ↓ renal function, breast-feeding
Drug Interactions:	Disulfiram-like intolerance of alcohol; loop diuretics and aminoglycosides ↑ nephrotoxicity; probenecid ↓ renal elimination
Key Points:	Can ↑ effect of anticoagulants (↑ bleeding) and nephrotoxic drugs

CEFTAZIDIME

Trade Names:	**Fortaz, Ceptaz**
Indications:	Prophylaxis against *Pseudomonas* spp. and other gram-(−) organisms in combination with aminoglucoside (3rd-generation cephalosporin)
Pharmacokinetics:	Onset: <10 min; peak: <1 h; protein binding: 5–24%; duration: 8–12 h; Vd: 0.23 L/kg; Cl: 1.05 mL/min/kg; $T_{1/2}$ β: 1.5–2 h (↑ 35 h with ↓ CrCl); no metabolism, excreted 1° in urine
Pharmacodynamics:	Inhibits bacteria cell wall synthesis
CNS:	Seizures, fever, headache, dizziness
GI:	Pseudomembranous colitis, nausea/vomiting, diarrhea, cramps, ↑ LFTs
Other:	Bone marrow suppression, thrombophlebitis, vaginitis, rash
Dosage:	0.5–2 g q 8–12 h (max. 6 g/d); 30–50 mg/kg q 8 h (children); ↓ dose by 50% and ↑ interval to q 24–48 h with ↓ CrCl
Contraindications:	β-lactam or penicillin allergic, breast-feeding, ↓ renal function
Drug Interactions:	Aminoglycosides ↑ risk of nephrotoxicity; chloramphenicol ↓ effect; quinolones ↑ effect
Key Points:	In presence of renal impairment (CrCl <30 mL/min), ↓ dosage by 50% and ↑ dosing interval to q 24–48 h

CEFTRIAXONE

Trade Name:	**Rocephin**
Indications:	Infections with aerobic gram-(+) and enteric gram-(−) organisms and some anaerobes (3rd-generation cephalosporin)

CEFTRIAXONE *continued*

Pharmacokinetics:	Onset: <10 min; peak: 1–4 h; protein binding: 90%; duration: 12 h; Vd: 0.16 L/kg; Cl: 0.24 mL/min/kg; $T_{1/2}$ β: 5–11 h; minimally metabolized, excreted 1° in urine
Pharmacodynamics:	Inhibits bacterial cell wall synthesis
GI:	Pseudomembranous colitis, diarrhea, ↑ LFTs
Other:	Bone marrow suppression, rash, infection pain, eosinophilia
Dosage:	1–2 g/d or 0.5–1 g q 12 h (max. 4 g/d): 250 mg IM (gonorrhea); 25–50 mg/kg q 12 h, or 80 mg/kg q 12 h (×3), then q 24 h (max. 4 g/d) (children)
Contraindications:	β-lactam and penicillin allergic, breast-feeding
Drug Interactions:	Aminoglycosides ↑ antimicrobial activity; probenecid ↓ elimination
Key Points:	Dosage adjustment required in the presence of hepatorenal impairment (max. 2 g/d)

CEFUROXIME

Trade Names:	**Zinacef, Kefurox, Ceftin**
Indications:	Infections with aerobes gram-(+) and gram-(−) anaerobic gram-(+) cocci and gram-(−) bacilli, gonorrhea, Lyme disease
Pharmacokinetics:	Onset: <10 min (IV); peak: 0.5–2 h; protein binding: 40%; duration: 8–12 h; Vd: 0.19 L/kg; Cl: 0.94 mL/min/kg; $T_{1/2}$ β: 1–2 h; no metabolism, 1° urinary excretion
Pharmacodynamics:	Inhibits bacterial cell wall synthesis
GI:	Pseudomembranous colitis, nausea, anorexia, vomiting, diarrhea
GU:	Nephrotoxicity (↑ BUN/Cr)
Other:	Bone marrow suppression (pancytopenia), rash, sterile abscesses
Dosage:	0.75–1.5 g IM/IV q 8 h (gonorrhea); 125–500 mg PO bid (Lyme disease); 70–80 mg/kg IM/IV q 8 h (meningitis) (children)
Contraindications:	β-lactam allergic, breast-feeding, renal failure
Drug Interactions:	Food ↑ absorption; aminoglycosides and diuretics ↑ risks of nephrotoxicity; probenecid ↓ renal elimination
Key Points:	For perioperative prophylaxis, give 1.5 g IV 30–60 min before surgery, then 750 mg q 8 h (×48 h)

CHLORAMPHENICOL

Trade Name:	**Chloromycetin**
Indications:	Infections with gram-(+) and gram-(−) cocci and bacilli (including anaerobes), *Rickettsia* spp., mycoplasma, chlamydia
Pharmacokinetics:	Onset: <30 min; peak: 1–3 h; protein binding: 55%; duration: 12 h; Vd: 1 L/kg; Cl: 2.4 mL/min/kg; therapeutic level: 10–20 µg/mL; $T_{1/2}$ β: 4.0 h; metabolized in liver, excreted in urine
Pharmacodynamics:	Inhibition of protein synthesis and peptide bond formation
CNS:	Headache, confusion, peripheral neuropathy, optic neuritis
CV:	Circulatory instability in newborns (gray syndrome)
GI:	Nausea, vomiting, stomatitis, enterocolitis, diarrhea, jaundice
Other:	Bone marrow suppression, hemoglobinuria, lactic acidosis, urticaria
Dosage:	50–100 mg IV qid; 25–50 mg/kg/d IV (children)
Contraindications:	Pregnancy, bone marrow suppression, AIP, G6PD deficiency
Drug Interactions:	↓ Metabolism of phenytoin, tolbutamide, warfarin, dicumarol, and chlorpropamide; penicillin ↓ bactericidal activity
Key Points:	Prolonged administration of nitrous oxide should be avoided due to potential bone marrow depression; avoid etomidate due to ↓ metabolism

CIPROFLOXACIN

Trade Names:	**Cipro, Cipro XR, Ciprodex**
Indications:	Infections with aerobic gram-(+) and gram-(−) microorganisms
Pharmacokinetics:	Onset: <30 min; bioavailability: 75%; peak: 1–2 h; protein binding: 30%; duration: 12 h; Vd: 1.8 L/kg; Cl: 6 mL/min/kg; $T_{1/2}$ β: 8 h; hepatic metabolism, renal excretion
Pharmacodynamics:	Fluoroquinolone antibiotic interferes with DNA synthesis
CNS:	Seizures, headache, dizziness, insomnia, confusion, paresthesia
CV:	Palpitations, arrhythmias

CIPROFLOXACIN *continued*

GI:	Nausea, vomiting, pseudomembranous colitis, diarrhea, oral candidiasis, dyspepsia, flatulence, ↑ LFTs, cholestatic jaundice
GU:	Interstitial nephritis, crystalluria, ↑ BUN/Cr, urethral bleeding, vaginitis
Other:	Rash, photosensitivity, toxic epidermal necrolysis, thrombophlebitis, arthralgia, myalgias, respiratory arrest, hiccups

Dosage: 250–750 mg PO bid, 250–500 mg IV q 12 h

Contraindications: CNS disorders (seizures), pregnancy, breast-feeding

Drug Interactions: Antacids ↓ absorption; ↓ clearance of warfarin, theophylline, caffeine; synergism against Pseudomonas aeruginosa with imipenem or anti-Pseudomonas penicillin; probenecid ↓ renal excretion; cyclosporine ↑ Cr

Key Points: Monitor carefully in patient receiving concomitant anticoagulant (warfarin) or bronchodilation (theophylline) therapy; ciprodex (0.3%) otic suspension contains dexamethasone 0.19%

CLARITHROMYCIN

Trade Name: **Biaxin**

Indications: Infections caused by sensitive aerobic gram-(+) and gram-(−) cocci, chlamydias, mycoplasma, mycobacteria, anaerobic gram-(+) bacteria

Pharmacokinetics: Onset: <1 h; bioavailability: 50%; peak: 2 h; duration: 12 h; $T_{1/2}$ β: 3–7 h (↑ with ↓ CrCl); hepatic metabolism to form active metabolite, excreted in urine

Pharmacodynamics:	Macrolite antibiotic inhibits protein synthesis
CNS:	Headache
CV:	QT prolongation, arrhythmias
GI:	Diarrhea, nausea, bad taste, dyspepsia, ↑ LFTs
Other:	Cholestatic hepatitis, ↑ BUN/Cr

Dosages: 250–500 mg PO bid; 15 mg/kg/d PO q 12 h (children)

Contraindication: Cardiac arrhythmias, concomitant use of ergot drugs, cisapride, astemizole, pimozide, terfenadine; sensitivity to microlides

Drug Interactions: ↑ Levels of carbamazepine, digoxin, theophylline, ranitidine, terfenadine, omeprazole, HMG-CoA reductase inhibitors

CLARITHROMYCIN *continued*

Key Points:	Monitor ECG carefully in presence of electrolyte disturbances

CLINDAMYCIN

Trade Name:	**Cleocin**
Indications:	Infections with anaerobic and aerobic gram-(+) cocci (1st-line); *Streptococcus pneumoniae*, pneumococcus (3rd-line); penicillin-resistant *Staphylococcus* sp.; *Corynebacterium diphtheriae*; *Campylobacter jejuni*; *Mycoplasma pneumoniae*
Pharmacokinetics:	Onset: <15 min; peak: 45–60 min; protein binding: 93%; duration: 6–12 h; Vd: 1.1 L/kg; Cl: 4.7 mL/min/kg; $T_{1/2}$ β: 2–3 h (7–14 h with hepatorenal disease); hepatic metabolism, urinary excretion
Pharmacodynamics:	Lincomycin-like bacteriostatic inhibition of protein synthesis
GI:	Pseudomembranous colitis, esophagitis, nausea/vomiting, jaundice
Other:	Rash, urticaria, pruritus, bone marrow suppression, vaginitis
Dosage:	75–300 mg PO qid; 300–600 mg (IV/IM) q 6 h; 3–5 mg/kg IV/IM q h or 5–7 mg/kg q 8 h (children)
Contraindications:	Chronic GI disorders, atopic reactions, asthma
Drug Interactions:	Kaolin ↓ absorption; erythromycin ↓ effect
Key Points:	Can ↑ muscle relaxants and ↑ need for reversal drugs

CLOFAZIMINE

Trade Name:	**Lamprene**
Indications:	Leprosy, atypical mycobacterial infections
Pharmacokinetics:	Onset: <1 h; bioavailability: 45–62%; peak: 1–6 h; duration: 8–12 h; $T_{1/2}$ β: <70 d
Pharmacodynamics:	Iminophenazine dye with bactericidal activity
CNS:	Conjunctival and corneal pigmentation, eye irritation
GI:	Epigastric pain, nausea, vomiting, diarrhea
Other:	Eosinophilia, skin pigmentation, ichthyosis
Dosage:	100–200 mg/d PO
Contraindications:	NK
Drug Interactions:	Dapsone, isoniazid ↓ effect
Key Points:	Check LFTs and electrolyte panel preoperatively

CLOTRIMAZOLE

Trade Names:	**Lotrimin, Mycelex**
Indications:	Candidiasis
Pharmacokinetics:	NK
Pharmacodynamics:	Fungistatic and fungicidal activity
CNS:	Dizziness, paresthesia
GI:	Nausea, diarrhea, ↑ LFTs
Other:	Erythema, blistering/peeling, edema, pruritus, urticaria
Dosage:	100–500 mg/d PO, 5 g % cream for 2–4 wk
Contraindications:	Sensitivity to clotrimazole, betamethasone dipropionate, other corticosteroids or imidazoles
Drug Interactions:	NK
Key Points:	Preparations containing betamethasone (e.g., Lotrisone) may suppress the hypothalamic-pituitary-adrenal axis; consider supplemental hydrocortisone during perioperative period

CLOXACILLIN, DICLOXACILLIN

Trade Names:	**Dycil, Dynapen, Pathocil**
Indications:	Penicillinase-producing staphylococci organisms, gram-(+) aerobic and anaerobic bacilli
Pharmacokinetics:	Onset: <1 h; bioavailability: 50%; peak: 2 h; protein binding: 95%; duration: 6 h; $T_{1/2}$ β: 0.5–1 h (2.5 with ↓ CrCl); partially metabolized and excreted in urine
Pharmacodynamics:	Bactericidal activity, penicillinase resistant
CNS:	Lethargy, hallucinations, seizures, confusion, dizziness
GI:	Nausea, vomiting, diarrhea, pseudomembranous colitis, ↑ LFTs, black "hairy" tongue, dyspepsia
GU:	Interstitial nephritis, nephropathy
Other:	Pancytopenia, rash, urticaria, anaphylaxis
Dosages:	*Cloxacillin*: 250–500 mg PO qid; 50–100 mg/kg/d PO (children) *Dicloxacillin*: 125–500 mg PO qid; 12.5 mg/kg/d PO (children)
Contraindications:	Sensitive to penicillins and cephalosporins
Drug Interactions:	Aminoglycosides ↑ bactericidal effects; probenecid ↓ renal elimination
Key Points:	Overdosage may ↑ anesthetic requirement due to CNS stimulation

DAPTOMYCIN

Trade Name:	**Cubicin**
Indications:	Aerobic gram-(+) bacteria
Pharmacokinetics:	Peak: 0.5 h; protein binding: 92%; Vd: 0.1 L/kg; Cl: 8 mL/kg/h; $T_{1/2}$ β: 8–9 h; hepatic metabolism, renal excretion
Pharmacodynamics:	Binds to bacterial membranes and causes rapid depolarization of membrane potential, inhibiting protein synthesis
CNS:	Headache, dizziness, paresthesias
CV:	Hypotension, hypertension
GI:	Diarrhea, pseudomembranous colitis, ↑ LFTs
GU:	UTI
Other:	Rash, pruritis, anemia, myalgias, arthralgia, local reactions
Dosage:	4 mg/kg/d IV over 30 min for 7–14 d
Contraindications:	NK
Drug Interactions:	NK
Key Points:	Avoid use in absence of documented sensitivity; ↑ dosing interval with renal dysfunction

ERTAPENEM

Trade Name:	**Invanz**
Indications:	Infections with aerobic and anaerobic gram-(+) and gram-(−) organisms
Pharmacokinetics:	Onset: <2 min; bioavailability: 90%; peak: 0.5–2 h; highly protein bound; duration: 24 h; Vd: 8 L; $T_{1/2}$ β: 4 h; metabolized by kidney, excreted in urine
Pharmacodynamics:	Carbapenem that inhibits bacterial cell wall synthesis
CNS:	Fatigue, headache, insomnia, dizziness, confusion, fever
CV:	Thrombophlebitis
GI:	Nausea, vomiting, diarrhea, pseudomembranous colitis
Dosage:	1 g/d IM/IV for 10–14 d (↓ dose by 50% if CrCl <30 mL/min)
Contraindications:	Sensitive to β-lactams and amide-type local anesthetics
Drug Interactions:	Probenecid ↓ renal clearance
Key Points:	Check electrolytes and volume status prior to induction of anesthesia, as GI side effects (e.g., diarrhea) may lead to dehydration

ERYTHROMYCIN

Trade Names:	**Ilosone, Ilotycin**
Indications:	Infections with aerobic gram-(+) and gram-(−) organisms (except methicillin-resistant staph), chlamydias, mycoplasma
Pharmacokinetics:	Onset: <1 h; peak: 1–4 h; protein binding: 85%; duration: 6–8 h; Vd: 0.78 L/kg; Cl: 9.1 mL/min/kg; $T_{1/2}\ \beta$: 1–2 h; metabolized in liver, excreted 1° in bile
Pharmacodynamics:	Macrolide that inhibits bacterial protein synthesis
CNS:	Fever, hearing loss, blurred vision
CV:	Arrhythmias, QT prolongation, thrombophlebitis
GI:	Cholestatic jaundice, dyspepsia, cramps, nausea, vomiting, diarrhea
Other:	Eosinophilia, urticaria, rash, pruritus, anorexia
Dosage:	250 mg qid PO; 250–500 mg IV q 6 h (4–5 mg/kg IV q 6 h); 30–50 mg/kg/d PO; 4–5 mg/kg IV q 6 h (children)
Contraindications:	Pregnancy, hepatic dysfunction, use of fluoroquindones and sparfloxacin
Drug Interactions:	↑ Effects of carbamazepine, corticosteroids, phenytoin, cyclosporine, digoxin, theophylline, warfarin; clindamycin/lincomycin ↓ effect
Key Points:	Can ↑ sedative effects of benzodiazepines

FLUCONAZOLE

Trade Name:	**Diflucan**
Indications:	Cryptococcal and candidal infections, candidiasis prophylaxis
Pharmacokinetics:	Onset: <30 min; bioavailability: high; peak: 1–2 h; protein binding: 12%; duration: 24 h; $T_{1/2}\ \beta$: 30 h; excreted unchanged in urine
Pharmacodynamics:	Bis-triazole inhibitor of fungal P_{450} demethylation
CNS:	Dysesthesias, headaches, hallucinations, seizures
GI:	Nausea, vomiting, abdominal pain, diarrhea, ↑ LFTs
Other:	Alopecia, exfoliative skin rash (Stevens-Johnson syndrome), hypercholesterolemia, blood dyscrasias
Dosage:	150–200 mg PO, followed by 100 mg/d (candidal); 400 mg PO, followed by 200 mg/d (cryptoccal); 3–12 mg/kg (children)
Contraindications:	Sensitivity to azole derivatives

FLUCONAZOLE *continued*

Drug Interactions:	Oral hypoglycemics ↑ hypoglycemia; ↑ levels of tolbutamide, phenytoin, cyclosporine, theophylline, warfarin; rifampin and cimetidine ↓ levels
Key Points:	Check PT and glucose levels when patients are receiving anticoagulants and oral hypoglycemic drugs, respectively

GATIFLOXACIN, LEVOFLOXACIN, LOMEFLOXACIN

Trade Names:	**Tequin (gatifloxacin), Levaquin, Quixin (levofloxacin), Maxaquin (lomefloxacin)**
Indications:	Infections with aerobic gram-(+) and gram-(−) organisms
Pharmacokinetics:	Onset: <30 min; peak: 1–2 h; protein binding: 20%; duration: 24 h; $T_{1/2}$ β: 6–8 h; excreted 1° unchanged in urine
Pharmacodynamics:	Fluoroquindone inhibits DNA gyrase and topoisomerase
CNS:	Headache, dizziness, insomnia, tremor, paresthesia, tinnitus, agitation
CV:	Palpitations, angina, peripheral edema, ↑ BP
GI:	Nausea, vomiting, diarrhea, glossitis, bitter taste, pseudomembranous colitis
GU:	Hematuria, vaginitis, dysuria
Other:	Rash, myalgias, photosensitivity, hypoglycemia, sweating, chills
Dosages:	*Gatifloxacin*: 400 mg/d PO for 7–14 d *Levofloxacin*: 500–750 mg/d PO/IV for 7–14 d; 1–2 drops q 2 h *Lomefloxacin*: 400 mg/d PO for 10–14 d
Contraindications:	QT interval prolongation, uncorrected hypokalemia
Drug Interactions:	Antacids ↓ absorption; oral hypoglycemics ↑ hypoglycemia; antipsychotics, TCAs, Class IA and III antiarrhythmics prolong QT interval; ↑ effect of warfarin and digoxin; NSAIDs ↑ risk of CNS stimulation; probenecid ↑ level (due to ↓ renal secretion)
Key Points:	Laser surgery may ↑ risk of photosensitivity; can ↑ effect of anesthetic drugs on QT interval

GEMIFLOXACIN

Trade Name:	**Factive**
Indications:	Pneumonia, chronic bronchitis

GEMIFLOXACIN *continued*

Pharmacokinetics:	Onset: rapid; bioavailability: 71%; peak: 0.5–2 h; Vd: 4 L/kg; Cl: 4 L/h; $T_{1/2}$ β: 7 h; limited hepatic metabolism, excreted unchanged in feces (62%) and urine (36%)
Pharmacodynamics:	Synthetic broad-spectrum antibacterial agent
CNS:	Headache, tremors, dizziness, hallucinations
CV:	↑ QT intervals, ↓ HR, angina
GI:	Diarrhea, nausea, cramps, unusual taste, ↑ ALT
GU:	↑ BUN/Cr
Other:	Rash, tendinitis, phototoxicity
Dosage:	320 mg/d PO (for 5–7 d)
Contraindications:	Allergy to quinolone-type antibiotics, advanced heart block, prolonged QT interval (with Class IA and Class III antiarrhythmics), pregnancy, breast-feeding
Drug Interactions:	Antacids, iron, zinc, sucralfate, didonosine ↓ absorption; probenecid ↓ clearance, antiarrhythmics and erythromycin, TCAs, ↑ QT prolongation
Key Points:	Potential for prolonged QT-induced arrhythmias

GENTAMICIN

Trade Names:	**Garamycin, Gentacidin**
Indications:	Infection with aerobic gram-(−) bacillus; neonatal infections
Pharmacokinetics:	Onset: <2 min; peak: 30–90 min; protein binding: minimal; duration: 8–24 h; Vd: 0.31 L/kg; $T_{1/2}$ β: 2–3 h (↑ 24–60 h with ↓ CrCl); no metabolism, urinary excretion unchanged
Pharmacodynamics:	Aminoglycoside inhibits ribosomal protein synthesis
CNS:	Ototoxicity, dizziness, lethargy, encephalopathy, headache, seizures, peripheral neuropathy, blurred vision
CV:	↓ BP, ↑ HR
GI:	Vomiting, nausea
Renal:	Nephrotoxicity, ↓ sensitivity of kidney to ADH
Other:	Myasthenia-like syndrome, bone marrow depression, electrolyte disturbances, rash, pruritus, photosensitivity
Dosage:	1.5–3 mg/kg IV q 8 h for 7–10 d; 1–1.7 mg/kg (after hemodialysis); max. 5 mg/kg/d (life-threatening infections); 2–2.5 mg/kg q 8–12 h for 7–10 d (children)
Contraindications:	Sensitivity to aminoglycosides (neomycin), pregnancy

GENTAMICIN *continued*

Drug Interactions:	Synergistic with bactericidal drugs (e.g., penicillin or ampicillin against enterococcus, nafcillin against *Staphylococcus* sp., and ticarcillin against *Pseudomonas* sp.); ↓ bacteriostatic drugs (e.g., tetracycline, erythromycin, sulfonamide); diuretics, NSAIDs, vancomycin, cyclosporine, amphotericin ↑ toxicity
Key Points:	Can ↑ neuromuscular blocking drugs and worsen renal function; antiemetic and antivertigo drugs can mask ototoxicity.

GRISEOFULVIN

Trade Names:	**Fulvicin, Grifulvin, Grisactin**
Indications:	Tineal infections
Pharmacokinetics:	Onset: 1–2 h; peak: 4–8 h; duration: 24 h; $T_{1/2}$ β: 9–24 h; absorbed in duodenum (25%–70%); metabolized in liver, excreted 1° in urine
Pharmacodynamics:	Disrupts fungal cells mitotic spindle; interferes with cell division
CNS:	Headache, fatigue, dizziness, paresthesia, transient ↓ hearing
GI:	Nausea/vomiting, bleeding, flatulence, dyspepsia, oral thrush
Other:	Granulocytopenia, rash or urticaria, angioedema, photosensitivity, SLE, proteinuria, menstrual irregularities
Dosage:	0.5–1 g/d PO; 125–500 mg/d (children)
Contraindications:	Porphyria, hepatic failure, pregnancy
Drug Interactions:	↓ Levels of cyclosporine and salicylates; ↓ effects of warfarin and hormonal contraceptives; sun exposure ↑ photosensitivity
Key Points:	Can ↑ CNS depressant effects of alcohol

IMIPENEM-CILASTATIN SODIUM

Trade Name:	**Primaxin**
Indications:	Anaerobic and broad-spectrum aerobic coverage, including gram-(+) and gram-(−) organisms
Pharmacokinetics:	Onset: <1 h; peak: 1–2 h; duration: 6–8 h; Vd: 0.23 L/kg; Cl: 3 mL/min/kg; $T_{1/2}$ β: 0.9 h; metabolized by kidney, urinary excretion

IMIPENEM-CILASTATIN SODIUM *continued*

Pharmacodynamics:	Inhibits bacterial cell wall synthesis, cilastatin inhibits imipenem's renal metabolism
CNS:	Seizures, drowsiness, paresthesias, encephalopathy, fever
CV:	↓ BP, thrombophlebitis, palpitations, ↑ HR
GI:	Nausea, vomiting, pseudomembranous colitis, ↑ LFTs
Other:	Agranulocytosis, thrombocytosis, (+) Coombs' test, rash, pruritis, urticaria, renal impairment
Dosage:	0.5–1 g q 6–8 h (max. 4 g/d), 25–50% reduction in dosage with ↓ CrCl <30 mL/min
Contraindications:	Sensitivity to β-lactam or amide-type local anesthetic, renal failure or seizure disorder
Drug Interactions:	Antagonistic with other β-lactams; synergistic with aminoglycosides versus *Pseudomonas* sp.; probenecid ↓ renal elimination; ganciclovir ↓ seizure threshold
Key Points:	Can ↑ CV depression during general anesthesia

ISONIAZID (INH)

Trade Names:	**Laniazid, Nydrazid**
Indications:	Prophylaxis and treatment of tuberculosis (TB)
Pharmacokinetics:	Onset: <1 h; bioavailability: high; peak: 1–2 h; duration: 12–24 h; $T_{1/2}$ β: 1–4 h (depending on acetylation rate); crosses placental barrier and enters breast milk; metabolized in liver, excreted in urine
Pharmacodynamics:	Inhibits cell wall synthesis by interfering with lipid and DNA synthesis
CNS:	Peripheral neuropathy, seizures, toxic encephalopathy (psychosis), fever
GI:	Nausea, vomiting, dyspepsia
Hepatic:	↑ LFTs, cholestatic jaundice
Other:	Hyperglycemia, metabolic acidosis, pyridoxine deficiency, ↓ Ca, ↓ phosphate, pancytopenia, rheumatic and lupus-like syndromes, gynecomastia
Dosage:	300–900 mg/d PO in divided doses; 10–40 mg/kg/d (children)
Contraindications:	Hepatitis, seizure disorders, pregnancy, breast-feeding
Drug Interactions:	↓ Bioavailability with food and antacids; ↑ acetaminophen toxicity; ↑ levels of carbamazepine, phenytoin, valproate, warfarin; rifampin ↓ levels; cycloserine ↑ CNS toxicity; pyridoxine (50 mg/d) prevents peripheral neuropathy

ISONIAZID (INH) *continued*

Key Points: ↓ Benzodiazepine metabolism can delay early recovery
                            from anesthesia; peripheral neuropathic changes may
                            complicate regional anesthesia

ITRACONAZOLE

Trade Name: **Sporanox**

Indications: Dermatophytosis, blastomycosis, histoplasmosis,
                            aspergillosis, candidiasis, coccidioidomycosis,
                            onychomyosis, other mycoses

Pharmacokinetics: Onset: 1 h; peak: 2–3 h; protein binding: 99%; duration:
                            12–24 h; Vd: 796 L; $T_{1/2}$ β: 21 h; metabolized in liver,
                            excreted in urine and feces

Pharmacodynamics: Synthetic triazola inhibits cytochrome P_{450}-dependent
                            synthesis of ergosterol (component of fungal
                            cell wall)
  CNS: Malaise, asthenia, hallucinations, anxiety, depression
  CV: ↑ BP, orthostatic hypotension, edema
  GI: Nausea, vomiting, diarrhea, ↑ LFTs, dyspepsia
  Other: Angioedema, Stevens-Johnson syndrome,
                            myalgias

Dosage: 50–400 mg/d PO (mycoses); 600 mg/d IV (systemic
                            infection)

Contraindications: Heart failure (or LV dysfunction), pregnancy,
                            breast-feeding

Drug Interactions: ↓ Metabolism of terfenadine, cisapride, astemizole,
                            cyclosporine, warfarin, benzodiazepines; H_2-blockers,
                            isoniazid, phenytoin, rifampin, grapefruit juice ↓ effect;
                            CCB may cause edema

Key Points: Can ↑ sedative effect of benzodiazepines due to ↓
                            metabolism; produces arrhythmias with nonsedative
                            antihistamines

KETOCONAZOLE

Trade Name: **Nizoral**

Indications: Treatment of candidiasis, dermatophytosis,
                            coccidioidomyocosis, paracoccidioidomycosis,
                            histoplasmosis, dermatophytoses

Pharmacokinetics: Onset: 1–2 h; peak: 2–4 h; protein binding: 90%;
                            duration: 12–24 h; $T_{1/2}$ β: 2–8 h; metabolized in liver,
                            excreted in feces and urine

KETOCONAZOLE *continued*

Pharmacodynamics:	Inhibits demethylation of danosferol and inhibits purine transport
GI:	Nausea, vomiting, abdominal pain, diarrhea, ↑ LFTs
Other:	Pruritus
Dosage:	200–400 mg/d PO; 3–6 mg/kg/d (children)
Contraindications:	Triazolam ↑ CV depression, pregnancy, breast-feeding
Drug Interactions:	Antacids and H_2 blockers ↓ absorption; ↑ level of carbamazepine, donepezil, quinidine, indinavir, midazolam, triazolam, cyclosporin, tacrolimus; ↑ effect of phenytoin, coumarin, oral hypoglycemic agents; isoniazid and rifampin ↑ metabolism
Key Points:	Prolongs sedative effect of benzodiazepines and other CNS depressants; alcohol can precipitate disulfiram-like reaction

LORACARBEF

Trade Name:	**Lorabid**
Indications:	Infections with aerobes gram-(+) and gram-(−) organisms
Pharmacokinetics:	Onset: <30 min; peak: 0.5–1 h; protein binding: 25%; $T_{1/2}$ β: 1 h; no metabolism; excreted in urine
Pharmacodynamics:	β-lactam antibiotic that inhibits cell-wall synthesis
CNS:	Headache, somnolence, nervousness, dizziness, anorexia
CV:	Vasodilation
GI:	Nausea, vomiting, diarrhea, abdominal pain, pseudomembranous colitis
Other:	Thrombocytopenia, leukopenia, rash, pruritus, urticaria
Dosage:	200–400 mg PO bid (↓ dose if CrCl <30 mL/min); 7.5 mg/kg bid (children)
Contraindications:	Sensitivity to cephalosporins, pseudomembranous colitis
Drug Interactions:	Probenecid ↑ level due to ↓ renal elimination
Key Points:	No known interactions with anesthetic drugs

METRONIDAZOLE

Trade Name:	**Flagyl**
Indications:	Protozoal amebiasis, trichomoniasis, anaerobic organisms, PID, peptic ulcer disease with *Helicobacter pylori*

METRONIDAZOLE *continued*

Pharmacokinetics:	Onset: <5 min; bioavailability: 80%; peak: 1–2 h; protein binding: 20%; duration: 6–10 h; Vd: 0.74 L/kg; Cl: 0.3 mL/min/kg; $T_{1/2}$ β: 6–8 h; metabolized in liver to active metabolite, excreted in urine and feces
Pharmacodynamics:	Nitroimidazole disrupts DNA and inhibits nucleic acid synthesis.
CNS:	Headache, peripheral neuropathy
CV:	ECG changes (↓ T-wave)
GI:	Cramps, nausea, vomiting, anorexia, dry mouth, metallic taste
GU:	Dark urine, cystitis, dyspareunia, vaginal dryness
Other:	Transient bone marrow suppression, arthralgias, rash, furry tongue, neutropenia, weakness
Dosage:	15 mg/kg IV, followed by 7.5 mg/kg PO q 6 h
Contraindications:	Pregnancy, breast-feeding, Crohn's disease, blood dyscrasia, alcoholism
Drug Interactions:	Disulfiram-like reaction to alcohol, ↑ lithium and warfarin levels
Key Points:	CNS stimulants may ↓ seizure threshold; N_2O should be avoided in prolonged procedures

MOXIFLOXACIN, NORFLOXACIN, OFLOXACIN, TROVAFLOXACIN

Trade Names:	**Avelox (moxifloxacin), Noroxin (norfloxacin), Floxin, Ocuflox (ofloxacin), Trovan (trovafloxacin)**
Indications:	Infections with aerobic gram-(+) and gram-(−) organisms
Pharmacokinetics:	Onset: <30 min; bioavailability: variable; peak: 1–3 h; protein binding: 10–50%; duration: 12–24 h; $T_{1/2}$ β: 3–12 h; limited metabolism, excreted 1° as unchanged drugs in urine and feces
Pharmacodynamics:	Fluoroquindones inhibit bacterial topoisomerase (DNA gyrase)
CNS:	Dizziness, headache, insomnia, anxiety, confusion, tremor, paresthesia
CV:	QT prolongation (moxifloxacin), ↑ HT, ↑ BP, edema
GI:	Nausea, vomiting, diarrhea, anorexia, pseudomembranous colitis, cholestatic jaundice, ↑ LFTs
Pulmonary:	Dyspnea
Other:	Neutropenia, thrombocytopenia, hyperhidrosis, photosensitivity, bitter taste, vaginitis, arthralgias, myalgias, rash

MOXIFLOXACIN, NORFLOXACIN, OFLOXACIN, TROVAFLOXACIN *continued*

Dosages:	*Moxifloxacin*: 400 mg/d PO for 5–10 d *Norfloxacin*: 400 mg PO bid for 10–21 d; ophthalmic: 0.3% *Ofloxacin*: 200–400 mg q 12 h for 10 d *Trovafloxicin*: 200–300 mg/d for 10–14 d
Contraindications:	Prolonged QT interval, seizure disorders
Drug Interactions:	Antacids, sucralfate, didanosine, metal cations ↓ absorption; probenecid ↑ drug level; ↑ effect of cyclosporine, warfarin, theophylline; photosensitivity with sun exposure; antipsychotics, erythromycin, TCAs ↑ effect; NSAIDs ↑ CNS stimulation
Key Points:	Avoid using NSAIDs and drugs known to prolong QT interval during perioperative period

NAFCILLIN

Trade Names:	**Nafcil, Nallpen, Unipen**
Indications:	Penicillinase-resistant penicillin for *Staphylococcus* sp. in abscesses, bacteremia, endocarditis, pneumonia, meningitis, osteomyelitis
Pharmacokinetics:	Onset: <5 min; peak: 0.25–0.5 h; protein binding: 80%; duration: 4–8 h; Vd: 0.35 L/kg; Cl: 7.5 mL/min/kg; $T_{1/2}$ β: 1–2 h; crosses placental barrier; metabolized in liver, excreted 1° in bile
Pharmacodynamics:	Inhibits bacterial cell wall synthesis (penicillin-binding proteins)
CNS:	Myoclonic twitching, seizures
GI:	Nausea, vomiting, diarrhea, pseudomembranous colitis
Other:	Uticaria, pruritus, hypotension, bronchospasm
Dosage:	0.25–2 g PO/IM/IV q 4–8 h (max. 20 g/d); 10–25 mg/kg IM q 8–12 hr; 10–20 mg/kg IV, max. 200 mg/kg/d (children)
Contraindications:	β-lactam allergic (penicillin, cephalosporin, imipenem), jaundice
Drug Interactions:	Synergistic with aminoglycosides against Streptococcus aureus, ↓ cyclosporine levels
Key Points:	Can ↑ airway resistance and ↑ pain on injection of IV anesthetics (e.g., methohexital, propofol) and analgesics (e.g., ketorolac)

NEOMYCIN

Trade Names:	**Mycifradin, Neo-Fradin**
Indications:	Infectious diarrhea due to *E. coli*, intestinal bacteria suppression; adjunct in hepatic coma, burns, topical bacterial infections
Pharmacokinetics:	Onset: <1 h; bioavailability: low; peak: 1–4 h; duration: 8 h; $T_{1/2}$ β: 2–3 h (12–24 h with ↓ CrCl); crosses placental barrier; no metabolism, excreted 1° unchanged in feces
Pharmacodynamics:	Aminoglycoside that inhibits bacterial protein synthesis
CNS:	Ototoxicity
GI:	Nausea, vomiting, diarrhea, colitis, malabsorption syndrome
GU:	Nephrotoxicity
Other:	Rash, urticaria, contact dermatitis
Dosage:	50 mg/kg/d in divided dose; 50–100 mg/kg/d (children)
Contraindications:	Intestinal obstruction
Drug Interactions:	↑ Digoxin and methotrexate levels, ↑ effects of anticoagulants
Key Points:	Enhances effects of neuromuscular blockers; ↑ requirement for reverse drugs, especially if dependent on renal elimination (e.g., pancuronium)

NITAZOXANIDE

Trade Name:	**Alinia**
Indications:	Diarrhea (due to *Cryptosporidium parvum*, *Giardia lamblia*)
Pharmacokinetics:	Onset: 1–2 h; peak: 2–4; protein binding: 99%; metabolized rapidly and excreted in urine, bile, feces
Pharmacodynamics:	Antiprotozoal ↓ sporozoites and oocysts
CNS:	Malaise, fever
GI:	Nausea, anorexia, flatulence, abdominal pain, enlarged salivary glands, ↑ SGPT
Other:	↑ BUN/Cr, pruritus, eye discoloration, rhinitis
Dosage:	100–200 mg PO q 12 h (×3 d)
Contraindications:	Compromised renal or hepatic function
Drug Interactions:	Highly protein-bound drugs ↑ effect
Key Points:	Consider use of prophylactic antiemetic drug

PENICILLIN G, PENICILLIN V

Trade Names:	**Bicillin, Wycillin, V-Cillin**
Indications:	Infections with nonpenicillinase-producing gram-(+) and gram-(−) aerobic cocci, spirochetes, and bacilli
Pharmacokinetics:	Onset: <1 h; peak: 1–2 h; protein binding: 60%; duration: 4–6 h; Vd: 0.35 L/kg; Cl: 1.8 g; $T_{1/2}$ β: 0.5–1 h (adult), 3 h (neonate); renal excretion
Pharmacodynamics:	Inhibits bacterial cell wall synthesis
CNS:	Myoclonic twitching, seizures, dizziness, tinnitus, headache, confusion, hallucinations, fatigue, hyperreflexia, fever
GI:	Nausea, vomiting, entercolitis, pseudomembranous colitis
GU:	Interstitial nephritis, ↑ K^+ (high doses)
Other:	Thrombophlebitis, bone marrow suppression, sterile abscess
Dosage:	1–5 million U q 4–6 h (↓ with CrCl <10 mL/min); 1–2 million U q 2 h or IV infusion, max. 3–4 million U/h (meningococcal meningitis); 30,000 U/kg q 12 h, max. 400,000 U/d (children)
Contraindications:	β-lactam allergic (e.g., cephalosporin, imipenem), renal failure
Drug Interactions:	Synergistic with aminoglycosides and clavulanate; probenecid and NSAIDs ↓ elimination
Key Points:	Use with heparin and oral anticoagulants ↑ risk of perioperative bleeding; ↑ risk of ↑ K^+ with high-dose penicillin G

PYRIMETHAMINE

Trade Name:	**Daraprim**
Indications:	Malaria, toxoplasmosis
Pharmacokinetics:	Onset: <1 h; bioavailability: 90%; peak: 1.5–8 h; protein binding: 80%; duration: 2 wk; $T_{1/2}$ β: 2–6 d; metabolized in liver, excreted in urine
Pharmacodynamics:	Inhibits conversion of dihydro- to tetrahydrofolate (folic acid antagonist)
CNS:	Seizures
GI:	Anorexia, vomiting, atrophic glossitis
Other:	Pancytopenia
Dosage:	25 mg/wk (prophylaxis); 6.25–12.5 mg/wk (children); 50 mg/d (treatment) 25 mg/d (children)

PYRIMETHAMINE *continued*

Contraindications:	Megaloblasmic anemia (folic acid deficiency), breast-feeding
Drug Interactions:	Cotrimoxazole, sulfonamides ↑ adverse effects; folic acid, PABA ↓ effects
Key Points:	High doses can cause CNS stimulation and ↑ anesthetic requirement; lorazepam ↑ hepatotoxicity

QUINUPRISTIN AND DALFOPRISTIN

Trade Name:	**Synercid**
Indications:	Infections involving vancomycin-resistant *Enterococcus faecium, Streptococcus pyogenes, S. aureus*
Pharmacokinetics:	Onset: <30 min; peak: 1–2 h; protein binding: moderate; duration: 8–12 h; Vd: 0.45 L/kg; $T_{1/2}$ β: 0.8 h (quinupristin), 0.7 h (dalfopristin); both drugs converted to active metabolites, excreted 1° in feces
Pharmacodynamics:	Streptogramin inhibitor of bacterial cell-wall synthesis
CNS:	Headache
GI:	Nausea, vomiting, diarrhea, pseudomembranous colitis, ↑ LFTs
Other:	Myalgia, rash, pruritus, thrombophlebitis
Dosage:	7.5 mg/kg IV infusion over 1 h q 8–12 h
Contraindications:	None known
Drug Interactions:	↑ Effect of CCB, carbamazepine, cyclosporine, delavirdine, diazepam, disopyramide, HMG-CoA reductase inhibitors, indinavir, lidocaine, midazolam, ritonavir, tacrolimus; ↑ QT interval with quinidine- and cytochrome P_{450}–metabolized drugs
Key Points:	Inhibits cytochrome P_{450} in liver; ↑ levels of IV anesthetics (e.g., propofol) and benzodiazepines (e.g., midazolam) in postoperative period

RIFAMPIN

Trade Names:	**Rifadin, Rimactane**
Indications:	Tuberculosis, meningococcal carriers, leprosy
Pharmacokinetics:	Onset: <1 h; peak: 1–2 h; protein binding: 90%; duration: 12–24 h; $T_{1/2}$ β: 1–5 h; crosses placental barrier; metabolized in liver, enterohepatic recirculation, excreted in feces

RIFAMPIN *continued*

Pharmacodynamics:	Inhibits DNA-dependent RNA polymerase
CNS:	Headache, fatigue, confusion, dizziness, ataxia, blurred vision, peripheral neuropathy
GI:	Nausea, vomiting, dyspepsia, diarrhea, flatulence, stomatitis, pseudomembranous colitis, pancreatitis, ↑ LFTs
Pulmonary:	Wheezing, dyspnea
Other:	Hemolytic anemia, acute tubular necrosis, yellow eyes or skin, weakness, hyperuricemia, osteomalacia, pruritus, urticaria
Dosage:	600 mg/d PO; 10 mg/kg/d (children)
Contraindications:	Severe hepatic dysfunction
Drug Interactions:	↑ Metabolism of glycosides, quinidine, β-blockers, verapamil, theophylline, phenytoin, PPIs, warfarin, narcotics, diazepam, midazolam, hormonal contraceptives; isoniazid ↑ hepatotoxicity
Key Points:	Decreased levels of anesthetic drugs (due to ↑ metabolism); can necessitate ↑ dosage requirements

STREPTOMYCIN, TOBRAMYCIN

Trade Names:	**Streptomycin, Nebcin (tobramycin)**
Indications:	Infections with aerobic gram-(−) and some gram-(+) organisms (e.g., tuberculosis, tularemia, plague, brucellosis, enterococcal, streptococcal endocarditis)
Pharmacokinetics:	Onset: <30 min; peak: 0.5–2 h; protein binding: 36%; duration: 8 h; $T_{1/2}$ β: 2–3 h (↑ to 110 h with CrCl <10 mL/min); crosses placental barrier; no metabolism, excreted 1° in urine
Pharmacodynamics:	Inhibit bacterial protein synthesis (at ribosomal subunit)
CNS:	Headache, confusion, seizures, ototoxicity, blurred vision
GI:	Nausea, vomiting, diarrhea
GU:	Nephrotoxicity, ↑ BUN/Cr
Other:	Bone marrow suppression, cough, pharyngitis, ↓ muscle tone, angioedema
Dosages:	*Streptomycin:* 1–2 g IM q 12 h; 20–40 mg/kg/d IM (children) *Tobramycin:* 3 mg/kg IV/IM q 8–12 h; 0.3% ophthalmic solution: 1–2 gtt q 4–6 h
Contraindications:	Sensitivity to aminoglycosides, labyrinthine disease; renal insufficiency, neuromuscular disorders

STREPTOMYCIN, TOBRAMYCIN *continued*

Drug Interactions:
Amphotericin B, cephalosporins, cisplastin, polymyxin B, vancomycin, other aminoglycosides ↑ nephrotoxicity, neurotoxicity, ototoxicity; incompatible with penicillins; bumetanide, ethacrynic acid, furosemide ↑ ototoxicity

Key Points:
With general anesthesia, ↑ neuromuscular blockers; ↑ requirement for reversal drugs at the end of surgery

SULFADIAZINE

Trade Name: **Same**

Indications:
Infections with aerobic gram-(+) bacteria, chlamydia, toxoplasmosis, *Plasmodium falciparum*, nocardiosis, meningococcal carriers

Pharmacokinetics:
Onset: 1–2 h; peak: 4–6 h; protein binding: 45%; duration: 4–8 h; $T_{1/2}$ β: 24–72 h; crosses placental barrier; metabolized in liver, excreted 1° in urine

Pharmacodynamics:
Inhibits bacterial synthesis of folic acid (from PABA)
CNS:
Headache, depression, seizures, hallucinations, anorexia
GI:
Nausea/vomiting, cramps, diarrhea, stomatitis, ↑ LFTs
GU:
Nephrotoxicity (i.e., oliguria, crystalluria, hematuria)
Other:
Bone marrow suppression, photosensitivity, Stevens-Johnson syndrome, epidermal necrolysis

Dosage:
2–4 g/d PO (in divided doses); 75–150 mg/kg/d in divided doses, max. 6 g/d (children)

Contraindications:
Sensitivity to sulfonamides, porphyria, pregnancy, breast-feeding

Drug Interactions:
↑ Effects of anticoagulants, oral antidiabetics; synergistic with pyrimethamine and trimethoprim; sun exposure ↑ photosensitivity; PABA ↓ effects

Key Points:
May increase risk of perioperative bleeding and hypoglycemia

TETRACYCLINE

Trade Name: **Topicycline**

Indications:
Infections with gram-(+) cocci, gram-(−) bacilli, rickettsia, brucellosis, Lyme disease, spirochetes, mycoplasma, chlamydia

TETRACYCLINE *continued*

Pharmacokinetics:	Onset: <1 h; bioavailability: 80%; peak: 2–4 h; protein binding: 45%; duration: 6–12 h; Vd: 1.5 L/kg; CrCl: 2 mg/min/kg; $T_{1/2}$ β: 6–12 h; no metabolism; excreted 1° unchanged in urine
Pharmacodynamics:	Reversible inhibition of bacterial protein synthesis
CNS:	Dizziness, headache, phototoxicity, vertigo, ataxia, fatigue, ↑ ICP
CV:	Arrhythmias, pericarditis, cardiac arrest, thrombophlebitis
GI:	Anorexia, dysphagia, nausea/vomiting, dyspepsia, stomatitis, glossitis, enterocolitis
Pulmonary:	Respiratory arrest
Other:	Dental discoloration, bone marrow suppression, ↑ skin pigmentation, muscle weakness
Dosage:	10–20 mg/kg bid (max. 2 g/d); 4 mg/kg, then 2 mg/kg q 12 h (children)
Contraindications:	Hepatorenal dysfunction, children (<8 yr), parturients
Drug Interactions:	Antacids ↓ absorption; sun exposure ↑ phototoxicity, ↑ digoxin and warfarin levels
Key Points:	Potential nephrotoxicity in patients administered sevoflurane; ↑ nondepolarizing muscle relaxants

TICARCILLIN

Trade Names:	**Ticar, Timentin (with clavulanate)**
Indications:	Broad-spectrum coverage for *P. aeruginosa*, *Enterobacter* and *Proteus* spp. (in UTI)
Pharmacokinetics:	Onset: <5 min; peak: 30–60 min; protein binding: 50%; duration: 4–6 h; Vd: 0.21 L/kg; Cl: 2.0 mL/min/kg; $T_{1/2}$ β: 1.3 1 h (↑ to 3 h with ↓ CrCl); crosses placental barrier; minimal metabolism, 1° urinary excretion
Pharmacodynamics:	Inhibits bacterial cell wall synthesis; binds irreversibly to β-lactamases
CNS:	Headache, myoclonic twitching, seizures
CV:	CHF, thrombophlebitis, edema
GI:	Nausea, vomiting, diarrhea, stomatitis, dyspepsia, flatulence, pseudomembranous colitis, ↑ LFTs, bad taste
Renal:	Fluid retention, hypokalemia, hypernatremia, interstitial nephritis
Other:	Platelet dysfunction, (+) Coombs' test, pruritus, chills, fever

TICARCILLIN *continued*

Dosage:

3 g IV initially, then 3 g q 3–6 h, 25–37.5 mg/kg q 3 h, 33.3–50 mg/kg q 4 h, or 50–75 mg/kg q 6 h; with ↓ renal function, 2 q 8–24 h (max. 500 mg/kg/d); 100 mg/kg initially, then 75 mg/kg q 8 h, followed by 100 mg/kg q 4 h (children)

Contraindications:

β-Lactam allergic (e.g., cephalosporin), impaired renal function

Drug Interactions:

Synergism with aminoglycoside (vs *Pseudomonas* sp.); probenecid ↑ levels; ↓ effect of hormonal contraceptives

Key Points:

Do not mix with an aminoglycoside antibiotic

TRIMETHOPRIM-SULFAMETHOXAZOLE

Trade Names:

Bactrim, Septra

Indications:

Prophylaxis and treatment of UTI with gram-(+) and gram-(−) organisms, with *Pneumocystis carinii*, shigellosis, enterotoxigenic *E. coli, Nocardia* sp., traveler's diarrhea

Pharmacokinetics:

Onset: <10 min; peak: 1–4 h; duration: 8–12 h; crosses placental barrier; Vd: 0.2–1.8 L/kg; Cl: 2–3 mL/min/kg; $T_{1/2}$ β: 8–12 h; metabolized in liver; excreted 1° in urine

Pharmacodynamics:

Inhibition of dihydrofolate reductase (↓ folic acid synthesis)

CNS:
Peripheral neuropathy, fever

GI:
Glossitis, stomatitis, dyspepsia, nausea/vomiting, diarrhea, ↑ LFTs

Other:
Pancytopenia, exfoliative dermatitis, toxic epidermal necrolysis, pruritus, Stevens-Johnson syndrome, methemoglobinemia

Dosages:

Trimethoprim: 20 mg/kg/d
Sulfamethoxazole: 100 mg/kg (pneumocystis); 8 mg/kg and 40 mg/kg IV bid, respectively (children)

Contraindications:

Megaloblastic anemia (due to folate deficiency), pregnancy, breast-feeding, infants (<2 mo), severe hepatorenal insufficiency

Drug Interactions:

Sulfamethoxazole ↓ resistance; ↑ thrombocytopenia with concomitant use of thiazides; ↓ metabolism of phenytoin

Key Points:

No known interactions with anesthetic drugs

VANCOMYCIN

Trade Names:	**Vancocin, Vancoled**
Indications:	Treatment for methicillin-resistant *S. aureus* and *C. difficile* in antibiotic-associated pseudomembranous colitis; *Flavobacterium meningosepticum* in meningitis; endocarditis prophylaxis (if penicillin allergic), *Enterococcus* sp., bacteremia septicemia
Pharmacokinetics:	Onset: <1 h; peak: 1–2 h; duration: 6–12 h; Vd: 0.39 kg; Cl: 0.79 mL/min/kg; $T_{1/2}$ β: 4–6 h (↑ to 20–146 h if CrCl <30); excreted in urine and in feces
Pharmacodynamics:	Inhibits cell wall synthesis and glycopeptide polymerization
CNS:	↑ ICP, ototoxicity, tinnitus
CV:	↓ BP (due to histamine release), thrombophlebitis
GI:	Nausea
Pulmonary:	Wheezing, dyspnea
Renal:	Nephrotoxicity, ↑ BUN/Cr
Other:	Red-man syndrome, neutropenia, eosinophilia, fever, chills
Dosage:	0.5–1 g IV q 6–12 h; 10–15 mg/kg IV q 6–12 h (children); 125–500 mg PO q 6–8 h for 7–10 d, 40 mg/kg PO q 6–8 h for 7–10 d (children)
Contraindications:	Severe hepatorenal impairment, elderly, hearing loss
Drug Interaction:	Nephrotoxicity with aminoglycosides, amphotericin B, cisplatin, colistin, polymyxin B; ↓ BP and histamine release (red-man syndrome) minimized by infusing slowly (<500 mg/h)
Key Points:	Enhances neuromuscular blockade; muscle relaxants that require renal excretion (e.g., pancuronium or dimethyltubocurarine) ↑ risk of nephrotoxicity; rapid IV infusion ↓ BP if volume depleted

13

Antineoplastics

ABARELIX

Trade Name:	**Plenaxis**
Indications:	Prostate cancer (with metastases)
Pharmacokinetics:	Onset: slow; peak: 3 d; protein binding: 98%; Vd: 60 L/kg; Cl: 208 L/d; $T_{1/2}$ β: 13 d, 13% excreted in urine
Pharmacodynamics:	LH-releasing hormone antagonist inhibits gonadotropin (Gn) and related androgen (testosterone) production by blocking GnRH receptors in pituitary gland
CNS:	Insomnia, dizziness, headache, pain
CV:	Peripheral edema, ↑ QT interval
GI:	Constipation
Other:	Hot flashes, allergic reactions, gynecomastia, dysuria, URI
Dosage:	100 mg IM q 2–4 wk
Contraindications:	NK
Drug Interactions:	NK
Key Points:	Monitor ECG when administering drugs that ↑ QT interval

ALDESLEUKIN

Trade Name:	**Proleukin**
Indications:	Metastatic renal cell carcinoma, metastatic melanoma
Pharmacokinetics:	Onset: 4 wk; duration: <12 mo; $T_{1/2}$ β: 85 min; metabolized by kidneys, excreted in urine
Pharmacodynamics:	Lymphokine, interleukin-2 (IL-2), ↑ lymphocyte mitogenesis
CNS:	Headache, seizures, dizziness, fatigue
CV:	Hypotension, arrhythmias, MI, pericardial effusion, edema
GI:	Nausea, vomiting, stomatitis, jaundice, diarrhea, ↑ LFTs
GU:	Oliguria, hematuria, UTI
Pulmonary:	Edema, pleural effusion, dyspnea
Other:	Bone marrow suppression, electrolyte imbalance, hyperuremia, dermatitis, coagulation disorders, petechiae, fever, chills
Dosage:	600,000 IU/kg IV q 8 h for 5 d
Contraindications:	Organ allografts, abnormal (+) thallium stress test and PFTs
Drug Interactions:	Antihypertensives ↑ risk of hypotension; ↑ side effects of cardiotoxic, hepatotoxic, myelotoxic, nephrotoxic drugs; corticosteroids ↓ effect

ALDESLEUKIN *continued*

Key Points: Muscle relaxants and anesthetic adjuvants that require
                           renal elimination should be carefully titrated during
                           surgery

AMINOGLUTETHIMIDE

Trade Name: **Cytadren**

Indications: Breast and prostatic carcinoma, Cushing's syndrome

Pharmacokinetics: Onset: <1 h; bioavailability: >90%; peak: 3–4 h;
                           protein binding: 23%; duration: 6–8 h; Vd: 76 L;
                           Cl: 3.5 L/h; $T_{1/2}$ β: 15.5 h; hepatic metabolism,
                           excreted in urine

Pharmacodynamics: Inhibition of conversion of cholesterol to pregnenolone;
                           inhibits estrogen production from androgens
  CNS: Lethargy, vertigo, nystagmus, ataxia, headache
  CV: Orthostatic hypotension, ↑ HR
  GI: Vomiting, ↑ LFTs, nausea, anorexia
  Other: Leukopenia, agranulocytosis, hypothyroidism,
                           myalgias, rash

Dosage: 250 mg PO qid

Contraindications: Pregnancy, breast-feeding

Drug Interactions: ↓ Levels of dexamethasone, warfarin, theophylline,
                           digitoxin

Key Points: Potential adrenocortical hypofunction during
                           perioperative period; consider supplemental hydrocorti-
                           sone and mineralocorticoids during anesthesia

ASPARAGINASE

Trade Name: **Elspar**

Indications: Acute lymphocytic leukemia (ALL) in children

Pharmacokinetics: Onset: <2 min; peak: <14 h; duration: 23–33 d;
                           $T_{1/2}$ β: 8–30 h; minimal distribution outside vascular
                           compartment

Pharmacodynamics: Inactivating asparagine to aspartic acid and ammonia,
                           interferes with protein, DNA, and RNA synthesis
  CNS: Confusion, drowsiness, hallucinations, depression,
                           nervousness
  CV: ↓ BP, angina
  GI: Nausea, vomiting, cramps, anorexia, hemorrhage,
                           pancreatitis, ↑ LFTs

ASPARAGINASE *continued*

Pulmonary:	Laryngeal constriction, wheezing
Renal:	Uric acid nephropathy, azotemia ($\uparrow$ BUN/Cr)
Other:	Pancytopenia, $\downarrow$ blood clotting, $\downarrow$ albumin, hyperthermia, hyperglycemia, glycosuria/polyuria, rash, pruritus
Dosage:	10,000 IU IV in combination with mannitol (80 mg), then 1000 IU/kg/d ($\times$10 d)
Contraindications:	Pancreatitis, severe hepatic impairment
Drug Interactions:	$\downarrow$ Efficacy of methotrexate; prednisone $\uparrow$ glucose; vincristine $\uparrow$ neuropathy
Key Points:	With prolonged use of N_2O, consider administering folinic acid or vitamin B_{12} at end of anesthesia

BEVACIZUMAB

Trade Name:	**Avastin**
Indications:	Metastatic colorectal carcinoma
Pharmacokinetics:	NK
Pharmacodynamics:	Prevents interaction of VEGF to receptors on endothelial cells, $\downarrow$ microvascular growth of metastasis
CV:	$\uparrow$ BP, CHF, thromboembolism
GI:	Perforation (after surgery), diarrhea, vomiting
Other:	Wound dehiscence, hemorrhage, proteinuria, pain
Dosage:	5 mg/kg IV q 2 wk
Contraindications:	Recent surgery (<1 mo), severe CHF, uncontrolled hypertension, pregnancy
Drug Interactions:	Do not administer with dextrose solution
Key Points:	Avoid for minimum of 28 d after major surgery

BICALUTAMIDE

Trade Name:	**Casodex**
Indications:	Advanced prostate cancer
Pharmacokinetics:	Onset: <1 h; peak: 4–5 h; protein binding: 96%; duration: 24 h; extensively metabolized in liver, excreted in urine and feces
Pharmacodynamics:	Nonsteroidal antiandrogen that competitively inhibits androgen binding to cytospandrogen receptors
CNS:	Asthenia, headache, dizziness, paresthesia, insomnia

BICALUTAMIDE *continued*

CV:	↑ BP, angina, "hot flashes," peripheral edema
GI:	Nausea, vomiting, abdominal pain, ↑ LFTs, constipation, diarrhea
GU:	UTI, impotence, urinary incontinence, nocturia
Pulmonary:	Dyspnea
Other:	Anemia, leukopenia, rash, diaphoresis, gynecomastia, myalgia

Dosage: 50 mg/d PO

Contraindications: Severe hepatic impairment

Drug Interactions: Displaces coumadin from binding sites; ↑ risk of bleeding

Key Points: Carefully check coagulation status prior to major surgery

BLEOMYCIN

Trade Name: **Blenoxane**

Indications: Squamous cell cancer of skin, vulva, cervix, head, neck; testicular cancer; Hodgkin's disease; malignant pleural effusions

Pharmacokinetics: Onset: <30 min; peak: 0.5–1 h; minimal protein binding; duration: 24–72 h; Vd: 0.27 L/kg; Cl: 1.1 mL/min/kg; $T_{1/2}$ β: 2–4 h; excreted in urine

Pharmacodynamics:	Cytotoxic antibiotic acts by inhibition of DNA synthesis
GI:	Stomatitis, anorexia, nausea, vomiting, diarrhea
Pulmonary:	Interstitial pneumonitis
Other:	Hyperpigmentation, rash, fever and chills, hyperuricemia

Dosage: 5–15 U/m²/d (max. 400 U); 30 U/m² (max. 250 U) (children)

Contraindications: Pregnancy, breast-feeding

Drug Interactions: Cyclophosphamide ↑ pulmonary toxicity; cisplatin ↓ clearance and ↑ levels; ↓ absorption of phenytoin and digoxin

Key Points: Minimize supplemental oxygen use during perioperative period; avoid fluid overload to minimize postoperative pulmonary edema

BORTEZOMIB

Trade Name: **Velcade**

Indications: Multiple myeloma

BORTEZOMIB *continued*

Pharmacokinetics:	Protein binding: 83%; Cl: 30–170 mL/min; $T_{1/2}$ β: 9–15 h; metabolized by hepatic cytochrome P_{450}; excretion unknown
Pharmacodynamics:	Reversible inhibitor of chymotrypsin-like activity of proteasome, disrupting intracellular homeostasis
CNS:	Malaise, peripheral neuropathy, headache, insomnia
CV:	Arrhythmias, orthostatic hypotension
GI:	Nausea, vomiting, diarrhea, constipation
Other:	Thrombocytopenia, fever, ↓ appetite/asthenia
Dosage:	1.3 mg/m² IV (with 35 mg mannitol) biweekly (×2 wk)
Contraindications:	Hypersensitivity to bortezomib, boron, or mannitol
Drug Interactions:	Oral hypoglycemics, unstable glucose levels; cytochrome P_{450} enzyme inhibitors ↓ metabolism
Key Points:	Carefully monitor glucose levels and maintain adequate hydration; check for peripheral neuropathic symptoms

BUSULFAN

Trade Names:	**Busulfex, Myleran**
Indications:	Chronic myelogenous leukemia (CML), myelofibrosis, stem cell transplantation
Pharmacokinetics:	Onset: 1–2 wk; peak: 1–2 h; Vd: 0.6–1.4 L/kg; Cl: 95–197 mL/min/m²; $T_{1/2}$ β: 1.5–2.3 h; metabolized in liver, excreted in urine
Pharmacodynamics:	Alkylation, cross-linking of DNA strands, interferes with DNA replication and RNA transcription
CNS:	Weakness, fatigue, cataracts
GI:	Nausea, vomiting, cheilosis, glossitis, anhydrosis, ↑ LFTs
Pulmonary:	Interstitial pulmonary fibrosis ("busulfan lung")
Other:	Gynecomastia, asthenia-like wasting, pancytopenia, hyperuricemia, fever, chills
Dosage:	4–8 mg/d PO or 0.8 mg/kg IV q 6 h
Contraindications:	Pregnancy, myoblastic crisis
Drug Interactions:	NK
Key Points:	Pulmonary fibrosis may be delayed for 4–6 mo; supplemental oxygen concentrations should be minimized during perioperative period; adequate hydration and urinary alkalinization to minimize hyperuricemia

CARMUSTINE

Trade Names:	**BiCNU, Gliadel**
Indications:	Brain tumor, multiple myeloma, Hodgkin's disease, malignant lymphomas
Pharmacokinetics:	Onset/peak/duration: NK; Vd: 3.25 L/kg; Cl: 56 mL/min/m^2; T$_{1/2}$ β: 30 min; metabolized in liver to active metabolites, excreted 1° in urine
Pharmacodynamics:	Metabolites interfere with DNA and RNA function
CNS:	Ataxia, drowsiness, dementia, ocular toxicity, flushing
GI:	Severe nausea (delayed 2–6 h), vomiting, LFTs
GU:	Azotemia, nephrotoxicity
Pulmonary:	Pulmonary fibrosis, interstitial pneumonitis
Other:	Pancytopenia, hypothyroidism, flulike symptoms
Dosage:	75–100 mg/m^2/d IV
Contraindications:	Pregnancy, breast-feeding
Drug Interactions:	Amphotericin B ↑ efficacy; H$_2$-blockers and cimetidine ↑ toxicity; anticoagulants and ASA ↑ risk of bleeding
Key Points:	Pulmonary toxicity is more likely in smokers and worsened by prolonged exposure to high inspired oxygen concentration

CETUXIMAB

Trade Name:	**Erbitux**
Indications:	Metastatic colorectal carcinoma
Pharmacokinetics:	Vd: 203 L/m^2; Cl: 0.05 L/h/m^2; T$_{1/2}$ β: 97 h
Pharmacodynamics:	Recombinant monoclonal antibody binds to epidermal GF receptor, inhibits kinase phosphorylation
CV:	↓ BP
GI:	Diarrhea, nausea, abdominal pain
Pulmonary:	Interstitial lung disease, bronchospasm, stridor
Other:	Urticaria, acneiform rash, asthenia/malaise
Dosage:	400 mg/m^2 IV initially, 250 mg/m^2 q wk
Contraindications:	Hypersensitivity to murine proteins
Drug Interactions:	Premedication with H$_1$ antagonist ↓ side effects
Key Points:	Check PFTs and consider bronchodilator prophylaxis

CHLORAMBUCIL

Trade Name:	**Leukeran**
Indications:	Chronic lymphocytic leukemia (CLL), malignant lymphomas
Pharmacokinetics:	Onset: <1 h; peak: 1 h; protein binding: 99%; duration: 24 h; $T_{1/2}$ β: 1.5 h; metabolized in liver to active metabolites, excreted in urine
Pharmacodynamics:	Cross-links strands of cellular DNA and RNA in tumor cells
CNS:	Agitation, confusion, seizures, peripheral neuropathy, tremor
GI:	Nausea, vomiting, diarrhea, stomatitis, ↑ LFTs
Pulmonary:	Interstitial pneumonitis
Other:	Bone marrow suppression, infertility, rash
Dosage:	0.1–0.2 mg/kg/d PO for 3–6 wk
Contraindications:	Seizure disorder, head trauma, sensitivity to other alkylating agents
Drug Interactions:	Anticoagulants and ASA ↑ bleeding
Key Points:	Ketamine and enflurane can produce seizure-like activity

CISPLATIN

Trade Name:	**Platinol**
Indications:	Metastatic testicular and ovarian tumors, advanced bladder cancer
Pharmacokinetics:	Onset/peak/duration: NA; detected up to 6 mo after last dose; extensively and irreversibly bound to plasma proteins; $T_{1/2}$ β: 58–78 h; excreted in urine
Pharmacodynamics:	Cross-links DNA strands and interferes with RNA synthesis
CNS:	"Glove-and-stocking" peripheral neuropathy; seizures, aphasia, ototoxicity, tinnitus, vestibular toxicity
CV:	Arrhythmias, postural hypotension, thrombotic microangiopathy (MI, CVA), cerebral arteritis, Raynaud's phenomenon
GI:	Nausea, vomiting (delayed 1–4 h), ↓ taste, anorexia, ↑ LFTs
GU:	Severe renal toxicity, hyperuricemia, ↑ BUN/Cr
Other:	Myelosuppression, hyperuricemia, electrolyte disturbances

CISPLATIN *continued*

Dosage:	20 mg/m^2 with bleomycin and vinblastine (metastatic testicular tumors); 50 mg/m^2 with doxorubicin (metastatic ovarian tumors); 50–70 mg/m^2 IV (bladder cancers)
Contraindications:	Severe renal or hearing impairment, myelosuppression
Drug Interactions:	Aminoglycosides ↑ nephrotoxicity; loop diuretics ↑ ototoxicity; aspirin ↑ risk of bleeding; ↓ phenytoin level
Key Points:	Adequate hydration may reduce both renal and ototoxicity; carefully titrate drugs eliminated by the kidney, consider use of prophylactic antiemetics

CYCLOPHOSPHAMIDE

Trade Names:	**Cytoxan, Neosar**
Indications:	Malignant lymphomas; breast, head, neck, lung, ovarian tumors; multiple myeloma, CLL, AUL, neuroblastoma, adenocarcinoma
Pharmacokinetics:	Onset: <1 h; bioavailability: >75%; peak: 1–3 h; protein binding: 50%; duration: 12–24 h; Vd: 0.34–1.2 L/kg; Cl: 1.3 mL/min/kg; T$_{1/2}$ β: 3–10 h; metabolized in liver, excreted by kidney
Pharmacodynamics:	Active metabolites are alkylating agents that prevent cell division by cross-linking DNA strands
CV:	Myocarditis, pericarditis
GI:	Anorexia, nausea, vomiting (<6 h), stomatitis, ↑ LFTs
GU:	Hemorrhagic cystitis, infertility, renal impairment
Pulmonary:	Interstitial fibrosis, pneumonitis
Other:	Bone marrow suppression, ↑ ADH, alopecia, hyperuricemia, hyponatremia, secondary malignancies, amenorrhea
Dosage:	1–5 mg/kg/d PO or 2–3 mg/kg/d (children); 40–50 mg/kg/ IV bid
Contraindications:	Depressed bone marrow function, severe hepatorenal impairment
Drug Interactions:	Doxorubicin ↑ cardiotoxicity; steroids and barbiturates ↓ effect
Key Points:	Prolonged use of N$_2$O ↑ bone marrow suppression; use of β-stimulants (or mixed α and β agonists) ↑ cardiotoxicity; ↓ plasma pseudocholinesterase and renal impairment ↑ sensitivity to muscle relaxants

DACARBAZINE

Trade Name:	**DTIC-Dome**
Indications:	Malignant melanoma, Hodgkin's lymphomas
Pharmacokinetics:	Onset/peak/duration: NK; Vd: 0.2 L/kg; Cl: 15.4 mL/kg/min; $T_{1/2}$ β: 5 h (10 h with ↓ CrCl); excreted 1° in urine as unchanged drug
Pharmacodynamics:	Inhibition of DNA and RNA synthesis (alkylation), antimetabolite for purine synthesis, binding with protein sulfydryl group
CNS:	Somnolence, facial paresthesia
CV:	Postural hypotension, vasculitis
GI:	Severe nausea, vomiting, anorexia, stomatitis
Hepatic:	Hepatic vein thrombosis
Other:	Myalgias; ↓ Mg^{+2}, Ca^{+2}, K^+; myelosuppression; flulike syndrome
Dosage:	2–4.5 mg/kg IV for 10 d, repeat q 4 wk (malignant melanoma); 150 mg/m² for 5 d, repeat q 4 wk (Hodgkin's lymphomas)
Contraindications:	Impaired bone marrow function
Drug Interactions:	Anticoagulants and ASA ↑ risks of bleeding; amphotericin B ↑ nephrotoxicity; with azathioprine or 6-mercaptopurine ↑ toxicity
Key Points:	With prolonged use of N_2O, administer folinic acid or vitamin B_{12} at end of surgery

DACTINOMYCIN

Trade Name:	**Cosmegen**
Indications:	Uterine and testicular carcinomas; rhabdomyosarcoma; Wilms', Ewing's, Kaposi's tumors
Pharmacokinetics:	Onset/peak/duration: NK; $T_{1/2}$ β: 36 h; widely distributed but does not cross blood-brain barrier; minimal metabolism, excreted in urine and bile
Pharmacodynamics:	Intercalates between DNA base pairs; inhibits messenger RNA synthesis and uncoiling the DNA helix
CNS:	Fatigue, anorexia
GI:	Nausea, vomiting, diarrhea, stomatitis, proctitis, ↑ LFTs
Other:	Bone marrow suppression, hyperuricemia, ↓ Ca^{2+}, myalgia, erythematosus, rash, esophagitis
Dosage:	500 μg/d × 5 d (max. 600 μg/m²/d); 15 μg/kg/d IV × 5 d (children)
Contraindications:	Chickenpox or herpes zoster

DACTINOMYCIN *continued*

Drug Interactions:	Vitamin K ↓ efficacy; bone marrow suppressants ↑ toxicity
Key Points:	Due to protracted emetic symptoms, consider use of prophylactic antiemetics

DAUNORUBICIN

Trade Names:	**DaunoXome, Cerubidine**
Indications:	HIV-related Kaposi's sarcoma, acute lymphocytic and nonlymphocytic leukemia
Pharmacokinetics:	Onset/peak/duration: NK; $T_{1/2}$ β: 4–18 h; widely distributed into body tissues, does not cross blood-brain barrier; metabolized in liver to active metabolites, excreted 1° in bile
Pharmacodynamics:	Cytotoxic activity by intercalating between DNA base pairs and uncoiling DNA helix; inhibits DNA synthesis
CNS:	Headache, neuropathy, dizziness, fatigue, ataxia, confusion, seizures, blurred vision, tinnitus
CV:	Cardiomyopathy, ↑ BP, palpitations, arrhythmias, pericardial effusion (tamponade), pulmonary hypertension, flushing, edema, CHF
GI:	Nausea, vomiting, diarrhea, stomatitis, dry mouth, GI hemorrhage, esophagitis, melena, tenesmus, ↑ LFTs
GU:	Dysuria, red urine, polyuria (nocturia)
Pulmonary:	Cough, dyspnea, hemoptysis, pulmonary infiltration
Other:	Dehydration, hyperuricemia, bone marrow suppression, alopecia, rash, myalgias, arthralgia, seborrhea, folliculitis
Dosage:	30–45 mg/m² IV qod 6 ×; 25 mg/m² IV q wk × 6 (children)
Contraindications:	Severe myelosuppression and cardiac disease, previous use of anthracycline (doxorubicin >300 mg/m²) or cyclophosphamide
Drug Interactions:	Doxorubicin and cyclophosphamide ↑ cardiotoxicity
Key Points:	Use with volatile anesthetics ↑ CV depression and hepatotoxic effects; careful evaluation of baseline cardiac function (e.g., echo) before major surgery

DOXORUBICIN

Trade Names:	**Doxil, Adriamycin, Rubex**
Indications:	Bladder, breast, lung, ovarian, stomach, and thyroid tumors; osteogenic sarcoma; Hodgkin's disease; ALL, AML

DOXORUBICIN *continued*

Pharmacokinetics:	Onset/peak/duration: NK; protein binding: 80%; Vd: 25 L/kg; Cl: 17 mL/kg/min; elimination 1° via liver and biliary system
Pharmacodynamics:	Intercalates between DNA base pairs and uncoils DNA helix, interfering with DNA-directed RNA synthesis
CNS:	Peripheral neuropathy, dizziness, confusion, fatigue, anxiety
CV:	CHF, angina, cardiomyopathy (ECG changes), pedal edema
GI:	Mouth ulceration (mucositis), nausea, vomiting, diarrhea, dyspepsia, dysphagia, stomatitis, esophagitis, ↑ LFTs
GU:	Infertility, red urine, hyperuricemia, albuminuria
Pulmonary:	Cough, dyspnea, pneumonia
Other:	Bone marrow suppression, alopecia, hyperpigmentation, rash, diaphoresis, asthenia
Dosage:	60–75 mg/m^2 IV q 21–28 d
Contraindications:	Severe cardiovascular disease, myelosuppression, anthracycline dose >550 mg/m^2, breast-feeding
Drug Interactions:	Cyclophosphamides ↑ cardiotoxicity; cyclosporin, verapamil, streptozocin ↑ effect; ↓ digoxin levels; incompatible with aminophylline, cephalothin, dexamethasone, diazepam, fluorouracil, furosemide, heparin, hydrocortisone
Key Points:	Preoperative cardiac evaluation (e.g., echo) is recommended; avoid high concentration volatile agents, β-stimulants, indirect sympathomimetics during surgery

EPIRUBICIN

Trade Name:	**Ellence**
Indications:	Breast cancer
Pharmacokinetics:	Binds to plasma protein, concentrates in RBCs; extensively metabolized in liver, excreted 1° in bile
Pharmacodynamics:	Inhibits DNA, RNA, and protein synthesis by intercalcating between nucleotide base pairs
CNS:	Lethargy, keratitis (blurred vision)
CV:	Cardiomyopathy, arrhythmias
GI:	Nausea, vomiting, diarrhea, anorexia, mucositis
Other:	Pancytopenia, alopecia, photosensitivity, amenorrhea, hot flashes

EPIRUBICIN *continued*

Dosage:	100–120 mg/m^2 IV over 3–5 min q 3–4 wk
Contraindications:	Sensitivity to anthracyclines, recent MI, CHF, hepatic insufficiency
Drug Interactions:	Cimetidine ↑ level; cytotoxic drugs ↑ hematologic toxicity; CCBs, ↑ CV depression; radiation therapy ↑ effect; sun exposure ↑ photosensitivity
Key Points:	Carefully evaluate cardiac function and hydration status preoperatively; potential myelosuppressive effect of N$_2$O following prolonged exposure

ETOPOSIDE

Trade Names:	**VePesid, Toposar**
Indications:	Refractory testicular tumors, small-cell lung cancer, AIDS-related Kaposi's sarcoma
Pharmacokinetics:	Onset/peak/duration: NK; Vd: 10–15.7 L/m^2; Cl: 27–39 mL/min/m^2; T$_{1/2}$ β: 4–11 h; minimal metabolism, excreted 1° unchanged in urine
Pharmacodynamics:	Inhibition of DNA synthesis in metaphase and premitosis
CNS:	Ataxia, peripheral neuropathy, somnolence
CV:	↓ BP, angina
GI:	Nausea, vomiting, anorexia, diarrhea, stomatitis, ↑ LFTs
Other:	Bone marrow suppression, alopecia, weakness
Dosage:	50–100 mg/m^2 PO/IV qd
Contraindications:	Sensitivity to etoposide and teniposide; previous cytotoxic or radiation therapy
Drug Interactions:	Cisplatin ↑ cytotoxicity; warfarin ↑ PT and INR
Key Points:	Careful neurologic evaluation prior to regional nerve block procedures

EXEMESTANE

Trade Name:	**Aromasin**
Indications:	Breast cancer
Pharmacokinetics:	Onset: <1 h; peak: 1–2 h; protein binding: 90%; duration: 24 h; T$_{1/2}$ β: 24 h; metabolized in liver by cytochrome P$_{450}$, excreted in urine and feces

EXEMESTANE *continued*

Pharmacodynamics:	Irreversible, steroidal aromatase inactivator, $\downarrow$ conversion of androgens to estrogens
CNS:	Depression, insomnia, anxiety, fatigue, headache, dizziness, paresthesia, confusion
CV:	$\uparrow$ BP, edema, angina
GI:	Nausea, vomiting, dyspepsia, anorexia, $\uparrow$ appetite
Pulmonary:	Dyspnea, cough, URI, pharyngitis, rhinitis, sinusitis
Other:	Pathologic fractures, arthralgia, rash, alopecia, $\uparrow$ diaphoresis, hot flashes
Dosage:	25 mg/d PO
Contraindications:	Pregnancy, breast-feeding
Drug Interactions:	Cytochrome P_{450} inducers $\downarrow$ level; estrogens $\downarrow$ efficacy
Key Points:	No known adverse interaction with anesthetic drugs

FLUOROURACIL (5-FU)

Trade Name:	**Adrucil**
Indications:	Colon, rectal, breast, stomach, pancreatic, bladder, prostate, ovarian, cervical, endometrial, lung tumors; actinic/solar keratoses
Pharmacokinetics:	Onset/peak/duration: NK; converted in tissues to active metabolite; metabolized 1° in liver, excreted in lungs (CO_2) and urine
Pharmacodynamics:	Antimetabolite that inhibits thymidine synthesis
CNS:	Acute cerebellar syndrome, nystagmus, headache, confusion
CV:	Myocardial ischemia, angina, arrhythmias, thrombophlebitis
GI:	Ulcerative stomatitis, esophagopharyngitis, GI bleeding, nausea and vomiting, diarrhea, protein malabsorption, anorexia, $\uparrow$ LFTs
Pulmonary:	Cough, dyspnea
Other:	Leukopenia, thrombocytopenia, fever, alopecia, dermatitis, weakness
Dosage:	12 mg/kg/d IV, then 6 mg/kg/d; topical 0.5–5%
Contraindications:	Depressed bone marrow function, serious systemic infections
Drug Interactions:	Leucovorin $\uparrow$ toxic effects
Key Points:	No known adverse interactions with anesthetic drugs

FLUTAMIDE

Trade Name:	**Eulexin**
Indications:	Metastatic prostatic carcinoma
Pharmacokinetics:	Onset: <1 h; peak: 2 h; protein binding: 95%; duration: 8 h; $T_{1/2}$ β: 7.8 h; extensively metabolized to active metabolite (hydroxyflutamide), excreted 1° in urine
Pharmacodynamics:	Inhibits androgen activity, ↓ testosterone level
CNS:	Drowsiness, confusion, nervousness
CV:	↑ BP, peripheral edema
GI:	Nausea, vomiting, diarrhea, ↑ LFTs
Other:	Pancytopenia, impotence, rash, photosensitivity, gynecomastia, cystitis, proctitis, hematuria
Dosage:	125–250 mg PO q 8 h
Contraindications:	Severe hepatic impairment
Drug Interactions:	Anticoagulants ↑ risk of bleeding
Key Points:	Check PT and INR prior to surgery

GEFITINIB

Trade Name:	**Iressa**
Indications:	Lung cancer
Pharmacokinetics:	Onset: slow; bioavailability: 60%; peak: 3–7 h; Vd: 20 L/kg; Cl: 9 mL/kg/min; $T_{1/2}$ β: 48 h; extensive hepatic metabolism, excreted via feces
Pharmacodynamics:	Inhibits phosphorylation of tyrosine kinases on cell surfaces
GI:	↑ LFTs, diarrhea, nausea, vomiting
Pulmonary:	Interstitial lung disease
Other:	Rash, acne, dry skin, pruritus, anorexia
Dosage:	250–500 mg/d PO
Contraindications:	Pregnancy
Drug Interactions:	↑ Warfarin anticoagulant effect
Key Points:	Obtain baseline PFTs prior to major surgery

HYDROXYUREA

Trade Names:	**Droxia, Hydrea**
Indications:	Solid tumors, head and neck cancers, sickle-cell crisis

HYDROXYUREA *continued*

Pharmacokinetics:	Onset: <1 h; peak: 2 h; duration: 24 h; $T_{1/2}$ β: 3–4 h; crosses blood-brain barrier; metabolized in liver, excreted in lungs (CO_2) and urine
Pharmacodynamics:	Inhibits DNA synthesis
CNS:	Hallucinations, headache, dizziness, seizure, drowsiness
GI:	Nausea, vomiting, stomatitis, pancreatitis, ↑ LFTs, diarrhea/constipation
Other:	Bone marrow suppression, rash, alopecia, fever, anorexia
Dosage:	80 mg/kg IV q 3 d (cancer); 15 mg/kg/d (max. 35 mg/kg/d) (sickle-cell)
Contraindications:	Severe bone marrow suppression, impaired renal function
Drug Interactions:	Didanosine, indinavir, and stavudine ↑ risk of pancreatitis; fluorouracil ↑ neurotoxicity
Key Points:	No known adverse interaction with anesthetic drugs

IDARUBICIN

Trade Name:	**Idamycin**
Indications:	AML
Pharmacokinetics:	Onset/peak/duration: NK; $T_{1/2}$ β: 22 h; extensive extrahepatic metabolism, excreted 1° in bile
Pharmacodynamics:	Inhibits nucleic acid synthesis by intercalation in DNA strands and interaction with topoisomerase II
CNS:	Headache, peripheral neuropathy, seizures
CV:	Cardiomyopathy (CHF), arrhythmias, angina, edema
GI:	Nausea, vomiting, cramps, diarrhea, mucositis, ↑ LFTs
Other:	Myelosuppression, nephrotoxicity, dyspnea, hyperuricemia, alopecia, rash
Dosage:	12 mg/m^2 IV over 10–15 min for 3 d
Contraindications:	NK
Drug Interactions:	NK
Key Points:	No known adverse interactions with anesthetic drugs

MECHLORETHAMINE (NITROGEN MUSTARD)

Trade Name:	**Mustargen**
Indications:	Hodgkin's and non-Hodgkin's lymphomas, bronchogenic tumors

MECHLORETHAMINE
(NITROGEN MUSTARD) *continued*

Pharmacokinetics:	Onset: <5 min; duration: 24 h; rapid chemical transformation in body fluids, combines with reactive cellular compound cells
Pharmacodynamics:	Alkylation causes cross-linking DNA strands, inhibits protein synthesis
CNS:	Weakness, dizziness, tinnitus, deafness, aphasia, peripheral neuropathy
CV:	Thrombophlebitis, hemorrhagic diathesis, pedal edema
GI:	Nausea, vomiting, anorexia, ↑ LFTs
GU:	Menstrual irregularities, infertility
Other:	Leukopenia, thrombocytopenia, rash, alopecia, hyperuricemia, amyloidosis
Dosage:	0.4 mg/kg IV/IM or 0.1 mg/kg/d (×4); 6.0 mg/m² (MOPP)
Contraindications:	Infectious diseases
Drug Interactions:	Glutathione-depleting agents ↑ alkylating activity
Key Points:	Peripheral neurologic exam should be performed before regional anesthesia; if low granulocyte count, avoid N_2O

MERCAPTOPURINE (6-MP)

Trade Name:	**Purinethol**
Indications:	ALL, chronic myelocytic leukemia
Pharmacokinetics:	Onset: <1 h; bioavailability: 50%; peak: 2 h; duration: >24 h; Vd: 0.9 L/kg; Cl: 719 mL/min/m²; $T_{1/2}$ α: 0.9 h; metabolized extensively in liver (1st pass), excreted in urine
Pharmacodynamics:	Converted intracellularly to active antimetabolite, ↓ purine synthesis
GI:	Anorexia, nausea, vomiting, mucositis, stomatitis, profound diarrhea, pancreatitis, jaundice, ↑ LFTs
Other:	Leukopenia, thrombocytopenia, anemia, hyperuricemia, rash, hematuria, crystalluria, hyperpigmentation
Dosage:	2.5 mg/kg/d PO (to 5 mg/kg/d)
Contraindications:	Pregnancy, severe hepatorenal impairment
Drug Interactions:	Allopurinol ↑ toxicity; ↓ anticoagulant effects of warfarin
Key Points:	Avoid N_2O because of potential detrimental effects on bone marrow

METHOTREXATE

Trade Names:	**Folex, Mexate**
Indications:	Trophoblastic tumors, ALL, meningeal leukemia, severe psoriasis, rheumatoid arthritis
Pharmacokinetics:	Onset: <1 h; peak: 1–2 h; protein binding: 50%; Vd: initial, 0.18 L/kg; Cl: 70–100 mL/min; $T_{1/2}$ β: 3–10 h; slightly metabolized in liver, excreted 1° in urine as unchanged drug
Pharmacodynamics:	Inhibits dihydrofolic acid reductase, ↓ purine metabolism
CNS:	Arachnoiditis, leukoencephalopathy (blurred vision, confusion, dizziness, drowsiness, headache, seizures, and ↑ ICP)
GI:	Stomatitis, anorexia, ulceration, enteritis, nausea, vomiting, diarrhea, ↑ LFTs
GU:	Nephropathy, hematuria, cystitis, menstrual irregularity
Pulmonary:	Pulmonary fibrosis, pneumonitis, cough, pharyngitis
Other:	Pancytopenia, hyperpigmentation, hyperuricemia, alopecia, rash, fever, osteoporosis
Dosage:	15–30 mg/d PO/IM (×5); 3.3 mg/m^2/d for 4–6 wk
Contraindications:	Pregnancy, breast-feeding, severe hepatic impairment
Drug Interactions:	Salicylates, sulfonamides, NSAIDs, PABA ↑ levels; antibiotics ↓ absorption; azathioprine, retinoids, sulfasalazine, alcohol ↑ hepatoxicity; ↑ warfarin anticoagulant effect; ↓ phenytoin level; antidote is leucovarin
Key Points:	Adequate hydration and urinary alkalinization during surgery minimize renal damage

MYCOPHENOLATE

Trade Name:	**Myfortic**
Indications:	Prophylaxis for organ rejection (in combination with cyclosporine and steroids)
Pharmacokinetics:	Onset: 0.5 h; peak: 2 h; protein binding: >98%; Vd: 1–2 L/kg; Cl: 140 mL/min; $T_{1/2}$ β: 8–16 h; hepatic metabolism, excreted 1° in urine
Pharmacodynamics:	Inhibitor of IMP dehydrogenase, ↓ guanosine nucleotide synthesis, cytostatic effect on lymphocytes
GI:	Constipation, diarrhea, nausea
Other:	Nasopharyngitis, anemia, leucopenia, UTI, insomnia

MYCOPHENOLATE *continued*

Dosage:	360–720 mg PO bid
Contraindications:	Hypersensitivity to drug or 1° metabolite (mycophenolic acid); live vaccines; pregnancy
Drug Interactions:	Antacids and food ↓ absorption; cholestyramine ↓ enterohepatic recirculation
Key Points:	No known interactions with anesthetic drugs

PEMETREXED

Trade Name:	**Alimta**
Indications:	Malignant pleural mesothelioma
Pharmacokinetics:	Protein binding: 81%; Vd: 16 L; Cl: 90 mL/min; $T_{1/2}$ β: 3.5 h; excreted 1° unchanged in urine
Pharmacodynamics:	Blocks folate-dependent metabolic processes (antifolate)
CNS:	Fatigue, peripheral neuropathy, depression
GI:	Nausea, vomiting, constipation
Pulmonary:	Dyspnea, chest pain
Other:	Pancytopenia, ↑ BUN/Cr, rash, infections
Dosage:	500 mg/m² IV q 3–4 wk
Contraindications:	NK
Drug Interactions:	NSAIDs ↑ toxicity; premedication with corticosteroids/vitamins ↓ toxicity
Key Points:	Administer folic acid if N_2O is used during surgery

PROCARBAZINE

Trade Name:	**Matulane**
Indications:	Hodgkin's disease, lymphomas, brain and lung tumors
Pharmacokinetics:	Onset: <1 h; bioavailability: 100%; duration: 12–24 h; $T_{1/2}$ β: 60 min; crosses blood-brain barrier; metabolized by liver, excreted in urine
Pharmacodynamics:	Inhibits incorporation of DNA precursors, ↓ RNA and protein synthesis
CNS:	Depression, nervousness, dizziness, hallucinations, insomnia, peripheral neuropathy, confusion, weakness
GI:	Nausea, vomiting, diarrhea, anorexia, stomatitis, dysphagia
GU:	Hematuria, urinary frequency, nocturia
Pulmonary:	Pneumonitis, pleural effusion, cough
Other:	Myelosuppression, hemolytic anemia, infertility

PROCARBAZINE *continued*

Dosage:	50–100 mg/m²/d PO; 2–4 mg/kg/d, then 4–6 mg/kg/d, followed by 1–2 mg/kg/d PO
Contraindications:	Inadequate bone marrow reserve
Drug Interactions:	↑ CNS effects of barbiturates, antihistamines, opiates, phenothiazines; ↓ metabolism of ester-type local anesthetics; MAOIs, ↑ ephedrine and neosynephrine toxicity; avoid TCAs, tyramine-rich foods, alcohol
Key Points:	↑ CNS depression produced by sedative-hypnotics and opioid analgesics, careful neurologic exam should precede regional nerve block techniques; with prolonged use of N_2O, supplement with vitamin B_{12} or folinic acid

TAMOXIFEN

Trade Name:	**Nolvadex**
Indications:	Breast tumors and ductal carcinoma
Pharmacokinetics:	Onset: 1–2 h; peak: 5 h; $T_{1/2}$ β: >7 d; extensively metabolized in liver, excreted 1° in feces
Pharmacodynamics:	Binds to estrogen receptors, inhibits DNA synthesis
CNS:	Depression, dizziness, headache, confusion, blurred vision
GI:	Nausea, vomiting, diarrhea, ↑ LFTs
Pulmonary:	Emboli
Other:	Bone pain, hypercalcemia, "hot flashes," menstrual irregularity, uterine sarcoma, ↑ thyroxine, ↑ lipids, thrombocytopenia and leukopenia, ↑ fertility in women, Stevens-Johnson syndrome, weight gain, rash
Dosage:	20–40 mg/d PO in divided doses
Contraindications:	Use of coumadin, history of DVT, pulmonary edema
Drug Interactions:	Bromocriptine ↑ levels, coumadin ↑ risk of bleeding; cytotoxic drugs ↑ risk of thromboembolic complications
Key Points:	Assess coagulation status prior to regional blocks

THIOTEPA

Trade Name:	**Thioplex**
Indications:	Breast and ovarian carcinoma; bladder tumors; neoplastic effusions; Hodgkin's disease, lymphomas

THIOTEPA *continued*

Pharmacokinetics:	Onset: <15 min; peak: 1 h; duration: 24 h; Vd: 0.25 L/kg; Cl: 186 mL/min/m^2; T$_{1/2}$ β: 125 min; extensively metabolized in liver, excreted in urine
Pharmacodynamics:	Alkylating agent, cross-linking strands of DNA, inhibits protein synthesis
CNS:	Confusion, blurred vision, headache, dizziness, fatigue
GI:	Nausea, vomiting, anorexia, stomatitis, abdominal pain, ↑ LFTs
GU:	Dysuria, amenorrhea, infertility, urinary retention
Pulmonary:	Wheezing, laryngeal edema
Other:	Alopecia, rash, urticaria, pancytopenia, fever, weakness
Dosage:	0.2–0.4 mg/kg/d IV at 1- to 4-wk intervals
Contraindications:	Severe hepatic, renal, or bone marrow dysfunction
Drug Interactions:	Anticoagulants and ASA ↑ risk of bleeding; ↑ platelet toxicity with sargramostim; prolonged apnea after succinylcholine
Key Points:	Avoid use of succinylcholine due to risk of ↓ pseudocholinesterase

TOPOTECAN

Trade Name:	**Hycamtin**
Indications:	Metastatic ovarian carcinoma, small-cell lung cancer
Pharmacokinetics:	Onset: <1 min; protein binding: 35%; duration: 24 h; T$_{1/2}$ β: 2–3 h; undergoes pH-dependent hydrolysis to form active metabolite, excreted in urine
Pharmacodynamics:	Binds to topoisomerase I complex, interrupting DNA synthesis
CNS:	Fatigue, asthenia, headache, paresthesia, insomnia
GI:	Nausea, vomiting, cramping, stomatitis, anorexia, ↑ LFTs
Pulmonary:	Dyspnea, cough, hoarseness
Other:	Bone marrow suppression, alopecia, rash, angina, fever
Dosage:	1.5 mg/m^2/d IV for 5 d
Contraindications:	Severe bone marrow suppression, pregnancy, breast-feeding
Drug Interactions:	Cisplatin ↑ myelosuppression, G-CSF prolongs effect
Key Points:	Prolonged use of N$_2$O should be avoided due to bone marrow suppression

TOSITUMOMAL

Trade Name:	**Bexxar**
Indications:	Non-Hodgkin's lymphoma
Pharmacokinetics:	Cl: 68 mg/h; excreted by kidneys
Pharmacodynamics:	^{131}I IgG lambda monoclonal antibody directed against lymphocytes, inducing cellular apoptosis
CNS:	Headache, asthenia, pain
GI:	Nausea, vomiting, diarrhea, cramps
Pulmonary:	Bronchospasm, pneumonia, pleural effusions
Other:	Pancytopenia, sepsis, angioedema, hypothyroidism
Dosage:	450 mg IV, then 5 mCi I-131 + 35 mg tositumomab
Contraindications:	Hypothyroidism, hypersensitivity to murine proteins, pregnancy, breast-feeding
Drug Interactions:	NK
Key Points:	Check thyroid function prior to major surgery

VALRUBICIN

Trade Name:	**Valstar**
Indications:	Bladder tumor *in situ*
Pharmacokinetics:	Penetrates directly into bladder wall after instillation; metabolites found in blood, excreted 1° by voiding
Pharmacodynamics:	Inhibits incorporation of nucleosides into nucleic acids
CNS:	Asthenia, headache, tremor, somnolence, tinnitus, blurred vision, dizziness, fatigue
CV:	Vasodilation, ↑ BP, angina, peripheral edema
GI:	Nausea, vomiting, dyspepsia, diarrhea, flatulence, pancreatitis, ↑ LFTs, anorexia
GU:	Cystitis, dysuria, urinary retention/frequency/incontinence
Pulmonary:	Dyspnea, pneumonia, pharyngitis
Other:	Anemia, thrombocytopenia, alopecia, rash, hyperglycemia, myalgia, ecchymosis
Dosage:	800 mg/wk for 6 wk (topical)
Contraindications:	UTI, sensitivity to anthracyclines or cremophor EL
Drug Interactions:	NK
Key Points:	No known adverse interactions with anesthetic drugs

VINBLASTINE

Trade Name:	**Velban**
Indications:	Hodgkin's disease; lymphocytic lymphoma; mycosis fungoides; Kaposi's sarcoma; histiocytosis X; choriocarcinoma; breast, testicular, lung tumors
Pharmacokinetics:	Onset: <10 min; peak: <1 h; duration: 1–2 wk; Vd: 27.3 L/kg; Cl: 0.74 L/kg/h; $T_{1/2}$ β: 2–25 h; crosses blood-brain barrier; metabolized in liver, excreted 1° in feces
Pharmacodynamics:	Blocking mitosis and interference with amino acid metabolism
CNS:	Peripheral neuropathy, malaise, headache, neuritis, vocal cord paralysis, cranial nerve paralysis, seizures, paresthesias
CV:	↑ BP, MI, phlebitis
GI:	Nausea, vomiting, constipation, ileus, ↑ LFTs, anorexia, stomatitis, rectal bleeding
Pulmonary:	Wheezing, dyspnea, pharyngitis
Other:	Myelosuppression, alopecia, hyperuricemia
Dosage:	0.1–0.5 mg/kg/wk IV
Contraindications:	Pregnancy, severe leukopenia/granulocytopenia, bacterial infection
Drug Interactions:	Erythromycin ↑ toxicity; mitomycin causes SOB and wheezing; ↑ efficacy of bleomycin; ↓ phenytoin levels
Key Points:	Careful neurologic exam and acceptable coagulation parameters prior to regional anesthetic techniques

VINCRISTINE

Trade Name:	**Oncovin**
Indications:	Hodgkin's disease, leukemias, Ewing's sarcoma, rhabdomyosarcoma, Wilms' tumor, lung cancer
Pharmacokinetics:	Onset: <10 min; peak: <1 h; protein binding: 75%; duration: 1 wk; Vd: 8.4 L/kg; $T_{1/2}$ β: 2–85 h; extensively metabolized in liver, excreted 1° in feces
Pharmacodynamics:	Binds to the microtubular proteins and blocks mitosis
CNS:	Peripheral neuropathy, cranial nerve neuropathy, headache, ataxia, seizures, doplopia, photophobia, ptosis
CV:	Orthostatic hypotension, ↑ HR
GI:	Anorexia, dysphagia, stomatitis, cramps, intestinal necrosis, nausea, vomiting, diarrhea, constipation

VINCRISTINE *continued*

GU:	Dysuria, urine retention, polyuria
Pulmonary:	Vocal cord paralysis, wheezing, dyspnea
Other:	Bone marrow suppression, hyperuricemia, hyponatremia, rash

Dosage: $1.4–2 \ mg/m^2$ IV q wk × 4

Contraindications: Pregnancy, breast-feeding, Charcot-Marie-Tooth disease

Drug Interactions: ↓ Digoxin level; nifedipine, asparaginase, mutamycin ↑ toxicity

Key Points: Rehydration should precede induction of anesthesia, and careful neurologic exam is recommended before regional anesthesia

14

Antivirals

ACYCLOVIR

Trade Name:	**Zovirax**
Indications:	HSV, encephalitis, other viral infections
Pharmacokinetics:	Onset: <1 h; peak: 2–5 h; Vd: 0.7 L/kg; Cl: 0.4 mL/min/kg; $T_{1/2}$ β: 2–3 h; metabolized intracellularly to its active form, excreted in urine
Pharmacodynamics:	Antiviral action via inhibition of DNA synthesis
CNS:	Encephalopathy, tremor, agitation, vertigo, headache, hallucinations
GI:	Diarrhea, nausea, vomiting, anorexia
GU:	Hemolytic-uremic syndrome, renal failure, hematuria
Other:	Myalgia, rash, thrombocytopenic purpura, DIC, edema
Dosage:	0.4–1.2 g/d PO, 10 mg/kg q 8 h infused over 1 h
Contraindications:	Renal insufficiency
Drug Interactions:	↑ Toxicity with interferon and methotrexate; probenecid ↑ level
Key Points:	↑ CNS stimulant effects of anesthetic drugs (e.g., enflurane, ketamine, lidocaine)

ADEFOVIR DIPIVOXIL

Trade Name:	**Hepsera**
Indications:	HIV infection
Pharmacokinetics:	Onset: rapid; peak: 1–2 h; protein binding: 45%; duration: 24 h; Vd: 0.4 L/kg; $T_{1/2}$ β: 7–8 h; prodrug converted to adefovir; metabolized in liver and excreted in urine
Pharmacodynamics:	Nucleotide analog with antiretroviral activity
CNS:	Malaise
GI:	Nausea, vomiting, diarrhea
GU:	Proteinuria, ↑ BUN/Cr, Fanconi's syndrome
Dosage:	60–120 mg/d PO (with L-carnitine)
Contraindications:	Severe renal failure
Drug Interactions:	Other nephrotoxic drugs and probenecid ↓ clearance
Key Points:	Consider use of prophylactic antiemetic drugs during surgery

AMANTADINE

Trade Name:	**Symmetrel**
Indications:	Parkinsonism, prophylaxis and treatment of influenza A

AMANTADINE *continued*

Pharmacokinetics:	Onset: <30 min; peak: 1–4 h; protein binding: 60%; duration: 12 h; Vd: 5 l/kg; $T_{1/2}$ β: 10–12 h; minimal metabolic breakdown, excreted unchanged in urine
Pharmacodynamics:	↑ Dopamine release in the substantia nigra; prevents influenza type A viral assembly and replication; interferes with uncoating of RNA in lysosomes
CNS:	Dizziness, insomnia, anxiety, mental aberrations
CV:	CHF, orthostatic hypotension, pedal edema
GI:	Nausea, dry mucous membranes
Other:	Neutropenia, urinary retention
Dosage:	100 mg PO bid (max. 400 mg/d); 4–8 mg/kg/d (children)
Contraindications:	Severe CHF, breast-feeding
Drug Interactions:	↑ Effects of anticholinergics
Key Points:	May predispose to postoperative postural hypotension; ↑ emetic symptoms on ambulation after surgery

ATAZANAVIR

Trade Name:	**Reyataz**
Indications:	HIV-1 infection in combination with other antiretrovirals
Pharmacokinetics:	Metabolized by hepatic cytochrome P_{450} enzymes
Pharmacodynamics:	Azapeptide inhibitor of HIV-1 protease
CNS:	Headache, depression
CV:	↑ Heart block (prolongs PR interval)
GI:	Nausea, jaundice, vomiting, diarrhea, ↑ LFTs
Other:	Fever, hyperglycemia, lactic acidosis syndrome
Dosage:	400 mg/d PO (with food)
Contraindications:	Use of ergot derivatives, benzodiazepines, pimozide, cisapride ↑ side effects, pregnancy
Drug Interactions:	↑ Levels of CCBs, warfarin, HMG-CoA inhibitors; H_2 antagonists, rifampin ↓ levels; antacids ↓ absorption
Key Points:	Check baseline ECG and blood glucose level; ↓ midazolam dose for premedication

CIDOFOVIR

Trade Name:	**Vistide**
Indications:	CMV retinitis, acyclovir-resistant herpes simplex infections
Pharmacokinetics:	Not metabolized, excreted unchanged in urine

CIDOFOVIR *continued*

Pharmacodynamics:	Inhibits CMV replication by selectively blocking DNA synthesis
CNS:	Malaise, seizures, headache, weakness, paresthesia, blurred vision
CV:	Orthostatic hypotension, ↑ HR
GI:	Nausea, vomiting, diarrhea, anorexia, dysphagia, oral candidiasis
GU:	Nephrotoxicity, UTI
Other:	Rash, alopecia, hyperglycemia, diaphoresis, hypokalemia, chills
Dosage:	5 mg/kg IV over 1 h bimonthly with probenecid
Contraindications:	Sensitivity to sulfa drugs, renal impairment
Drug Interactions:	↑ Nephrotoxicity of aminoglycosides, amphotericin B, foscarnet, pentamidine
Key Points:	Avoid anesthetic adjuvants dependent on renal elimination

DIDANOSINE

Trade Name:	**Videx**
Indications:	HIV and hepatitis B infections
Pharmacokinetics:	Onset: <30 min; peak: 30–60 min; duration: 12–24 h; Vd: 1 L/kg; $T_{1/2}$ β: 1.5 h; crosses blood-brain barrier; excreted in urine
Pharmacodynamics:	Inhibits the activity of HIV-1 reverse transcriptase, ↓ DNA replication
CNS:	Peripheral neuropathy, drowsiness, headache, seizures
GI:	Pancreatitis, nausea, vomiting, ↑ LFTs
Other:	Myopathy, bone marrow suppression, rash, blood dyscrasias, anemia, hepatitis, fever, chills
Dosage:	400 mg/d or 200 mg PO bid; 120 mg/m^2 bid (children)
Contraindications:	Pancreatitis, peripheral neuropathy, hyperuricemia
Drug Interactions:	↑ Confusion with benzodiazepines; ↑ adverse effects of antacids; allopurinol ↑ levels
Key Points:	Prolongs CNS depressant effect of anesthetic drugs; neurologic assessment prior to performing a regional nerve block

ENFUVIRTIDE

Trade Name:	**Fuzeon**
Indications:	HIV-1 infection in combination with other antiretrovirals

ENFUVIRTIDE *continued*

Pharmacokinetics:	Onset: <3 h; bioavailability: 84%; peak: 8 h; protein binding: 92%; Vd: 6 L; Cl: 25–30 mL/kg/h; $T_{1/2}$ β: 4 h; hepatic metabolism (deamidated metabolite), excretion unknown
Pharmacodynamics:	Synthetic peptide that inhibits fusion of HIV-1 with cellular membranes, blocking viral entry into cells
CNS:	Guillain-Barré syndrome, peripheral neuropathy, unusual taste, insomnia
GI:	Constipation, pancreatitis, ↓ appetite
GU:	Glomerulonephritis
Pulmonary:	Pneumonia (bacterial)
Other:	Local injection site reactions, nodules, ecchymosis
Dosage:	90 mg SC bid
Contraindications:	Hypersensitivity reactions (1° immune complex reaction)
Drug Interactions:	Synergistic with antiretrovirals (e.g., zidovudine, lamivudine, nelfinavir, indinavir, efavirenz)
Key Points:	Perform neurologic exam prior to peripheral block

FAMCICLOVIR

Trade Name:	**Famvir**
Indications:	Herpes zoster infection
Pharmacokinetics:	Onset: <30 min; bioavailability: 77%; peak: 1 h; protein binding: 21%; duration: 8 h; metabolized in liver to active metabolite (penciclovir), excreted in urine
Pharmacodynamics:	Penciclovir inhibits DNA polymerase, ↓ viral DNA synthesis and replication
CNS:	Headache, fatigue, dizziness, paresthesia
GI:	Nausea/vomiting, diarrhea
Other:	Arthralgia, pruritus
Dosage:	500 mg PO tid for 7 d
Contraindications:	NK
Drug Interactions:	Probenecid ↑ drug level
Key Points:	Neurologic assessment before regional nerve block

FOSCARNET

Trade Name:	**Foscavir**
Indications:	CMV, HSV infections
Pharmacokinetics:	Onset: <30 min; peak: <1 h; protein binding: 15%; duration: 8–12 h; Vd: 0.41 l/kg; Cl: 5 L/h; $T_{1/2}$ β: 3 h; excreted unchanged in urine
Pharmacodynamics:	Analog of pyrophosphate inhibits viral replication by blocking DNA polymerase and reverse transcriptases
CNS:	Headache, seizures
CV:	Arrhythmias
GI:	Diarrhea, nausea, vomiting, anorexia
Other:	Hypocalcemia, hypophosphatemia, hypokalemia, nephrotoxicity, anemia
Dosage:	90 mg/kg infused over 1–2 h q 12 or 40–60 mg/kg IV q 8 h for 2–3 wk
Contraindications:	Sensitivity to phosphoric acid, renal impairment
Drug Interactions:	↑ Toxicity of pentamidine and amphotericin B, zidovudine ↑ anemia
Key Points:	Assess electrolyte panel and fluid status before surgery; maintain adequate hydration and urine output during anesthesia to minimize renal damage

GANCICLOVIR

Trade Name:	**Cytovene**
Indications:	CMV, HSV, EBV, HIV infections
Pharmacokinetics:	Onset: <1 h; peak: 1–3 h; minimal protein binding; duration: 8–24 h; Vd: 0.74 L/kg; excreted in urine as unchanged drug
Pharmacodynamics:	Purine nucleoside analog of guanine, inhibits viral replication
CNS:	Headache, seizures, depression, blurred vision
GI:	Diarrhea, nausea, vomiting, ↑ LFTs
Other:	Neutropenia, anemia, thrombocytopenia, diaphoresis, local injection pain, fever, hemorrhage, vitreous detachment, cataracts
Dosage:	5 mg/kg infused over 1 h q 12 h for 2–3 wk, then 5 mg/kg infused over 1 h qd, or 1000 mg PO tid
Contraindications:	Sensitivity to acyclovir
Drug Interactions:	Probenecid ↓ clearance; ↑ toxicity with dapson, pentamidine, flucytosine, vincristine, vinblastine, adriamycin, amphotericin B, imipenem, trimethoprim/ sulfamethoxazole

GANCICLOVIR *continued*

Key Points:	With prolonged use of N_2O, administer folinic acid and avoid N_2O in patients with bone marrow suppression

NEVIRAPINE

Trade Name:	**Viramune**
Indications:	HIV infections
Pharmacokinetics:	Onset: 1–2 h; bioavailability: 93%; peak: 4 h; protein binding: 60%; duration: 12–24 h; Vd: 1.2 L/kg; $T_{1/2}$ β: 45 h; crosses placental barrier; metabolized in liver, excreted in urine
Pharmacodynamics:	Blocks RNA- or DNA-dependent DNA polymerase activity
CNS:	Headache, peripheral neuropathy
GI:	Nausea, diarrhea, ulcerative stomatitis, ↑ LFTs, abdominal pain
Other:	Neutropenia, fever, rash, Stevens-Johnson syndrome
Dosage:	200 mg/d PO for 2 wk, then 200 mg bid; 4 mg/kg/d, then 4 mg/kg bid (children)
Contraindications:	NK
Drug Interactions:	↓ Level of hormonal contraceptives, protease inhibitors, ketoconazole; St. John's Wort ↓ drug level
Key Points:	Careful neurologic exam should be done before regional nerve blocks are performed; check LFTs before surgery and avoid halothane due to potential hepatotoxicity

OSELTAMIVIR

Trade Name:	**Tamiflu**
Indications:	Influenza A and B infections
Pharmacokinetics:	Onset: 1 h; peak: 2–3 h; Vd: 23–26 L; Cl: 194 kg/h; metabolized to active carboxylase metabolite in liver, excreted 1° in urine
Pharmacodynamics:	Carboxylase inhibits enzyme neurominidase in viral particles
CNS:	Dizziness, insomnia, headache, fatigue, otitis media
GI:	Nausea, vomiting, abdominal pain, diarrhea
Pulmonary:	Cough
Dosage:	75 mg PO bid for 5 d; 30–60 mg PO bid (children)
Contraindications:	NK

OSELTAMIVIR *continued*

Drug Interactions: NK

Key Points: Use prophylactic antiemetic therapy during
                           perioperative period

RIBAVIRIN

Trade Names: **Rebetol, Virazole**

Indications: RSV, chronic hepatitis C infections

Pharmacokinetics: Onset: <0.5 h; bioavailability: 45%; peak: 1–1.5 h;
                           minimal protein binding; duration: 12 h; Vd: 10 L/kg
                           and 40 h; Cl: 38 L/kg/h; $T_{1/2}$ β: 9.5 h (oral); hepatic
                           metabolism, excreted 1° in urine

Pharmacodynamics: Inhibits RNA and DNA synthesis
  CNS: Fatigue, headache, dizziness, insomnia
  CV: Hypotension, cardiac arrest
  GI: Anorexia, nausea, dyspepsia
  Pulmonary: Dyspnea, bronchospasm, pulmonary edema
  Other: Hemolytic anemia, rash, pruritis, myalgia, eye edema

Dosage: 400–600 mg bid (inhalation)

Contraindications: Pregnancy

Drug Interactions: NK

Key Points: No adverse interactions during perioperative period

RITONAVIR

Trade Name: **Norvir**

Indications: HIV infection

Pharmacokinetics: Onset: <1 h; peak: 2–4 h; protein binding: 99%;
                           duration: 12 h; $T_{1/2}$ β: 3–5 h; metabolized in liver,
                           excreted in feces

Pharmacodynamics: HIV protease inhibitor, prevents cleavage of viral
                           polyproteins
  CNS: Asthenia, headache, paresthesia, dizziness, somnolence
  CV: Vasodilation, ↑ HR
  GI: Anorexia, nausea, vomiting, flatulence, ↑ LFTs
  Other: Thrombocytopenia, myalgia, sweating, hyperkalemia,
                           hyperglycemia

Dosage: 300–600 mg PO bid; 400 mg/m^2 bid (children)

Contraindications: NK

RITONAVIR *continued*

Drug Interactions:	Cytochrome P_{450} activators ↓ drug level; ↑ CNS depression with benzodiazepines, zolpidem; ↑ toxicity of amiodarone, bepridil, encainide, flecainide, desipramine, meperidine, piroxicam, quinidine; St. John's Wort ↓ level
Key Points:	↑ CNS depression associated with benzodiazepines and opioids; may cause prolonged recovery from anesthesia

SAQUINAVIR

Trade Names:	**Fortovase, Invirase**
Indications:	HIV infections
Pharmacokinetics:	Highly protein bound (98%); rapidly metabolized in liver, excreted in feces
Pharmacodynamics:	Inhibits activity of HIV protease, ↓ cleavage of HIV polyproteins
CNS:	Paresthesia, headache, confusion, asthenia
GI:	Diarrhea, nausea, abdominal pain, mucosal ulceration, pancreatitis
Pulmonary:	Bronchitis, dyspnea, hemoptysis, URI, cough
Other:	Hyperglycemia, myalgias
Dosage:	0.6–1.2 mg/kg PO tid
Contraindications:	Ergot alkaloid derivatives, benzodiazepines
Drug Interactions:	↑ Levels of midazolam, triazolam, terfenadine, astemizole; carbamazepine, phenobarital, phenytoin, dexamethasone, nevirapine, rifampin, garlic supplements, St. John's Wort ↓ drug level; delaverdine, indinavir, ritonavir, ketoconazole, saquinavir, sildenafil, grapefruit juice ↑ drug level; HMG-CoA reductase inhibitors ↑ risk of myopathy, rhabdomyolysis
Key Points:	Avoid use of benzodiazepines during anesthesia due to prolonged effect; carefully monitor reversal of neuromuscular blockade

STAVUDINE

Trade Name:	**Zerit**
Indications:	HIV infections
Pharmacokinetics:	Onset: <30 min; bioavailability: 86%; peak: 1 h; minimal protein binding; duration: 12 h; Vd: 58 L; $T_{1/2} \beta$: 1–2 h; no metabolism, excreted in urine
Pharmacodynamics:	Inhibits HIV reverse transcriptase and DNA synthesis

STAVUDINE *continued*

CNS:	Peripheral neuropathy, headache, malaise, insomnia
GI:	Pancreatitis, diarrhea, anorexia, nausea, vomiting, ↑ LFTs
Other:	Dyspnea, lactic acidosis, bone marrow suppression, arthralgia, fever, anemia, chills, myalgia, rash, pruritus
Dosage:	30–40 mg PO q 12 h; 1 mg/kg q 12 h (children)
Contraindications:	NK
Drug Interactions:	Zidovudine ↓ drug effect
Key Points:	Assess peripheral nerve function prior to performing regional block

TENOFOVIR

Trade Name:	**Viread**
Indications:	HIV infection
Pharmacokinetics:	Onset: <1 h; bioavailability: 25%; peak: 1–2 h; protein binding: 7%; duration: 24 h; Vd: 1.3 L/kg; not metabolized, excreted in urine
Pharmacodynamics:	Competitive antagonist of HIV reverse transcriptase
CNS:	Asthenia, headache
GI:	Anorexia, nausea/vomiting, diarrhea, flatulence
Other:	Hyperglycemia, neutropenia
Dosage:	300 mg/d PO
Contraindications:	Renal insufficiency
Drug Interactions:	Probenecid, acyclovir, cidofovir, ganciclovir ↑ drug level
Key Points:	No known interaction with anesthetic drugs

ZALCITABINE

Trade Name:	**Hivid**
Indications:	HIV infection
Pharmacokinetics:	Onset: <1 h; bioavailability: 80%; peak: 1–2 h; minimal protein binding; duration: 8 h; Vd: 0.5–1.2 L/kg; $T_{1/2}$ β: 2 h; crosses blood-brain barrier; excreted in urine
Pharmacodynamics:	Inhibits HIV replication by blocking DNA reverse transcriptase
CNS:	Peripheral neuropathy, dizziness, confusion, tremor, ototoxicity, headache
GI:	Pancreatitis, nausea, vomiting, glossitis, diarrhea, constipation

ZALCITABINE *continued*

Other:	Bone marrow suppression, rash, pruritis, arthralgia
Dosage:	0.375–0.75 mg q 8 h
Contraindications:	NK
Drug Interactions:	Antacids ↓ absorption; cimetidine and probenecid ↓ elimination; pentamidine ↑ risk of pancreatitis; amino-glycosides, foscarnet, amphotericin B ↑ nephrotoxicity; chloramphenicol, cisplatin, dapsone, didanosine, disulfiram, ethionamide, gold salts, hydralazine, iodoquinol, isoniazid, metronidazole, phenytoin, ribavirin, vincristine ↑ neurotoxicity
Key Points:	Neurologic exam recommended before major regional nerve blocks

ZIDOVUDINE (AZT)

Trade Name:	**Retrovir**
Indications:	HIV infection
Pharmacokinetics:	Onset: <30 min; bioavailability: 65%; peak: 0.5–1.5 h; protein binding: 36%; Vd: 1.6 L/kg; Cl: 400 mL/min; $T_{1/2}$ β: 1 h; undergoes 1st-pass hepatic metabolism, excreted in urine
Pharmacodynamics: *CNS:* *GI:* *Other:*	Inhibits activity of HIV reverse transcriptase Headache, malaise, insomnia Nausea, vomiting, anorexia, lactic acidosis Bone marrow suppression, fever, rash, myalgia
Dosage:	1 mg/kg infused over 1 h (max. 5–6 mg/kg), or 600 mg/d PO
Contraindications:	Severe bone marrow suppression, hepatorenal impairment
Drug Interactions:	Ganciclovir, cytotoxic agents, interferon-alpha ↑ hema-tologic toxicity; valporic acid and probenecid ↑ drug level
Key Points:	Avoid use of N_2O during surgery

15

Benzodiazepine
Agonists and
Antagonists

ALPRAZOLAM

Trade Name:	**Xanax**
Indications:	Anxiety disorder, panic disorder
Pharmacokinetics:	Onset: 15–30 min; peak: 1–2 h; protein binding: 80%; duration: 6–24 h; $T_{1/2}$ β: 11 h; metabolized in liver, "active" excreted in urine
Pharmacodynamics:	↑ γ-aminobutyric acid (GABA)–mediated neural inhibition
CNS:	Drowsiness, light-headedness, depression, dysarthria, headache, fatigue, ataxia, amnesia
CV:	↓ BP
GI:	Dry mouth, constipation, diarrhea, nausea, vomiting
Other:	Nasal congestion, blurred vision
Dosage:	0.25–2 mg PO tid, 0.5–3 mg/d ER
Contraindications:	Acute narrow-angle glaucoma, use with ketoconazole or itraconazole
Drug Interactions:	↑ TCA, cimetidine, CCPs, fluoxetine, propoxyphene ↑ levels; alcohol and herb kava ↑ CNS depression; smoking ↑ metabolism
Key Points:	Use prior to general anesthesia delays early recovery due to residual CNS depressant effects; abrupt withdrawal produces seizures

CHLORDIAZEPOXIDE

Trade Names:	**Librium, Mitran**
Indications:	Panic and anxiety disorders, alcohol withdrawal
Pharmacokinetics:	Onset: <30 min; peak: 1–1.5 h; duration: 3–5 h; Vd: 0.3 L/kg; Cl: 0.5 mL/kg/min; $T_{1/2}$ β: 5–30 h; metabolism conjugated in liver, excreted in urine
Pharmacodynamics:	Potentiation of GABA-mediated neural inhibition
CNS:	Anxiolysis, drowsiness, ataxia, confusion, extra-pyramidal reactions
CV:	↓ BP, pedal edema
GI:	Nausea, constipation, jaundice, ↑ LFTs
Pulmonary:	Upper airway obstruction, ↓ RR and hypoxic drive
Other:	Agranulocytosis, menstrual irregularities, ↓ libido, dermatitis
Dosage:	50–100 mg IM/IV, then 25–50 mg q 6–8 h; 5–25 mg PO q 6–8 h; 5 mg PO tid (children)
Contraindications:	Severe hepatic failure, pregnancy, critical illness
Drug Interactions:	Hepatic disease, advanced age, and cimetidine ↑ levels; antacids ↓ absorption

CHLORDIAZEPOXIDE *continued*

Key Points: ↑ Respiratory and CNS depressant effects with general anesthetics and opioid analgesics

CLONAZEPAM

Trade Name: **Klonopin**

See Chapter 7, "Anticonvulsants"

DIAZEPAM

Trade Name: **Valium**

Indications: Anxiety disorders, alcohol withdrawal, conscious sedation, muscle spasms, status epilepticus, preoperative medication

Pharmacokinetics: Onset: <5 min (IV), <30 min (oral); peak: 0.5–4 h; duration: 3–8 h; Vd: 0.7–1.7 L/kg; Cl: 0.2–0.5 mL/kg/min; $T_{1/2} \beta$: 20–50 h hepatic metabolism to "active" metabolite (desmethyldiazepam), excreted in urine

Pharmacodynamics: ↑ GABA-mediated neural inhibition
  CNS: Sedation, anxiolysis, ↓ $CMRO_2$, ↓ CBF, headache, confusion
  CV: ↓ HR, ↓ BP, ↓ SVR, thrombophlebitis
  Pulmonary: ↓ Tidal volume, ↓ minute volume, ↓ $PaCO_2$, ↓ hypoxic drive
  Other: Nausea, constipation, centrally-active muscle relaxant, rash

Dosage: 0.1–0.3 mg/kg PO (premedication); 2.5–5 mg IV q 2–4 h (sedation)

Contraindications: Acute narrow-angle glaucoma

Drug Interactions: Cimetidine, alcohol, smoking, advanced age ↓ clearance; antacids ↓ absorption; ↓ bupivacaine metabolism

Key Points: Use in combination with general and spinal anesthesia can potentiate respiratory and cardiovascular depression, postoperative sedation

FLUMAZENIL

Trade Name: **Romazicon**

Indications: Reverse benzodiazepine-induced sedation and amnesia

FLUMAZENIL *continued*

Pharmacokinetics:	Onset: 1–2 min; peak: 6–10 min; duration: 60–90 min; Vd: 0.6–1.6 L/kg; Cl: 10–20 mL/kg/min; $T_{1/2}$ β: 0.7–1.3 h; extensive hepatic metabolism, excreted in urine
Pharmacodynamics:	Competitively antagonizes benzodiazepine agonist activity
CNS:	Headache, anxiety, dizziness, agitation, tremor, seizures
CV:	Arrhythmias, palpitations, vasodilation ($\downarrow$ PVR)
GI:	Nausea, vomiting, constipation
Pulmonary:	Dyspnea, hyperventilation
Other:	Diaphoresis, pain on injection, blurred vision, urinary retention
Dosage:	0.2 mg q 1–2 min (max. 1 mg); resedation in 60–90 min; 12 µg/kg (children)
Contraindications:	Chronic benzodiazepine use, TCA overdose, status epilepticus
Drug Interactions:	$\uparrow$ Seizures in chronic benzodiazepine users and after TCA overdose
Key Points:	Resedation occurs approximately 60 min after reversal due to shorter duration of action compared with benzodiazepine agonists

FLURAZEPAM, TEMAZEPAM

Trade Names:	**Dalmane (flurazepam), Restoril (temazepam)**
Indications:	Insomnia
Pharmacokinetics:	Onset: <0.5 h; peak: 1–2 h; protein binding: 96%; duration: 8–12 h; $T_{1/2}$ β: 10–20 h; metabolized in liver, excreted in urine
Pharmacodynamics:	$\uparrow$ GABA effects on CNS, blocks cortical and limbic arousal
CNS:	Dizziness, drowsiness, ataxia, blurred vision, disorientation
GI:	Nausea, vomiting, heartburn, diarrhea, abdominal pain, $\uparrow$ LFTs
Other:	Psychological dependence, dry mouth, dyspnea
Dosages:	*Flurazepam* 15–30 mg PO h.s. *Temazepam* 7.5–30 mg PO h.s.
Contraindications:	Pregnancy, breast-feeding
Drug Interactions:	Antidepressants, antihistamines, barbiturates, alcohol, sedative-hypnotics, digoxin, MAOIs $\uparrow$ CNS depression; cimetidine, disulfizam, isoniazid, ritonavir, OCPs $\downarrow$ metabolism; $\uparrow$ phenytoin and levodopa levels; smoking and rifampin $\uparrow$ metabolism; theophylline $\downarrow$ CNS effect; herbals $\uparrow$ CNS effects

FLURAZEPAM, TEMAZEPAM *continued*

Key Points:	Use before surgery can ↑ CNS depressive effects and prolong recovery from anesthesia due to long-acting active metabolites

LORAZEPAM

Trade Name:	**Ativan**
Indications:	ICU sedation, alcohol withdrawal, anxiety, insomnia
Pharmacokinetics:	Onset: 5 min (IV); 15–30 min (IM), 1 h (oral); peak: 1–2 h; duration: 6–24 h; Vd: 0.8–1.3 L/kg; Cl: 0.8–1.8 mL/kg/min; $T_{1/2}$ β: 11–22 h; hepatic metabolism to glucuronide conjugate, excreted in urine
Pharmacodynamics:	↑ GABA-mediated neural inhibition
CNS:	Anxiolysis, drowsiness, dizziness, weakness, ataxia, amnesia,
CV:	Orthostatic hypotension (↓ SVR), ↑ HR
GI:	Nausea, abdominal discomfort, ↓ appetite
Pulmonary:	↑ RR (low-dose), ↓ RR (high-dose), upper airway obstruction
Other:	Acute withdrawal syndrome, spinally mediated muscle relaxation
Dosage:	0.02–0.04 mg/kg IV/IM (max. 2 mg), then 0.03–0.05 mg/kg PO q 6–8 h
Contraindications:	Pregnancy, acute narrow-angle glaucoma, hepatorenal impairment
Drug Interactions:	Antidepressants, antihistamines, MAOIs, phenothiazines ↑ CNS depression; cimetidine, disulfiram, alcohol, advanced age ↓ clearance; scopolamine ↑ confusion and irrational behavior
Key Points:	Use with anesthetics and opioid analgesics will enhance respiratory and CNS depressant effects, produces profound amnesic effect

MIDAZOLAM

Trade Name:	**Versed**
Indications:	Preoperative medication, "conscious" sedation, ICU sedation
Pharmacokinetics:	Onset: <5 min (IV), 15 min (IM), <30 min (oral); peak: <1 h; duration: 2–4 h; Vd: 1.4 L/kg; Cl: 7.5 mL/kg/min; $T_{1/2}$ β: 2–4 h; rapidly oxidized in liver, excreted in urine
Pharmacodynamics:	↑ GABA-mediated central neural inhibition

MIDAZOLAM *continued*

CNS:	Sedation-hypnosis, anxiolysis, delirium, amnesia, ↓ CBF, ↓ CMRO$_2$
CV:	↓ BP (↓ SVR), ↓ cardiac output, ↑ HR
Pulmonary:	↑ RR (low-dose), ↓ RR (high-dose); ↓ tidal volume, ↑ upper airway obstruction, ↓ hypoxic respiratory drive, apnea
Other:	Spinally mediated muscle relaxant properties, hiccups, headache

Dosage:	1–3 mg IV bolus (premedication), 0.25–1.5 µg/kg/min infusion (ICU sedation); 0.5–1 mg/kg PO (children)
Contraindications:	Acute narrow-angle glaucoma, coma, hypotension (shock)
Drug Interactions:	↓ Volatile anesthetic requirement; antidepressants, antihistamines, tranquilizers ↑ CNS depression; cimetidine, isoniazid, erythromycin, verapamil, sagunavir, alcohol, advanced age ↓ clearance; ↓ ketamine-induced delirium; aminophylline ↓ CNS effect; rifampin ↓ levels
Key Points:	Use with anesthetics or opioid analgesics enhances respiratory depression and ↑ sedative effects; potent amnesic effect lasts 1–2 h; large doses (>5 mg) prolong emergence from anesthesia

OXAZEPAM

Trade Name:	**Serax**
Indications:	Anxiety, alcohol withdrawal
Pharmacokinetics:	Onset: <1 h; peak: 2–4 h; protein binding: 90%; duration: 6–8 h; T$_{1/2}$ β: 5–20 h; metabolized in liver, excreted in urine
Pharmacodynamics:	Stimulates GABA receptors, blocks cortical and limbic arousal
CNS:	Drowsiness, dizziness, amnesia, tremor, headache, syncope
CV:	Pedal edema
GI:	Nausea, ↑ LFTs
Other:	Skin rash, ↓ libido
Dosage:	10–30 mg PO q 6–8 h
Contraindications:	Psychosis, breast-feeding
Drug Interactions:	Antacids ↓ absorption; antidepressants, antihistamines, MAOIs, phenothiazines, sedative-hypnotics, opioids ↑ CNS depression; cimetidine and disulfizam ↑ level; ↓ effect of levodopa
Key Points:	Use prior to surgery; ↑ CNS depression effects and can prolong emergence from general anesthesia

16

Beta-Blockers

ACEBUTOLOL

Trade Name: **Sectral**

                           See Chapter 4, "Antiarrhythmics"

ATENOLOL

Trade Name: **Tenormin**

Indications: Hypertension, angina, acute MI, tachyarrhythmias,
                           alcohol withdrawal

Pharmacokinetics: Onset: <5 min (IV), 1 h (oral); bioavailability: 55%;
                           peak: 2 h; duration: 12–24 h; Vd: 1.1 L/kg; $T_{1/2}$ β:
                           6–7 h; crosses placenta, secreted into breast milk;
                           no metabolism, excreted in urine

Pharmacodynamics: Selective $β_1$ antagonist
  CNS: Dizziness, fatigue, depression, headaches
  CV: ↓ HR, ↓ BP
  GI: Nausea, diarrhea
  Pulmonary: ↑ Airway resistance (with asthma or COPD)
  Renal: ↓ Plasma renin/aldosterone activity, ↓ RBF, ↓ GFR

Dosage: 25–100 mg/d PO; 1–5 mg IV over 5 min (acute
                           MI/tachyarrhythmia)

Contraindications: Severe myocardial impairment, advanced heart block

Drug Interactions: Antihypertensives ↑ hypotension; acute withdrawal
                           causes rebound ↑ HR and ↑ BP; masks signs of
                           hyperthyroidism and hypoglycemia; ↓ bronchodilation
                           by β-agonists

Key Points: Drug should not be discontinued before surgery because
                           of risk of postoperative myocardial ischemia,
                           hypertension, tachyarrhythmias

BETAXOLOL

Trade Names: **Kerlone, Betoptic (ophthalmic)**

Indications: Hypertension, chronic open-angle glaucoma, ocular
                           hypertension

Pharmacokinetics: Onset: <1 h; bioavailability: 85%; peak: 4 h; duration:
                           12–24 h; Vd: 7.5 L/kg; $T_{1/2}$ β: 14–22 h; hepatic
                           metabolism, excreted in urine and feces

Pharmacodynamics: Selective $β_1$ antagonist
  CNS: Dizziness, fatigue, depression, headache, ↓ IOP,
                           asthenia
  CV: ↓ HR, ↓ BP, CHF, pedal edema

BETAXOLOL *continued*

Pulmonary:	Bronchospasm, ↑ airway resistance (with asthma or COPD)
Other:	Nausea, toxic epidermal necrolysis
Dosage:	5–20 mg/d PO; 0.5% 1–2 gtt bid
Contraindications:	Severe myocardial impairment, advanced heart block, active bronchospastic disease, severe COPD, "brittle" diabetes
Drug Interactions:	CCB and catecholamine-depleting drugs ↑ hypotension
Key Points:	β-blockers should not be abruptly discontinued prior to surgery (due to risk of rebound ↑ HR, ↑ BP, angina); ↑ CV depressant effects of anesthetics

BISOPROLOL

Trade Name:	**Zebeta**
Indications:	Hypertension
Pharmacokinetics:	Onset: <1 h; bioavailability: 85%; peak: 1–4 h; duration: 24 h; $T_{1/2}$ β: 9–12 h; 1st-pass hepatic metabolism, excreted in urine
Pharmacodynamics:	Selective $β_1$ antagonist
CNS:	Dizziness, fatigue, depression, headache
CV:	↓ HP, ↑ BP, ↓ RBF
Pulmonary:	Wheezing, ↑ airway resistance (asthma or COPD), cough
Other:	Diarrhea
Dosage:	5–10 mg/d PO (max. 20 mg/d)
Contraindications:	Severe myocardial impairment, advanced heart block, asthma
Drug Interactions:	Antihypertensives ↑ hypotension; ↓ bronchodilation produced by β-agonists
Key Points:	Continue β-block therapy until day of surgery because acute withdrawal may cause rebound ↑ HR and ↑ BP; β-blockers may mask signs of hyperthyroidism and hypoglycemia under anesthesia

CARTEOLOL

Trade Name:	**Cartrol**
Indications:	Hypertension
Pharmacokinetics:	Onset: <1 h; bioavailability: 85%; peak: 1–3 h; protein binding: 25%; duration: 24 h; $T_{1/2}$ β: 6 h; minimal metabolism, excreted in urine

CARTEOLOL *continued*

Pharmacodynamics:	Long-acting, nonselective β-blocker with intrinsic sympathomimetic activity
CNS:	Fatigue, somnolence, paresthesia, ↓ sympathetic outflow
CV:	↓ HR, ↓ BP, ↓ CO
Pulmonary:	Wheezing, ↑ airway resistance (with asthma and COPD)
Other:	Muscle cramps, arthralgias, rash
Dosage:	2.5 mg PO initially, then 10 mg/d
Contraindications:	Myocardial impairment, advanced heart block, wheezing
Drug Interactions:	Antihypertensives ↑ hypotension; ↓ bronchodilation by β-agonists
Key Points:	Continue β-block therapy, as acute withdrawal can cause rebound ↑ HR and ↑ BP; β-blockers mask signs of hyperthyroidism and hypoglycemia under anesthesia

CARVEDILOL

Trade Name:	**Coreg**
Indications:	Hypertension, heart failure
Pharmacokinetics:	Onset: <1 h; bioavailability: 30%; peak: 1–2 h; duration: 7–10 h; extensively metabolized in liver, excreted in feces
Pharmacodynamics:	Nonselective β-blocker with α-blockade activity
CNS:	Malaise, headache, dizziness, fatigue, asthenia
CV:	↓ HR, AV block, pedal edema, orthostatic hypotension
Pulmonary:	Dyspnea, wheezing (with asthma and COPD)
Other:	Thrombocytopenia, diarrhea, impotence, hypercholesterolemia, gout, hyperglycemia
Dosage:	3–12 mg PO bid (max. 24 mg bid)
Contraindications:	Severe cardiac failure, bronchial asthma, advanced heart block
Drug Interactions:	CCBs, MAOIs, reserpine, clonidine ↑ bradycardia and hypotension; rifampin ↓ level; ↑ digoxin level
Key Points:	Adequate hydration prior to ambulation minimizes postural hypotension and PONV after surgery

ESMOLOL

Trade Name:	**Brevibloc**
Indications:	Hypertension, SVT, acute MI, perioperative tachycardia

ESMOLOL *continued*

Pharmacokinetics:	Onset: <5 min; peak: <30 min; duration: 30 min; Vd: 23 L/kg; Cl: 225 mL/min/kg; $T_{1/2}$ β: 8–12 min; metabolized by red blood cell esterases, excreted in urine
Pharmacodynamics:	Short-acting, selective $β_1$ antagonist
CNS:	Dizziness, somnolence, headache, confusion
CV:	↓ HR, ↓ BP, ↓ CO, ↓ RBF
GI:	Nausea, ↓ hepatic (and splancnic) blood flow
Pulmonary:	Bronchospasm (↑ airway resistance), pharyngitis
Dosage:	0.5–1 mg/kg IV, then 50–150 µg/kg/min infusion
Contraindications:	Myocardial impairment, advanced heart block, wheezing
Drug Interactions:	Antihypertensives ↑ hypotensive effects; ↓ bronchodilation by β-agonists
Key Points:	Useful adjunct for controlling transient acute autonomic responses during surgery; produces an anesthetic and analgesic-sparing effect; may mask signs of inadequate anesthesia and hypoglycemia

LABETALOL

Trade Names:	**Normodyne, Trandate**
Indications:	Hypertension, controlled hypotension during surgery, tetanus
Pharmacokinetics:	Onset: <5 min (IV), 20 min (oral); bioavailability: 35%; duration: 2–4 h (IV), 8–12 h (oral); Vd: 10 L/kg; $T_{1/2}$ β: 5–8 h; extensive 1st-pass hepatic metabolism, excreted in urine
Pharmacodynamics:	Nonselective $β_1$- and $β_2$-antagonist with $α_1$-antagonist activity
CNS:	Dizziness, fatigue
CV:	↓ HR, ↓ BP, ↓ CO, postural hypotension (↓ SVR)
GI:	Nausea, dyspepsia, vomiting, ↑ LFTs
Pulmonary:	↑ Airway resistance (may cause bronchospasm)
Other:	Hyperglycemia, agranulocytosis
Dosage:	5–20 mg IV initially, then 20–40 mg q 10–15 min, or 2 mg/min infusion; 100 mg PO bid, then 200–400 mg PO bid
Contraindications:	Severe myocardial impairment, advanced heart block, profound bradycardia, breast-feeding, acute wheezing
Drug Interactions:	Antihypertensives ↑ hypotensive effect; cimetidine ↑ levels; ↓ bronchodilation produced by β-agonists; ↑ Raynaud's phenomenon

LABETALOL *continued*

Key Points:	Useful adjuvant for controlling transient (acute) hyperdynamic responses during surgery in presence of adequate anesthesia and analgesia; adequate fluid replacement minimizes risk of postural hypotension

LEVOBUNOLOL

Trade Name:	**Betagan**
Indications:	Chronic open-angle glaucoma, ocular hypertension
Pharmacokinetics:	Onset: 1 h; peak: 2–6 h; duration: 24 h; minimal systemic absorption
Pharmacodynamics:	Nonselective β_1- and β_2-antagonist
CNS:	Headache, ↓ IOP, ataxia, dizziness
CV:	↓ HR, ↓ BP, chest pain
GU:	Nausea, diarrhea
Other:	Blepharoconjunctivitis, photophobia, bronchospasm
Dosage:	1–2 gtt/d; 0.25% and 0.5%
Contraindications:	Angle-closure glaucoma (unless combined with a miotic drug)
Drug Interactions:	Carbonic anhydrase inhibitors, epinephrine, pilocarpine ↓ IOP
Key Points:	No known adverse interactions with anesthetic drugs

METOPROLOL

Trade Names:	**Lopressor, Toprol XL**
Indications:	Hypertension, cardiac arrhythmias, angina, acute MI
Pharmacokinetics:	Onset: 5 min (IV), 15 min (oral); bioavailability: 50%; peak: <1 h; duration: 5–8 h (IV), 6v12 h (oral); $T_{1/2}$ β: 3–7 h; crosses placenta, blood-brain barrier and secreted into breast milk; extensive 1st-pass hepatic metabolism, excreted in urine
Pharmacodynamics:	Selective β_1-antagonist
CNS:	Fatigue, dizziness, depression, ↓ sympathetic outflow
CV:	↓ HR, ↓ BP, ↓ CO, orthostatic hypotension
GI:	Constipation, dyspepsia, nausea, diarrhea
Renal:	↓ Renin activity, ↑ Cr/BUN

METOPROLOL *continued*

Other:	Bone marrow suppression, wheezing, pruritus, rash
Dosage:	2.5–5 mg IV q 5 min, then 100 mg bid; 50–100 mg/d PO, then 100–450 mg/d
Contraindications:	Severe myocardial impairment, advanced heart block, profound bradycardia, active bronchospastic disease, breast-feeding
Drug Interactions:	Amiodarone and antihypertensives ↑ hypotension
Key Points:	Continue β-blocker therapy prior to surgery because acute withdrawal may result in rebound ↑ HR and ↑ BP; enhances CNS depressant effects of benzodiazepines; neostigmine produces marked ↓ HR when used for reversal of neuromuscular blockade; masks signs of intraoperative hyperthyroidism and hypoglycemia

NADOLOL

Trade Name:	**Corgard**
Indications:	Hypertension, angina, arrhythmias, vascular headaches
Pharmacokinetics:	Onset: 0.5–1 h; bioavailability: 35%; peak: 2–4 h; protein binding: 30%; duration: 12–24 h; $T_{1/2}$ β: 20 h; crosses placenta and blood-brain barrier and secreted into breast milk; not metabolized, excreted in urine
Pharmacodynamics: *CNS:* *CV:* *GI:* *Pulmonary:* *Other:*	Long-acting, nonselective β_1- and β_2-antagonist Dizziness, fatigue, anorexia ↓ HP, ↓ BP, ↓ CO Nausea, abdominal pain, diarrhea/constipation ↑ Airway resistance (wheezing) ↓ Free fatty acids and insulin (↑ glucose)
Dosage:	20–40 mg/d PO, increase to 40–80 mg/d
Contraindications:	Impaired myocardial function, 2nd- or 3rd-degree AV block, severe bradycardia, acute bronchospastic disease, breast-feeding
Drug Interactions:	Antihypertensives and curare ↑ hypotensive effect; ↓ bronchodilation by β-agonists and sympathomimetics; ↓ hypoglycemic effects of oral agents; ↑ theophylline levels
Key Points:	Airway stimulation with inadequate hypnosis (or relaxation) may trigger severe bronchospastic response; can mask signs of hypoglycemia, hyperthyroidism, inadequate anesthesia

PENBUTOLOL

Trade Name:	**Levatol**
Indications:	Hypertension
Pharmacokinetics:	Onset: <1 h; bioavailability: 100%; peak: 1–3 h; duration: 12–24 h; $T_{1/2}$ β: 5 h; hepatic metabolism, excretion in urine
Pharmacodynamics:	Nonselective $β_1$- and $β_2$-antagonist
CNS:	Headache, fatigue
CV:	↓ HP, ↓ BP, ↓ CO, arrhythmias
Pulmonary:	↑ Airway resistance (wheezing)
Dosage:	20 mg/d PO, then 20–40 mg/d
Contraindications:	Myocardial impairment, advanced heart block, wheezing
Drug Interactions:	Antihypertensives ↑ hypotension
Key Points:	β-blocker therapy should be continued to prevent rebound ↑ HR and ↑ BP associated with abrupt withdrawal; masks signs of hyperthyroidism and hypoglycemia under anesthesia

PINDOLOL

Trade Name:	**Visken**
Indications:	Hypertension, angina
Pharmacokinetics:	Onset: <30 min; bioavailability: 80%; peak: 1–2 h; protein binding: 98%; duration: 24 h; Vd: 1.6 L/kg; $T_{1/2}$ β: 3–7 h; crosses placenta and blood-brain barrier and secreted into breast milk; hepatic metabolism, excreted in urine
Pharmacodynamics:	Nonselective β-antagonist with intrinsic sympatho-mimetic activity
CNS:	Fatigue, dizziness, insomnia, anxiety, paresthesia
CV:	↓ HR, ↓ BP, ↓ PVR, ↓ CO, pedal edema
GI:	Nausea, abdominal discomfort, diarrhea, vomiting, ↑ LFTs
Pulmonary:	↑ Airway resistance (bronchospasm)
Other:	↓ Free fatty acids and insulin, myalgias, arthralgia
Dosage:	5 mg PO bid, then 10–30 mg/d; 15–40 mg/d (angina)
Contraindications:	Impaired myocardial function, 2nd- or 3rd-degree AV block, severe bradycardia, active bronchospastic disease
Drug Interactions:	CCB and antihypertensives ↑ hypotension; NSAIDs ↓ antihypertensive effect; ↑ lidocaine levels; thioridazine ↑ QT interval

PINDOLOL *continued*

Key Points: In asthmatic patients, ↑ risk of wheezing during anesthesia; reflex tachycardia due to intraoperative blood loss may be blunted, as well as autonomic signs of "light anesthesia," hypoglycemia, hyperthyroidism

PROPRANOLOL

Trade Name: **Inderal**

Indications: Hypertension, angina, ideopathic hypertrophic subaortic stenosis (IHSS), pheochromocytoma, thyrotoxicosis, migraine, acute MI, essential tremor

Pharmacokinetics: Onset: <2 min (IV), 30 min (oral); peak: 1–1.5 h (oral), <5 min (IV); duration: <10 min (IV), 12 h (oral); Vd: 43 L/kg; $T_{1/2}$ β: 3–5 h; crosses placental and blood-brain barrier and into breast milk; hepatic metabolism (to active metabolites), excreted in urine

Pharmacodynamics: Nonselective $β_1$- and $β_2$-antagonist
  CNS: Fatigue, dizziness, depression, insomnia, peripheral neuropathy
  CV: ↓ HR, ↓ BP, ↓ CO
  GI: Nausea/vomiting, cramping, diarrhea/constipation
  Pulmonary: ↑ Airway resistance (bronchospasm)
  Other: ↓ Glycogenolysis, ↓ renin activity, ↑ free fatty acids and insulin, agranulocytosis, thrombocytopenic purpura

Dosage: 0.5–3 mg IV, repeat q 2 min; 20–40 mg PO bid (or 60–80 mg/d), then 160–480 mg/d

Contraindications: Severe myocardial impairment, advanced heart block, profound bradycardia, bronchial asthma, breast-feeding

Drug Interactions: CCB and antihypertensives ↑ hypotension; anticholinergics ↑ HR; ↓ theophylline clearance, ↓ bronchodilation by β-agonists and sympathomimetic drugs; ↓ hypoglycemic effect of insulin and glyburide; antacids and alcohol ↓ absorption

Key Points: Higher doses ↑ neuromuscular blocking drugs; volatile anesthetics can ↑ arrhythmias; neostigmine can produce severe bradycardia during reversal of residual neuromuscular blockade

SOTALOL

Trade Name: **Betapace**

Indications: Ventricular arrhythmias, recurrent atrial fibrillation/flutter

SOTALOL *continued*

Pharmacokinetics:	Onset: <1 h; bioavailability: 95%; peak: 2–4 h; duration: 12 h; Vd: 1.5 L/kg; $T_{1/2}$ β: 12 h; not metabolized, excreted unchanged in urine
Pharmacodynamics:	Nonselective β_1- and β_2-antagonist
CNS:	Fatigue, dizziness, asthenia
CV:	↓ HR, ↓ BP, arrhythmias, ↑ QT interval (torsades de pointes)
GI:	Nausea, vomiting, dyspepsia
Pulmonary:	↑ Airway resistance (bronchospasm), dyspnea
Other:	↓ Free fatty acids and insulin (hyperglycemia)
Dosage:	80 mg PO bid, ↑ 160–320 mg/d (max. 480 mg/d)
Contraindications:	SA node dysfunction, advanced heart block, wheezing
Drug Interactions:	Antacids ↓ absorption; CCB and antihypertensives ↑ hypotension; ↓ bronchodilation by β-agonists; amiodarone ↓ HR and BP; TCAs ↑ QT interval
Key Points:	Avoid anesthetic drugs known to prolong QT interval; can prolong neuromuscular blockade produced by nondepolarizing blockers; volatile anesthetics may ↑ arrhythmias and ↑ myocardial depression

TIMOLOL

Trade Names:	**Blocadren, Timoptic (ophthalmic)**
Indications:	Hypertension, angina, acute MI, migraine headache, glaucoma
Pharmacokinetics:	Onset: <30 min; bioavailability: 90%; peak: 1–2 h; protein binding: 50%; duration: 6–12 h; $T_{1/2}$ β: 4 h; extensive 1st-pass hepatic metabolism, excreted in urine
Pharmacodynamics:	Nonselective β_1- and β_2-antagonist
CNS:	Fatigue, dizziness, ↓ IOP, headache
CV:	↓ HR, postural hypotension, heart block, angina, arrhythmia
GI:	Nausea, vomiting, abdominal discomfort, diarrhea, constipation
Pulmonary:	↑ Airway resistance (bronchospasm), dyspnea,
Other:	hyperglycemia
Dosage:	5–10 mg PO bid, then 10–40 mg/d; 0.25%–0.5% 1 gtt bid
Contraindications:	Bronchial asthma, severe COPD, advanced heart AV block, profound bradycardia, CHF, breast-feeding

TIMOLOL *continued*

Drug Interactions:

Digoxin, diltiazem, verapamil ↑ bradycardia and cardiac depression; ↑ muscle weakness in patients with myasthenia gravis

Key Points:

Anesthetic and opioid analgesics ↑ hypotension and bradycardia; use of volatile anesthetics ↑ arrhythmias and ↑ myocardial depression

17

Blood Substitutes and Volume Expanders

ALBUMIN

Trade Names:	**Albutein, Albuminar, Plasbumin, Albumin**
Indications:	Hypovolemia, hemodilution, adjunct to crystalloid for CPB pump, ARDS, hemodialysis, hypoproteinemia, severe burns, neonatal hyperbilirubinemia, ascites, nephrosis, pancreatitis
Pharmacokinetics:	Onset: <15 min; duration: 1–20 d; $T_{1/2}$ β: 24 h (intracellular) and 15–20 d (extracellular)
Pharmacodynamics:	Transport protein that binds therapeutic and toxic materials in circulation; 5% albumin is iso-oncotic with human plasma and ↑ blood volume equivalent to the amount infused; 25% albumin is oncotically equivalent to 5× the volume of plasma, an intravascular volume equal to 3.5× the amount infused
CNS:	Dizziness, headache
CV:	↑ BP, ↑ CVP, ↑ plasma volume, flushing
GI:	Nausea, vomiting
Other:	↓ Hematocrit, ↓ blood viscosity, dyspnea, binds bilirubin, fatty acids, hormones, enzymes, drugs, dyes, trace metals
Dosage:	2 g/kg/24 h IV (5% and 25% solutions)
Contraindications:	Severe anemia, CHF, pulmonary edema
Drug Interactions:	Incompatible with verapamil, alcohol-containing solutions, amino acid solutions, fat emulsions, protein hydrolysates
Key Points:	Use of 5% and 25% albumin for volume expansion should include hemodynamic monitoring to prevent circulatory overload

DEXTRAN

Trade Names:	**Dextran 40, Dextran 70**
Indications:	Hemodilution and volume expansion, venous thrombosis prophylaxis
Pharmacokinetics:	Variable due to wide range of molecular sizes; at 1 and 24 h after administration, 26% and 17% remained intravascular and 21% and 31% had been excreted in urine; biologic $T_{1/2}$ β: 12–24 h
Pharmacodynamics:	Low–molecular weight polymer of glucose
CV:	↑ Plasma volume, ↑ CVP, ↓ blood viscosity
Pulmonary:	Pulmonary edema
Other:	Bleeding disorder, impairs typing and cross-matching of blood products, anaphylactic reactions, ↑ ESR, ↑ bleeding time, ↓ Factors II, V, VIII, IX

DEXTRAN *continued*

Dosage:	20 mL/kg IV infusion of 10% dextran 40 or 6% dextran 70 in glucose-containing (or normal saline) solution
Contraindications:	Thrombocytopenia, hypofibrinogenemia, renal failure
Drug Interactions:	Incompatible with ampicillin and heparin; anticoagulants and antiplatelet drugs ↑ bleeding times
Key Points:	Central venous pressure (and/or pulmonary artery wedge pressure) should be monitored during rapid infusion to prevent volume overload

DEXTROSE

Other Names:	**$D_{2.5}W$, D_5W, $D_{10}W$, $D_{20}W$**
Indications:	Fluid replacement and caloric (glucose) supplementation
Pharmacokinetics:	Metabolized to carbon dioxide and water
Pharmacodynamics:	Calories and fluids, ↑ glycogen deposition and prevents ketosis
CNS:	Confusion, fever
CV:	Pulmonary edema, hypertension, CHF, phlebitis
GU:	Glycosuria, osmotic diuresis
Other:	Hyperglycemia, hyperosmolarity, dehydration
Dosage:	0.1–0.5 g/kg/h IV (2.5%, 5%, 10%, and 20% glucose in water)
Contraindications:	Diabetic coma, intracranial hemorrhage, anuria, hepatic coma
Drug Interactions:	May cause pseudoagglutination of transfused RBCs; corticosteroids and corticotropin ↑ serum glucose level; alters insulin and oral hypoglycemic drug requirements; causes vitamin B complex deficiency
Key Points:	Careful assessment of hydration status to avoid excess "free water"

F-DECALIN (FDC); F-TRIPROPYLAMINE (FTPA); F-*N*-METHYL-DECAHYDROISOQUINOLINE (FMIQ); PERFLUBRON (PFOB)

Trade Names:	**Fluosol-DA (FDC + FTPA), Oxyfluor, Oxygent (PFOB)**
Indications:	Myocardial protection during PTCA, isovolemic hemodilution, blood replacement therapy (Oxygent, Oxyfluor), ↑ tumor cell susceptibility to radiation and chemotherapy, ARDS, organ preservation

F-DECALIN (FDC); F-TRIPROPYLAMINE (FTPA); F-*N*-METHYL-DECAHYDROISOQUINOLINE (FMIQ); PERFLUBRON (PFOB)
continued

Pharmacokinetics:	$T_{1/2} \beta$: 4–65 d (PFOB, 4 d; FDC, 7 d; FTPA, 65 d); elimination via exhalation (low MW) and phagocytosis (high MW); excretion rate dependent on MW of fluorocarbon
Pharmacodynamics:	Fluorocarbon-based O_2 carriers; straight oxyhemoglobin-dissociation curve; O_2-carrying capacity dependent on concentration of fluorocarbon
CV:	Myocardial protection
Other:	Myalgias, flulike symptoms, phagocytosis of high-MW fluorocarbons by reticuloendothelial systems and "foamy" macrophages in liver and spleen
Dosage:	20% intravascular perfluorochemical emulsion consists of three components: (1) fluosol emulsion, (2) Solution #1, (3) Solution #2 (water-insoluble emulsions [0.1–0.3 μm diameter])
Contraindications:	NK
Drug Interactions:	Anaphylaxis to F-68 constituent in Fluosol-DA
Key Points:	May be alternative to blood transfusion in patient populations who refuse blood products (e.g., Jehovah's Witnesses)

HEMOGLOBIN-BASED OXYGEN CARRIER (HBOC)

Trade Name:	**Hemopure**
Indications:	Blood replacement therapy, isovolemic hemodilution, anemia
Pharmacokinetics:	Unmodified hemoglobin tetramer ($\alpha_2\beta_2$) rapidly dissociates into dimers ($\alpha\beta$) outside RBCs; $T_{1/2} \beta$: 1–2 h; intravascular retention times up to 36 h, binding of large molecules to α or β chains, polymerization via intermolecular cross-linking; cellular hemoglobin is stable for 3 y, has lower viscosity, and is compatible with all blood types
Pharmacodynamics:	Modified hemoglobin with oxygen carrying capacity
CNS:	Retinal changes
CV:	Interference with NO in heart, coronary vasoconstriction, MI, cardiac output during hemodilution, enzymatic changes in heart
GU:	Renal vasoconstriction, ↓ GFR, renal toxicity

HEMOGLOBIN-BASED
OXYGEN CARRIER (HBOC) *continued*

Pulmonary:	Enzymatic changes in lungs, pulmonary edema
Other:	Enzyme changes in spleen, abdominal pain, yellow discoloration
Dosage:	30 g IV initially, then 60 g (max. 300 g)
Contraindications:	Severe coronary artery disease; allergic to bovine-derived products
Drug Interactions:	↑ Immunogenicity of enlarged hemoglobin molecules
Key Points:	Investigational blood substitutes for emergency situations

HETASTARCH

Trade Name:	**Hespan**
Indications:	Acute isovolemic hemodilution, plasma volume expansion
Pharmacokinetics:	Onset: <5 min; $T_{1/2}$ β: 25 h; biologic $T_{1/2}$ β: 10–15 d (<10% detected intravascularly after 2 wk); larger molecules degraded by amylase in liver and spleen, small molecules (<50,000 D) excreted in urine
Pharmacodynamics:	Modified amylopectin polymer, non–O_2-carrying blood replacement therapy
CNS:	Headache, fever
CV:	↑ BP, ↑ cardiac index, ↑ CVP, ↑ plasma volume, ↑ PCWP
GI:	↑ Amylase, bilirubin levels, vomiting
Pulmonary:	Pulmonary edema
Other:	Myalgias, impaired reticuloendothelial system, ↑ PT, ↑ PTT, ↓ platelet function
Dosage:	6% hetastarch in 0.9% NaCl, max. 20 mL/kg/d IV (1500 mL)
Contraindications:	Bleeding disorders, CHF, renal failure, thrombocytopenia
Drug Interactions:	Rash, urticaria, anaphylactoid reactions
Key Points:	Do not use for upper abdominal procedures due to risk of postoperative pancreatitis; careful hemodynamic monitoring prevents circulatory overload

PENTASTARCH

Trade Name:	**Pentaspan**
Indications:	Isovolemic hemodilution and volume expansion, plasmaphoresis

PENTASTARCH *continued*

Pharmacokinetics:	Onset: <5 min; $T_{1/2}$ β: 2.5 h; hydrolyzed by plasma amylase (more rapid than hetastarch); excreted 1° in urine <24 h
Pharmacodynamics:	Low–molecular weight hydroxyethyl starch (HES) colloid solution
CNS:	Headache, fatigue
CV:	Pedal edema
GI:	Nausea
Other:	↓ Platelets, ↑ PT, ↑ aPTT, ↓ Factor VIII levels
Dosage:	500–1000 mL infusion (max. 2000 mL/d)
Contraindications:	CHF
Drug Interactions:	Rash, urticaria, anaphylactoid reactions
Key Points:	Shorter-acting alternative to hetastarch with lower risk of pancreatitis

PLASMA PROTEIN FRACTION

Trade Names:	**Plasmanate, Protenate**
Indications:	Shock, hypoproteinemia
Pharmacokinetics:	Liver, kidney, intestine provide elimination mechanisms
Pharmacodynamics:	Expands plasma volume using albumin, α-, β-, γ-globulins
CNS:	Headache
CV:	Vascular overload, ↑ HR, flushing
GI:	Nausea/vomiting, hypersalivation
Pulmonary:	Pulmonary edema, dyspnea
Other:	Rash, ↑ plasma protein, fever, myalgia
Dosage:	250–500 mL of 5% solution (max. 250 g/48 h); 22–33 mL/kg at 5–10 mL/min (children)
Contraindications:	Severe anemia, heart failure, CPB procedures
Drug Interactions:	NK
Key Points:	Avoid rapid IV infusion (<10 mL/min) in elderly and patients with myocardial impairment

RINGER LACTATE SOLUTION

Other Name:	**Lactated Ringer's solution**
Indication:	Maintenance of intravascular volume
Pharmacokinetics:	Intravascular $T_{1/2}$ β: 15 min; at 1 h after infusing this solution, only 6% remained intravascular

RINGER LACTATE
SOLUTION *continued*

Pharmacodynamics:	Electrolyte solution to ↑ plasma volume
CV:	↑ BP, ↑ CVP, ↑ intravascular volume
Pulmonary:	Pulmonary edema, dyspnea
Other:	Acidosis, ↓ renal function
Dosage:	5–20 mL/kg/h infusion
Contraindications:	CHF, ARF
Drug Interactions:	Incompatibility with ampicillin and nicardipine
Key Points:	With severe cardiac disease, CVP (or pulmonary artery wedge pressure) should be monitored during prolonged infusions to avoid volume "overloading"

SODIUM BICARBONATE

Trade Names:	**Soda mint, Neut**
Indications:	Lactic or ketoacidosis, hyperkalemia, renal tubular acidosis
Pharmacokinetics:	Bicarbonate is filtered and reabsorbed in kidney; <1% excreted in urine
Pharmacodynamics:	Bicarbonate buffers excess H^+ in the blood, ↑ plasma pH
CNS:	CSF acidosis, ↑ CVR, ↓ CBF, somnolence
CV:	↓ CO, ↑ arrhythmias
Metabolic:	Hypernatremia, hyperosmolality, shift oxyhemoglobin dissociation curve to left (less O_2 released to tissue at a given SpO_2)
Pulmonary:	↑ Ventilation, dyspnea
Dosage:	0.5–1 mEq/kg IV or 84 mg/mL
Contraindications:	Intractable vomiting, hypochloremic alkalosis
Drug Interactions:	Precipitates Ca^{2+} salts; ↑ digoxin toxicity; ↓ clearance of sympathomimetics; ↑ clearance of chlorpropamide, lithium, ASA tetracycline; ↑ activity of opioid and local anesthetics; incompatible with norepinephrine, dobutamine, glycopyrrolate, ceftazidime, nicardipine; steroids ↑ Na retention
Key Points:	When sodium bicarbonate infusions are used during surgery, electrolyte levels and SpO_2 should be monitored during perioperative period

SODIUM CHLORIDE

Trade Name:	**Normal saline**
Indications:	Fluid replacement, diluting drug for parenteral injection

SODIUM CHLORIDE *continued*

Pharmacokinetics:	NK
Pharmacodynamics:	NaCl solution for maintaining electrolyte balance
CNS:	Confusion
CV:	Pulmonary edema, ↑ intravascular volume
Other:	Febrile reactions, venous thrombosis
Dosage:	10–25 mL/kg/h; 0.9% saline
Contraindications:	NK
Drug Interactions:	Allergic to benzyl alcohol
Key Points:	In fasting patients, 20 versus 2 mL/kg was associated with ↓ postoperative side effects (e.g., dizziness, drowsiness, fatigue, thirst, nausea)

18

Bronchodilators

ALBUTEROL

Trade Names:	**Proventil, Ventolin**
Indications:	Bronchodilation with asthma and COPD, hyperkalemic familial periodic paralysis
Pharmacokinetics:	Onset: <30 min; peak: 1–3 h; duration: 3–4 h (inhaled), 6–12 h (oral); $T_{1/2}$ β: 4 h; extensively metabolized in liver, excreted 1° in urine
Pharmacodynamics:	β_2-selective bronchodilation
CNS:	Tremor, nervousness, headache, vertigo
CV:	↑ HR, ↑ BP
GI:	Nausea/vomiting, oropharyngeal edema, bad taste
Other:	Muscle cramps, hypokalemia (large doses)
Dosage:	2–4 mg PO q 6–8 h; 1–2 puffs (90 μg/puff) q 4–6 h
Contraindications:	CHF, dysrhythmias, CAD, hypertension, hyperthyroidism, seizure disorders
Drug Interactions:	β-adrenergic blockers ↓ effect; ↑ arrhythmias with sympathomimetics (theophylline), MAOIs, and TCAs
Key Points:	Check electrolyte levels before surgery; use of metered dose nebulizer requires activation during inspiration and breathholding for 10 sec

AMINOPHYLLINE

Trade Name:	**Same**
Indications:	Acute bronchospasm, COPD, paroxysmal nocturnal dyspnea (or periodic apnea), neonatal apnea
Pharmacokinetics:	Onset: <30 min; peak: 1–2 h; duration: 2–6 h; therapeutic level 10–20 μg/mL; hepatic metabolism, excreted in urine
Pharmacodynamics:	Aminophylline is converted to theophylline, a methylxanthine bronchodilator; inhibiting phosphodiesterase ↑ levels of cAMP
CNS:	Headaches, excitement, irritability, SIADH, insomnia
CV:	↓ BP, ↑ CO, ↓ PVR, angina, CHF, ↑ HR, arrhythmias
GI:	Nausea, vomiting, abdominal pain, diarrhea
Pulmonary:	Bronchodilation, tachypnea
Other:	Alopecia, rash
Dosage:	5 mg/kg IV (over 20 min), or 6 mg/kg PO, then 0.5–1.0 mg/kg/h infusion; 2–4 mg/kg PO q 6–12 h (children)

AMINOPHYLLINE *continued*

Contraindications:	Allergic to xanthines (caffeine, theobromine), active peptic ulcer, breast feeding, severe cardiac dysfunction, seizure disorders
Drug Interactions:	β-adrenergic blockers ↓ effects; sympathomimetics ↑ effects; ↑ toxicity with cimetidine, quinolones, allopurinol, contraceptives, β-blockers, corticosteroids, erythromycins; ↑ toxicity with liver insufficiency; ↑ dose required with rifampin, phenobarbital, phenytoin, hepatic enzyme-inducing agents, smoking
Key Points:	Avoid administering other drugs into same IV line because of numerous drug incompatabilities with aminophylline infusion

ATROPINE

Trade Name:	**Atropine**
	See Chapter 5, "Anticholinergics"

BECLOMETHASONE

Trade Names:	**Beclovent, Vanceril**
Indications:	Acute bronchospasm, prolonged asthma treatment, seasonal rhinitis
Pharmacokinetics:	Onset: <5 min; peak: <10 min; protein binding: 87%; duration: 4–6 h; biologic $T_{1/2}$: 15 h; rapid hepatic inactivation and metabolism by lung esterases, excreted 1° in feces
Pharmacodynamics:	Potent glucocorticoid with weak mineralocorticoid activity
GI:	Dry mouth, fungal infection involving mucous membranes
Other:	Headache, hypothalamic-pituitary-adrenal suppression, angioedema, rash, wheezing, nasopharyngeal irritation
Dosage:	42–84 mg (metered spray); 2 puffs tid, then 1 puff tid
Contraindications:	Acute bronchospasm, tuberculosis, fungal or bacterial infections
Drug Interactions:	Potassium-depleting diuretics (e.g., furosemide) may ↑ toxicity
Key Points:	Patients on maintenance therapy should receive perioperative IV steroid coverage; continue steroids to avoid acute adrenal insufficiency

BITOLTEROL

Trade Name:	**Tornalate**
Indications:	Treatment and prevention of bronchospasm
Pharmacokinetics:	Onset: 2–3 min; peak: 0.5–1 h; duration: 6–8 h; hydrolyzed by esterases to active metabolites, excreted 1° in urine
Pharmacodynamics:	Selectively stimulates β_2-adrenergic receptors
CNS:	Tremor, nervousness, headache, dizziness
CV:	↑ HR, angina, palpitations
GI:	Nausea, vomiting, throat irritation, ↑ LFTs
Other:	Bone marrow suppression, proteinuria ↑ ACT
Dosage:	1–2.5 mg PO tid (max. 8 mg); 0.2% solution 1–2 puffs
Contraindications:	Severe CAD, hyperthyroidism, hypertension, diabetes
Drug Interactions:	β-blocker ↓ effects; β-adrenergic agonists ↑ sympathomimetic effects; theophylline ↑ cardiotoxicity
Key Points:	↑ Dysrhythmias when used with volatile anesthetics, sympathomimetics, cardiac glycosides; with acute wheezing, administer over 15–20 min prior to induction of anesthesia and achieve deep anesthesia prior to tracheal intubation

CROMOLYN

Trade Name:	**Intal**
Indications:	Prevention of bronchospasm, allergic rhinitis, mastocytosis
Pharmacokinetics:	Onset: <5 min; peak: <10 min; duration: 6 h; $T_{1/2}$ β (lung): 1 h, $T_{1/2}$ β (plasma): 81 min; excreted in urine and bile
Pharmacodynamics:	↓ Release of histamine and SRS-A "degranulation" from mast cells
CNS:	Dizziness, headache
CV:	Angina (from propellant), arrhythmias
GI:	Nausea, throat dryness and irritation, ↑ LFTs
Pulmonary:	Bronchospasm, cough
Other:	Myalgias, swelling, rash, angioedema
Dosage:	800 µg/metered spray; 1–2 puff qid; 100–200 mg PO qid (mastocytosis)
Contraindications:	Status asthmaticus, severe cardiac disease with arrhythmias
Drug Interactions:	Use lactose-free preparations in lactase-deficient patients

CROMOLYN *continued*

Key Points:	Do not administer prior to induction of anesthesia due to potential airway irritating properties

EPHEDRINE

Trade Name:	Generic
	See Chapter 1, "Adrenergic Agonists and Antagonists"

EPINEPHRINE

Trade Name:	Adrenaline
	See Chapter 1, "Adrenergic Agonists and Antagonists"

FLUTICASONE-SALMETEROL

Trade Names:	Flonase (fluticasone alone), Advair Diskus (fluticasone ± salmetrol)
Indications:	Long-term therapy for asthma, seasonal allergic rhinitis
Pharmacokinetics:	Onset: <30 min; peak: 1–2 h; protein binding: 95%; duration: 12–24 h; $T_{1/2}$ β: 6–8 h; metabolized in liver, excreted in feces
Pharmacodynamics:	Anti-inflammatory activity with β_2-adrenergic stimulation
CNS:	Sleep disorders, tremors, headache
CV:	↑ HR, palpitations
GI:	Nausea/vomiting, diarrhea, oral ulcerations
Pulmonary:	Cough, URI (bronchitis)
Other:	Myalgia, diaphoresis, hyperglycemia, rash
Dosage:	50 μg/metered dose; 2 puff/d (250 μg fluticasone; 50 μg salmeterol bid)
Contraindications:	Status asthmatics, viral, fungal, or tubercular infections
Drug Interactions:	β-blockers ↓ CV effect of salmeterol; ketoconazole and inhibitors of P_{450} system ↑ fluticasone level; MAOIs and TCAs ↑ CV effects
Key Points:	Not recommended prior to induction of anesthesia due to upper airway irritation; volatile anesthetics ↑ risk of arrhythmias

IPRATROPIUM

Trade Name: **Atrovent**

                         See Chapter 5, "Anticholinergics"

ISOPROTERENOL

Trade Name: **Isuprel**

                         See Chapter 1, "Adrenergic Agonists and Antagonists"

METAPROTERENOL

Trade Names: **Alupent, Metaprel**

Indications: Bronchodilation (asthmatic attack), COPD (acute
                         exacerbation)

Pharmacokinetics: Onset: <30 min; peak: 1–3 h; duration: 2–5 h; hepatic
                         metabolism, excreted in urine

Pharmacodynamics: β_2-mediated bronchodilation and β_1 effects at high
                         doses
  CNS: Nervousness, headache, fatigue, vertigo, weakness,
                         tremor
  CV: ↑ HR, ↑ BP, palpitations, cardiac arrest
  GI: Dry mouth, dyspepsia, nausea, vomiting
  Pulmonary: Paradoxical bronchoconstriction, cough
  Other: Muscle cramps, rash

Dosage: 10–20 mg PO q 3–5 h; 0.4%–5% 2–3 puffs
                         (0.65 mg/metered dose) q 4–6 h

Contraindications: CHF, severe coronary artery disease, diabetes,
                         hypertension, hyperthyroidism, seizure activity

Drug Interactions: β-adrenergic blocker ↓ effects; sympathomimetics
                         (e.g., cardiac glycosides, levodopa, theophylline),
                         parabens and contrast dyes ↑ arrhythmias

Key Points: Increases arrhythmias with volatile anesthetics and ↓
                         splanchic blood flow ↓ hepatic and renal elimination

MONTELUKAST

Trade Name: **Singulair**

Indications: Prophylaxis and chronic treatment of asthma

Pharmacokinetics: Onset: <30 min; bioavailability: 64%; peak: 2–4 h;
                         protein binding: 99%; duration: 4–8 h; Vd: 8–11 L;
                         $T_{1/2}$ β: 4 h; hepatic cytochrome P_{450} metabolism,
                         excreted in urine

MONTELUKAST *continued*

Pharmacodynamics:	Inhibits cysteinyl leukotriene (LTD_4) receptors
CNS:	Headache
GI:	Gastroenteritis, dyspepsia, ↑ LFTs
Other:	URI, rash
Dosage:	4–10 mg/d PO
Contraindications:	Status asthmaticus
Drug Interactions:	Phenobarbital and rifampin ↑ clearance
Key Points:	Not indicated for treating wheezing in preoperative period

OMALIZUMAB

Trade Name:	**Xolair (rhuMAB-E25)**
Indications:	Allergic asthma, severe IgE-mediated seasonal allergies
Pharmacokinetics:	Onset: slow; peak: 7–8 d; duration: 1 mo; Vd: 78 mL/kg; $T_{1/2}$ β: 26 d; cleared by hepatic RE system
Pharmacodynamics:	Monoclonal anti-IgE antibody (blocks type-1 immune response) by forming complex with free IgE, blocking interaction with mast cells and basophils
Pulmonary:	↓ Bronchospasm, ↑ PFT, URI, sinusitis, pharyngitis
Other:	↓ Ocular and nasal secretions, anaphylaxis, local reactions
Dosage:	0.016 mg/kg SC q 4 wk (× 24 wk)
Contraindications:	NK
Drug Interactions:	↓ Corticosteroid requirement
Key Points:	No known interactions with anesthetic drugs

OXTRIPHYLLINE

Trade Name:	**Choledyl SA**
Indications:	Bronchial asthma, bronchospasm (due to chronic bronchitis/COPD)
Pharmacokinetics:	Onset: <1 h; peak: 2–3 h; duration: 6–8 h; metabolized to theophylline, excreted in urine
Pharmacodynamics:	Blocks adenosine receptors in bronchi, inhibits phosphodiesterase and ↑ level of cAMP (relaxing smooth muscle)
CNS:	Dizziness, headache, insomnia, restlessness, seizures, tremor
CV:	↑ HR, ↓ BP, arrhythmias, flushing
GI:	Nausea, vomiting, diarrhea, epigastric pain

OXYTRIPHILLINE *continued*

Other:	Rash, dyspnea
Dosage:	4.7 mg/kg PO q 6–8 h; 6.2 mg/kg PO qid (children)
Contraindications:	Tachyarrhythmias, sensitivity to xanthines (e.g., caffeine, theobromine), breast-feeding
Drug Interactions:	↓ Antiarrhythmic effect of adenosine; allopurinol, cimetidine, macrolides, propranolol, and quinones ↑ level; barbiturates, smoking, marijuana ↓ level; ↑ lithium excretion
Key Points:	Use with volatile anesthetics and β-agonists can ↑ risk of arrhythmias; enflurane or ketamine may ↑ incidence of seizures

TERBUTALINE

Trade Names:	**Brethine, Brethaire, Bricanyl**
Indications:	Acute bronchospasm (with COPD), premature labor (tocolytic)
Pharmacokinetics:	Onset: 30 min (oral), 15 min (SC); peak: 2–3 h (oral), 1–2 h (inhaled), 30–60 min (SC); duration: 4–8 h (oral), 1.5–4 h (SC); limited hepatic metabolism, excreted 1° unchanged in urine
Pharmacodynamics:	β_2-selective bronchodilation with β_1 effects (at high doses)
CNS:	Tremor, nervousness, vertigo, headache, drowsiness, tinnitus, seizures
CV:	↑ HR, palpitations, ↑ BP, arrhythmias, flushing
GI:	↓ Secretions, nausea, vomiting, dyspepsia, unusual taste
Pulmonary:	Bronchodilator, cough, ↓ secretions
Other:	Diaphoresis, hypokalemia, ↓ uterine contractions, muscle cramps
Dosage:	2.5–5 mg PO tid, 0.26 mg SC q 30 min (max. dose: 0.5 mg/4 h)
Contraindications:	Uncontrolled dysrhythmias, angina, CHF, diabetes, seizures, hypokalemia, hyperthyroidism
Drug Interactions:	↓ Effect with β-adrenergic blockers; ↓ pressor response with theophylline; ↑ pressor response with MAOIs and TCAs; ↑ hypokalemia with diuretics
Key Points:	↑ Dysrhythmias and CV depression when used with volatile anesthetics; paradoxical bronchospasm with prolonged use

THEOPHYLLINE

Trade Names:	**Accurbron, Elixophyllin, Theobid**
Indications:	Management of acute asthma and bronchospasm (dueto COPD and chronic bronchitis); cystic fibrosis
Pharmacokinetics:	Onset: 15 min (IV), 15–60 min (oral); peak: 15–30 min (IV), 1–2 h (oral); protein binding: 40%; duration: 6–12 h; Cl: 0.65 mL/kg/min; $T_{1/2} \beta$: 7–9 h; therapeutic level: 10–20 mg/mL; metabolized in liver, excreted in urine
Pharmacodynamics:	Inhibits phosphodiesterase, ↑ cyclic AMP, antagonizing adenosine receptors, relaxing bronchial smooth muscle
CNS:	↓ Seizure threshold, hyperactivity, anxiety, headache
CV:	↑ HR, ↓ BP, arrhythmias (PVCs), flushing
GI:	Vomiting, nausea, dyspepsia, ↑ LFTs
Pulmonary:	Tachypnea, dermatitis, urinary frequency
Dosage:	300 mg/d PO tid; 12–20 mg/kg/d (children)
Contraindications:	Sensitivity to xanthines, active PUD, seizure disorders, breast-feeding
Drug Interactions:	↑ Toxicity of digoxin; ↓ diazepam sedation; cimetidine and propranolol ↓ clearance; ephedra ↑ toxicity; St. John's Wort ↓ toxicity
Key Points:	Volatile anesthetic and β-stimulants can ↑ incidence of arrhythmias; antagonizes benzodiazepine-induced CNS depression

TIOTROPIUM

Trade Name:	**Spiriva**
	See Chapter 5, "Anticholinergics"

ZAFIRLUKAST

Trade Name:	**Accolate**
Indications:	Prophylaxis and chronic treatment of asthma, seasonal rhinitis
Pharmacokinetics:	Onset: <1 h; peak: 3 h; duration: 12 h; $T_{1/2} \beta$: 10 h; hepatic cytochromes P_{450} metabolism, excreted in feces
Pharmacodynamics:	Selective peptide leukotriene receptor antagonist
CNS:	Headache, dizziness, asthenia
GI:	Nausea, dyspepsia, vomiting, ↑ LFTs
Other:	Arthralgia, myalgia, eosinophilia
Dosage:	10–20 mg PO bid; 10 mg bid (children)

ZAFIRLUKAST *continued*

Contraindications:	Breast-feeding, severe hepatic impairment
Drug Interactions:	↑ PT with warfarin; aspirin ↑ level; erythromycin and theophylline ↓ levels
Key Points:	Avoid use of potentially hepatoxic drugs

ZILEUTON

Trade Name:	**Zyflo**
Indications:	Prophylaxis and treatment of asthma in adults and children
Pharmacokinetics:	Onset: <30 min; peak: 2 h; protein binding: 93%; duration: 4–8 h; Vd: 1.2 L/kg; $T_{1/2}$ β: 2.5 h; hepatic metabolism, excreted in urine
Pharmacodynamics:	Inhibitor of 5-lipoxygenase, ↓ leukotriene formation, ↓ inflammatory response
CNS:	Headache, asthenia, dizziness, fatigue
GI:	Dyspepsia, flatulence, nausea, abdominal pain
Other:	Myalgia, UTI, vaginitis
Dosage:	600 mg PO qid
Contraindications:	Active liver disease (with ↑ LFTs)
Drug Interactions:	↑ Theophylline and propranolol levels, ↓ PT with warfarin
Key Points:	Avoid potentially hepatotoxic anesthetic drugs (e.g., halothane)

19

Calcium Channel
Blockers

AMLODIPINE

Trade Name:	**Norvasc**
Indications:	Coronary vasospasm (Prinzmetal's angina), hypertension
Pharmacokinetics:	Onset: 1–2 h; bioavailability: 80%; peak: 6–12 h; protein binding: 93%; duration: 24 h; Vd: 21 L/kg; $T_{1/2}$ β: 30–50 h; extensively metabolized by hepatic cytochrome P_{450}, excreted in urine
Pharmacodynamics:	Class IV antiarrhythmic, long-acting dihydropyridine-type CCB
CNS:	Headache, fatigue, paresthesia, dizziness
CV:	↓ HR, ↓ BP, pedal edema, flushing, palpitations, angina
GI:	Nausea, abdominal pain
Dosage:	2.5–10 mg PO initially, then 5–10 mg/d
Contraindications:	Sick sinus syndrome, advanced heart block (without pacemaker), aortic stenosis, severe hepatic impairment, breast-feeding
Drug Interactions:	β-blocker ↑ hypotension; grapefruit ↑ levels
Key Points:	↓ Anesthetic concentrations to minimize myocardial depression due to peripheral vasodilation; opioid analgesics potentiate ↓ BP and ↑ fluid requirements

BEPRIDIL

Trade Name:	**Vascor**
Indications:	Chronic stable angina
Pharmacokinetics:	Onset: <1 h; bioavailability: 59%; peak: 2–3 h; protein binding: >99%; duration: 24 h; $T_{1/2}$ β: 42 h; secreted in breast milk; metabolized in liver, excreted 1° in urine
Pharmacodynamics:	Class I antiarrhythmic, blocks calcium and sodium channels
CNS:	Dizziness, nervousness, headache, asthenia, tremor
CV:	Arrhythmias, ↑ QT interval, pedal edema, palpitations
GI:	Nausea, constipation, diarrhea, dry mouth, ↑ LFTs
Other:	Dyspnea, rash
Dosage:	200–300 mg/d PO (max. 400 mg/d)
Contraindications:	Sick sinus syndrome; advanced heart block, recent MI, CHF, prolonged QT interval, breast-feeding
Drug Interactions:	TCAs, procainamide, quinidine, glycosides ↑ QT interval; β-blockers ↑ hypotension

BEPRIDIL *continued*

Key Points: ↓ Anesthetic concentrations to avoid severe hypotension due to ↑ vasodilation; avoid drugs that prolong QT interval

CLEVIDIPINE

Trade Name: **Clevelox (investigational)**

Indication: Perioperative hypertension

Pharmacokinetics: Onset: <5 min; peak: <10 min; protein binding: 99%; duration: 10–20 min; Vd: 0.15 L/kg; Cl: 150 mL/kg/min; $T_{1/2}$ β: 20 min; lipid emulsion; metabolized in blood (hydrolysis) and tissue (non-specific esterases), excreted in urine and feces

Pharmacodynamics: Ultra short-acting calcium (L-type) channel blocker
   CNS: Headache
   CV: ↓ BP, ↓ PVR, flushing
   GI: ↓ Gastric emptying, constipation
   GU: Mild natriuretic (diuretic)

Dosages: 0.3–3 µg/kg/min infusion (max. 16 µg/kg/min)

Contraindications: Sensitivity to CCB or soybean oil, pregnancy, breast-feeding

Key Points: Pseudocholinesterase deficiency ↓ clearance and prolongs recovery

DILTIAZEM

Trade Name: **Cardizem**

Indications: Angina, atrial tachyarrhythmias, hypertension, Raynaud's phenomenon

Pharmacokinetics: Onset: 3 min (IV), 30–60 min (oral); bioavailability: 40–55%; peak: 2–3 h; protein binding: 75%; duration: 6–24 h; $T_{1/2}$ β: 3.5–6 h; therapeutic serum level: 50–200 ng/mL; metabolized in liver, excreted in urine

Pharmacodynamics: Calcium ion channel influx inhibitor, coronary vasodilator
   CNS: Dizziness, headache, asthenia, tremor, paresthesia
   CV: ↓ PVR, ↓ SA node automaticity, ↓ AV nodal conduction, ↑ PR interval, arrhythmias, ↓ myocardial oxygen demand
   GI: Nausea, constipation, ↑ LFT
   Other: Pedal edema

Dosage: 30 mg PO qid (max. 360 mg/d); 60–240 mg bid; or 120–180 mg/d (max. 480 mg/d ER); 0.25 mg/kg IV followed by 15 mg/h infusion

DILTIAZEM *continued*

Contraindications:	Sick sinus syndrome; advanced heart block; recent MI; SVT (WPW, LGL), CHF, hypotension, pulmonary edema, breast-feeding
Drug Interactions:	↑ Levels of digoxin, carbamazepine, and cyclosporine; ↑ sedative effect of midazolam; β-blocker ↑ hypotension and bradyarrhythmias
Key Points:	↑ CV depressant effects of general anesthetics, opioid analgesics, and benzodiazepines; ↑ anesthetic-induced vasodilation

FELODIPINE

Trade Name:	**Plendil**
Indications:	Hypertension
Pharmacokinetics:	Onset: 1–3 h; bioavailability: 20%; peak: 3–5 h; protein binding: 99%; duration: 24 h; $T_{1/2}$ β: 14 h; hepatic metabolism, excreted in urine
Pharmacodynamics:	Class IV antiarrhythmic, dihydropyridine calcium channel blocker
CNS:	Dizziness, headache, asthenia, paresthesia, insomnia
CV:	Arrhythmias, pedal edema, flushing, angina
GI:	Dyspepsia, eructation, flatulence, nausea
Other:	Polyuria, dyspnea, cough, arthralgia, ↓ libido, gynecomastia
Dosage:	5 mg PO initially; ↑ 2.5–5 mg at 2-wk intervals (max. 20 mg/d)
Contraindications:	Pregnancy, breast-feeding, sick sinus syndrome, severe hypotension, acute MI, hepatic impairment
Drug Interactions:	↓ Metoprolol; digoxin, carbamazepine, cyclosporin clearance; hydantoins and barbiturates ↓ levels; erythromycin ↑ level
Key Points:	↑ CV depressant effects of general anesthetics; adequate hydration ↓ risk of hypotension in perioperative period

ISRADIPINE

Trade Name:	**DynaCirc**
Indications:	Hypertension
Pharmacokinetics:	Onset: <1 h; bioavailability: 20%; peak 1–2 h; protein binding: 95%; duration: 12 h; $T_{1/2}$ β: 8 h; extensive 1st-pass hepatic metabolism, excreted in urine and feces

ISRADIPINE *continued*

Pharmacodynamics:	Class IV antiarrhythmic, dihydropyridine-type CCB
CNS:	Dizziness, headache
CV:	↓ BP (↓ SVR), ↑ HR, palpitations, flushing
GI:	Nausea, diarrhea, vomiting, ↑ LFTs
Other:	Peripheral edema, dyspnea
Dosage:	2.5 mg PO bid, ↑ 5 mg/d; 5 mg/d q 2–4 wk (max. 20 mg/d)
Contraindications:	Ventricular dysfunction, CHF, pregnancy, breast-feeding
Drug Interactions:	Fentanyl and β-blockers ↓ BP; cimetidine ↑ level; rifampicin ↓ level
Key Points:	↑ CV depressant effects of anesthetic drugs (doses >10 mg/d), ↑ fluid requirement during perioperative period

NICARDIPINE

Trade Name:	**Cardene**
Indications:	Angina, hypertension, CHF
Pharmacokinetics:	Onset: <2 min (IV), 20 min (oral); bioavailability: 35%; peak: <5 min (IV), 1–2 h (oral); protein binding: 95%; duration: 12 h; $T_{1/2}$ β: 2–4 h; excreted in breast milk; therapeutic levels: 28–50 ng/mL; extensive 1st-pass hepatic metabolism, excreted
Pharmacodynamics:	Class IV antiarrhythmic, dihydropyridine-type CCB and vasodilator
CNS:	Dizziness, headache, asthenia, paresthesia
CV:	↓ BP, ↓ SVR, ↑ HR, pedal edema, angina, QT prolongation
GI:	Nausea, dry mouth
Other:	Rash, flushing, thrombophlebitis (IV)
Dosage:	0.625- to 2.5-mg IV boluses, then 0.5–5 mg/h; 20–60 mg PO bid
Contraindications:	Hepatorenal impairment, aortic stenosis, CHF, breast-feeding
Drug Interactions:	H_2-antagonists and grapefruit ↑ level; fatty meals ↓ levels; not compatible with $NaHCO_3$ or Ringer's solution
Key Points:	↑ Vasodilating properties of anesthetic and analgesic drugs; ↑ volume of fluids required during perioperative period; possesses anesthetic and opioid-sparing properties during surgery

NIFEDIPINE

Trade Names:	**Adalat, Procardia**
Indications:	Angina, hypertension, migraine headache, Raynaud's phenomenon, CHF, cardiomyopathy
Pharmacokinetics:	Onset: 20 min; bioavailability: 60%; peak: 5 h; protein binding: 95%; duration: 8–24 h; $T_{1/2}$ β: 2–5 h; therapeutic level: 25–100 ng/mL; metabolized in liver, excreted in urine and feces
Pharmacodynamics:	Inhibits influx of calcium ions into cardiac muscle, arteriolar dilator
CNS:	Dizziness, headache, asthenia, nervousness
CV:	↓ BP (↓ SVR), reflex ↑ HR, syncope, flushing, pedal edema
GI:	Nausea, dyspepsia, ↑ LFTs
Pulmonary:	Dyspnea, cough, wheezing, pulmonary edema
Other:	↓ Platelet aggregation ↑ bleeding time, hypokalemia, muscle weakness
Dosage:	10–30 mg PO tid, or 30–60 mg/d
Contraindications:	CHF, aortic stenosis, elderly, β-blocker use, breast-feeding
Drug Interactions:	Alcohol, grapefruit ↑ level; ↑ phenytoin levels; β-blockers ↓ BP
Key Points:	↑ Hypotensive effects of anesthetic and analgesic drugs

NIMODIPINE

Trade Name:	**Nimotop**
Indications:	Subarachnoid hemorrhage, migraine headache
Pharmacokinetics:	Onset: <30 min; bioavailability: 13%; peak: 1 h; protein binding: >95%; duration: 4 h; $T_{1/2}$ β: 1–2 h; extensive 1st-pass hepatic metabolism, excreted 1° in urine
Pharmacodynamics:	Dihydropyridine calcium channel blocker, dilates cerebral vessels
CNS:	Headache, psychiatric disturbances, dizziness, ↑ CBF
CV:	↓ BP, ↓ myocardial contractility, flushing
GI:	Nausea, abdominal discomfort, ↑ LFTs
Other:	Peripheral edema, dyspnea, rash, muscle cramps
Dosage:	30–60 mg PO q 4 h
Contraindications:	Severe hepatic impairment, breast-feeding
Drug Interactions:	Potentiates effects of other antihypertensive drugs; ↑ phenytoin levels

NIMODIPINE *continued*

Key Points:	Careful titration of inhalational anesthetics and vasodilators is necessary to avoid profound intraoperative hypotension

NISOLDIPINE

Trade Name:	**Sular**
Indications:	Hypertension
Pharmacokinetics:	Onset: 1–2 h; peak: 6–12 h; protein binding: 99%; duration: 24 h; $T_{1/2}$ β: 7–12 h; extensively metabolized in liver, excreted in urine
Pharmacodynamics:	Blocks calcium ion channels at vascular smooth muscle, causing arteriolar dilation
CNS:	Headache, dizziness
CV:	Vasodilation (↓ PVR), ↓ BP, pedal edema
Other:	Rash, nausea, sinusitis
Dosage:	20 mg/d PO, then 20–40 mg/d
Contraindications:	Sensitivity to other CCBs
Drug Interactions:	Cimetidine and grapefruit ↑ level; quinidine ↓ level
Key Points:	Potentiates CV depressant effects of anesthetics and opioid analgesics

VERAPAMIL

Trade Names:	**Calan, Isoptin, Verelan**
Indications:	Angina, hypertension, arrhythmias, SVT, hypertrophic cardiomyopathy, migraine headache
Pharmacokinetics:	Onset: <30 min; peak: 1–2 h; protein binding: 88%; duration: 2–10 h; Vd: 5–7 L/kg; $T_{1/2}$ β: 6–12 h; therapeutic level: 80–300 ng/mL; secreted in breast milk, metabolized in liver, excreted in urine
Pharmacodynamics:	Slow CCB, modulates the influx of calcium in arterial smooth muscle and in myocardial cells, dilates arterioles
CNS:	Dizziness, headache, asthenia
CV:	↓ BP (↓ SVR), arrhythmias, ↑ AV block, pulmonary and peripheral edema
GI:	Constipation, nausea, ↑ LFTs
Dosage:	5–10 mg IV boluses (0.075–0.15 mg/kg), repeat in 15–30 min; 40–80 mg PO initially, then 120–480 mg q 6–8 h

VERAMAPIL *continued*

Contraindications:	Sick sinus syndrome, CHF (LV dysfunction), tachyarrhythmias, advanced heart block, severe hypotension, β-blocker therapy
Drug Interactions:	↑ Levels of metoprolol, digoxin, carbamazepine, theophylline, cyclosporine; rifampin and sulfinpyrazone ↓ level; ↑ hypotension with quinidine, flesanide, disopyramide, dantrolcnc, β-blockers
Key Points:	↑ CNS depressant effects of anesthetics and analgesics; ↑ neuromuscular blockade

20

Central Stimulants

ALMOTRIPTAN, ELETRIPTAN, NARATRIPTAN, ZOLMITRIPTAN

Trade Names:	**Axert (almotriptan), Relpax (eletriptan), Amerge (naratriptan) , Zomig (zolmitriptan)**
Indications:	Migraine headache
Pharmacokinetics:	Onset: 1 h; bioavailability: 50%; peak: 1–3 h; protein binding: 30%–85%; duration: 3–4 h; Vd: 2 L/kg; $T_{1/2}$ β: 3–4 h; hepatic metabolism (active metabolites), excreted in urine
Pharmacodynamics:	Binds with high affinity to $5\text{-}HT_{1D}$, $5\text{-}HT_{1F}$, $5\text{-}HT_{1B}$ receptors
CNS:	Somnolence, vertigo, weakness, cerebral vasoconstriction, CVA
CV:	Angina, coronary vasospasm, palpitations, ↑ PVR, ↑ BP, tachyarrythmias
GI:	Dry mouth, dyspepsia, dysphagia, nausea
Other:	Myalgia, diaphoresis
Dosages:	*Almotriptan:* 6.24–12.5 mg, repeat after 2 h *Eletriptan:* 20–40 mg, repeat after 2 h *Naratriptan:* 1–2.5 mg, repeat after 4 h (max. 5 mg/d) *Zolmitriptan:* 2.5–5 mg, repeat after 2 h (max. 10 mg/d)
Contraindications:	Uncontrolled hypertension, ischemic heart disease; hepatic impairment, concurrent use of MAOIs, 5-HT agonists, or ergot derivatives
Drug Interactions:	Cimetidine ↑ effect; ergotamines ↑ vasospasm; SSRIs ↑ weakness, hyperreflexia, incoordination; OCPs and MAOIs ↑ toxicity
Key Points:	Use with sympathomimetic drugs (e.g., phenylephrine) ↑ PVR and ↑ hemodynamic instability during surgery

AMANTADINE

Trade Name:	**Symmetrel**
	See Chapter 14, "Antivirals"

BACLOFEN

Trade Name:	**Lioresal**
Indications:	Spasticity due to multiple sclerosis and spinal cord diseases, muscle spasms
Pharmacokinetics:	Onset: 4 h; peak: 2–4 h; duration: 6 h; excreted unchanged in urine

BACLOFEN *continued*

Pharmacodynamics: Analog of GABA depresses neurons both at spinal and supraspinal levels

CNS: Drowsiness, dizziness, syncope

CV: Chest pain (angina)

GI: Nausea, constipation

Other: Urinary frequency, dark urine, ↓ tendon reflexes, ovarian cysts

Dosage: 5–10 mg PO qid (max. 80 mg/d); 0.5–2 mg IM; 50 μg (IT)

Contraindications: Seizure disorders, spasticity for motor function (e.g., cerebral palsy)

Drug Interactions: ↑ Antidiabetic drug requirements; MAOIs and TCAs ↑ CNS depression

Key Points: Preoperative use will ↑ CNS depressant effects of anesthetic and analgesic drugs; abrupt withdrawal results in ↑ spasticity, pruritis, hypotension, paresthesias

BROMOCRIPTINE

Trade Name: **Parlodel**

Indications: Amenorrhea, galactorrhea, acromegaly, Parkinson's disease, Cushing's syndrome, hepatic encephalopathy, NMS

Pharmacokinetics: Onset: 2 h; peak: 8 h; protein binding 93%; duration: 24 h; hepatic metabolism, excreted 1° in feces

Pharmacodynamics: ↓ Prolactin release from anterior pituitary gland, dopamine receptor agonist, ↑ prolactin inhibitory factor

CNS: Drowsiness, dizziness, fatigue, seizures, hallucinations, confusion, dyskinesia

CV: ↓ BP, MI, ↑ HR

GI: Nausea, cramps, anorexia, ↑ LFTs

Other: Hyperuricemia, digital vasospasm

Dosage: 2.5–5 mg/d PO

Contraindications: Pregnancy, uncontrolled hypertension, sensitivity to ergot derivatives

Drug Interactions: ↓ Efficacy with phenothiazines, butyrophenones, vasopressors

Key Points: ↑ Hypotensive effects of anesthetic and analgesic drugs

CAFFEINE

Trade Names:	**Cafcit, NoDoz, Quick Pep, Slo-Bid, Vivarin**
Indications:	Fatigue, drowsiness, vascular headache, apnea of prematurity
Pharmacokinetics:	Onset: <1 h; peak: 1–2 h; protein binding: 30%; duration: 3–9 h; Vd: 0.5 L/kg; metabolized in liver, excreted in urine
Pharmacodynamics:	Antagonism of adenosine receptors, α_1 and α_2 subtypes
CNS:	Stimulates medullary respiratory center, excitement, dizziness
CV:	↑ HR, orthostatic hypotension
GI:	↓ GI motility, ↓ esophageal sphincter tone, dyspepsia, diarrhea, nausea, vomiting
Pulmonary:	Bronchodilation, ↑ vital capacity, ↑ diaphragmatic contraction
Other:	Diuresis, bladder/uterine relaxation, muscle tremor
Dosage:	200 mg PO tid; 2.5–10 mg/kg IV
Contraindications:	Active peptic ulcer disease, seizure disorders
Drug Interactions:	↑ Metabolism with smoking (nicotine), phenytoin, and phenobarbital, ↑ CNS depressants and β-agonists
Key Points:	Not recommended as antidote for CNS depressant effects of anesthetic drugs in postoperative period

CARISOPRODOL

Trade Name:	**Soma**
Indications:	Musculoskeletal pain
Pharmacokinetics:	Onset: 30 min; peak: 2–4 h; duration: 4–6 h; $T_{1/2}$ β: 8 h; metabolized by liver, excreted by urine
Pharmacodynamics:	Centrally acting muscle relaxant, blocks interneurons in spinal cord
CNS:	Sedation, dizziness, headache
CV:	↑ HR, postural hypotension, facial flushing
GI:	Epigastric distress, nausea, vomiting
Other:	Eosinophilia, erythema multiforme rash
Dosage:	350 mg PO qid
Contraindications:	Intermittent porphyria, severe hepatorenal impairment
Drug Interactions:	Additive CNS depressant effect with alcohol
Key Points:	Preoperative use ↑ CNS depressant effects of anesthetics and analgesics; can ↑ recovery from anesthesia

CYCLOBENZAPRINE

Trade Name:	**Flexeril**
Indications:	Musculoskeletal pain
Pharmacokinetics:	Onset: 1 h; peak: 3–8 h; duration: 12–24 h; protein binding: ~99%; $T_{1/2}$ β: 1–3 d; metabolized by liver, excreted in urine
Pharmacodynamics:	Central and peripheral anticholinergic activity
CNS:	Drowsiness, dizziness
CV:	↓ BP, reflex ↑ HR, arrhythmias
Dosage:	10–20 mg PO tid (max. 2–3 wk)
Contraindications:	Use of MAOIs, acute MI, heart block, CHF, hyperthyroidism
Drug Interactions:	↑ Effects of alcohol, barbiturates, and CNS depressants; ↓ effects of guanethidine; discontinue MAOIs (>2 wk)
Key Points:	↑ CNS depressant effects of anesthetics, benzodiazepines, opioid analgesics

DANTROLENE

Trade Name:	**Dantrium**
Indications:	Malignant hyperthermia, upper motor neuron spasms
Pharmacokinetics:	Duration: 3 h (postinfusion); $T_{1/2}$ β: 4–8 h; metabolized by liver, excreted in urine
Pharmacodynamics:	↓ Calcium release from sarcoplasmic reticulum, ↓ muscle tension
CNS:	Drowsiness, dizziness, seizure, insomnia
CV:	↑ HR, phlebitis, pericarditis
GI:	Anorexia, ↑ LFTs, metallic taste, cramping, diarrhea
GU:	Urinary frequency/retention/incontinence, hematuria, crystalluria
Pulmonary:	Pleural effusion
Other:	Myalgias, muscle weakness, anemia, diaphoresis
Dosage:	1 mg/kg IV (max. 10 mg/kg); 25–100 mg/d PO
Contraindications:	Spasticity needed for motor function; use of verapamil (malignant hyperthermia), severe hepatic impairment, breast-feeding
Drug Interactions:	Use with CCB, hyperkalemic cardiovascular collapse; estrogen ↑ hepatotoxicity
Key Points:	↑ Effects of nondepolarizing muscle relaxants, ↑ sedative effect of benzodiazepines and IV anesthetics

DISULFIRAM

Trade Name:	**Antabuse**
Indications:	Chronic alcoholism
Pharmacokinetics:	Onset: 1 h; peak: 3–12 h; duration: 7–14 d; metabolized in liver, excreted in urine
Pharmacodynamics:	Irreversibly inhibits aldehyde dehydrogenase, blocks oxidation of alcohol, ↑ acetaldehyde levels
CNS:	Headache, drowsiness, fatigue, ↓ seizure threshold, optic neuritis, mood changes, paresthesias
GI:	Nausea, vomiting, metallic taste, ↑ LFTs
Other:	Flushing, impotence, hypercholesterolemia
Dosage:	125–500 mg/d PO
Contraindications:	Acute alcohol intoxication, use of alcohol-containing products, pregnancy, angina
Drug Interactions:	Alfentanil ↓ clearance; ↑ anticoagulant effect of warfarin
Key Points:	↑ Sedative effect and ↑ recovery of barbiturates and benzodiazepines administered during perioperative period

DOXAPRAM

Trade Name:	**Dopram**
Indications:	Postoperative respiratory depression, hypercapnia (2° to drug overdose or COPD)
Pharmacokinetics:	Onset: 30 sec; peak: 1–2 min; duration: 5–12 min; metabolized in liver, excreted in urine
Pharmacodynamics:	Analeptic, direct stimulation of peripheral carotid chemoreceptors and medullary respiratory center
CNS:	Excitation, ↓ CBF, confusion, dizziness
CV:	↑ HR, ↑ BP, angina, thrombophlebitis, flushing
GI:	Nausea, vomiting, diarrhea
GU:	Urinary retention, bladder irritation
Pulmonary:	Hiccups, cough, dyspnea, wheezing
Other:	↓ Shivering, diaphoresis
Dosage:	0.5–1 mg/kg IV/IM, then 2–3 mg/min (max. 2 mg/kg)
Contraindications:	Seizure disorder, CNS tumor, head injury, CVA, coronary artery disease, CHF/hypertension, pheochromocytoma, asthma
Drug Interactions:	MAOIs, ↑ HR/BP and seizures, ↑ effect of vasopressors
Key Points:	When administered during anesthesia, ↑ risk of arrhythmias; respiratory stimulant effect very short-lasting

ENTACAPONE

Trade Name:	**Comtan**
Indications:	Parkinson's disease (adjunct to levodopa/carbidopa)
Pharmacokinetics:	Onset: <1 h; peak: 1 h; protein binding: 98%; duration: 6 h; Vd: 20 L; $T_{1/2}$ β: 2–3 h; hepatic metabolism, excreted in feces
Pharmacodynamics:	Selective and reversible inhibitor of peripheral catechol-O-methyltransferase (COMT), ↑ levodopa levels
CNS:	Dyskinesia, hyperkinesia, fatigue, hallucinations
GI:	Diarrhea, abdominal pain, nausea, constipation, ↑ LFTs
GU:	Urine discoloration
Dosage:	200–400 mg/d PO in divided doses (max. 1.6 g)
Contraindications:	Severe hepatic impairment, biliary obstruction
Drug Interactions:	Alcohol and drugs interfering with biliary excretion (e.g., brobenecid, cholestyramine, erythromycin, rifampicin, ampicillin, chroramphenicol) ↑ toxicity; ↑ levels of drugs metabolized by COMT (e.g., dobutamine, dopamine, epinephrine, isoproterenol, norepinephrine)
Key Points:	↑ CNS depressant effects of anesthetics and analgesics

ERGOTAMINE, DIHYDROERGOTAMINE, METHYSERGIDE

Trade Names:	**Wigrane, Cafergot (ergotamine), DHE (dihydroergotamine)**
Indications:	Migraine, cluster, and vascular headaches; coronary artery spasm (during angiography), diarrhea (2° to carcinoid)
Pharmacokinetics:	Onset: <10 min; peak: 1–2 h; protein binding: 90%; duration: 3–8 h; metabolized in liver, excreted 1° in feces
Pharmacodynamics:	Competitive serotonin antagonist, agonist/antagonist at α-adrenergic receptors
CNS:	Cerebral vasoconstriction, ↑ IOP
CV:	Vasoconstriction, vasospasm, edema
GI:	Severe nausea, vomiting, ↑ LFTs
Other:	Uterine contraction, extremity ischemia, gangrene, agranulocytosis, thrombocytopenia, fibrotic reactions
Dosages:	*Ergotamine:* 2–4 mg (with 100 mg caffeine) *Dihydroergotamine:* 0.5 mg IV

ERGOTAMINE, DIHYDROERGOTAMINE, METHYSERGIDE *continued*

Contraindications:	Hypertension, coronary artery disease, peripheral vascular disease, pregnancy, breast-feeding, Raynaud's phenomenon
Drug Interactions:	↑ Toxicity with vasoconstrictors; cimetidine, β-blockers ↑ vasospasm; CCBs ↓ vasospasm
Key Points:	Use of local anesthetics containing vasoconstrictors (e.g., epinephrine) ↑ vasoconstriction and may produce ischemia

LEVODOPA (L-DOPA), CARBIDOPA

Trade Names:	**Dopar, Larodopa (levodopa), Sinemet (L-dopa/carbidopa), Stalevo (L-dopa, carbidopa, entacapone)**
Indications:	Parkinson's disease, myoclonus
Pharmacokinetics:	Onset: 0.5–1 h; peak: 1–3 h; duration: 5 h; $T_{1/2}$ β: 1–3 h; decarboxylated in plasma L-amino acid decarboxylase, extensive 1st-pass hepatic metabolism, excreted in urine
Pharmacodynamics:	Converted to dopamine in basal ganglia, stimulates dopaminergic receptors in basal ganglia; *carbidopa* inhibits peripheral decarboxylation of L-dopa; entacapone inhibits COMT
CNS:	↓ Tremor, rigidity, and bradykinesia; prolactin secretion, anxiety, confusion, dizziness, fatigue, hallucinations, ↑ facial expression
CV:	Orthostatic hypotension, arrhythmias, flushing
GI:	↓ Gastric emptying, anorexia, nausea/vomiting, bruxism, dysphagia, sialorrhea, ↑ LFTs
Pulmonary:	Hyperventilation, hiccups
Dosage:	25/250 mg or 25/100 mg PO tid (max. 8/d)
Contraindications:	Use with MAOIs; severe cardiovascular disease, acute angle-closure glaucoma, melanoma
Drug Interactions:	Pyridoxine ↑ extracellular metabolism; antipsychotic drugs cause parkinsonism-like effect; MAOIs ↑ central hypertension and fever; antihypertensives ↑ hypotension; droperidol ↓ effect
Key Points:	Use with epinephrine and β-agonists; ↑ risk of arrhythmias with volatile anesthetics; discontinue L-dopa 6–8 h prior to elective surgery; use of anticholinergics ↑ efficacy, while benzodiazepines, anticonvulsants ↓ efficacy

MEMANTINE

Trade Name:	**Namenda**
Indications:	Dementia, Alzheimer's disease
Pharmacokinetics:	Peak: 3–7 h; protein binding: 45%; Vd: 10 L/kg; $T_{1/2}$ β: 60–80 h; minimal metabolism, renal tubular secretion in urine
Pharmacodynamics:	Open-channel NMDA and 5-HT$_3$ antagonist
CNS:	Dizziness, syncope, TIA
CV:	↑ BP
GI:	Constipation
Other:	Hypothermia, allergic reactions
Dosage:	5 mg/d PO (max. 20 mg/d)
Contraindications:	NK
Drug Interactions:	Carbonic anhydrase inhibitors and sodium bicarbonate ↓ clearance; ↑ amantadine effect
Key Points:	May ↑ effect of NMDA antagonists (e.g., ketamine and dextromethorphan)

METHYLPHENIDATE, DEXTROAMPHETAMINE

Trade Names:	**Adderall, Desoxyn, Dexedrine (dextroamphetamine), Concerta, Metadate, Ritalin, Ritalin-SR (methylphenidate)**
Indications:	Attention-deficit hyperactivity disorder (ADHD), narcolepsy
Pharmacokinetics:	Onset: <30 min; peak: 2–4 h; duration: 24 h; $T_{1/2}$ β: 2–15 h; metabolized by liver, excreted in urine
Pharmacodynamics:	Blocks reuptake at dopaminergic neurons; CNS stimulation
CNS:	Enhanced concentration, ↓ seizure threshold, blurred vision
CV:	Arrhythmias, ↑ BP, ↑ HR, angina
GI:	Diarrhea, nausea, vomiting, cramps, anorexia
Other:	Fever, rash, thrombocytopenia, muscle cramps
Dosages:	*Methylphenidate:* 5–30 mg/d PO *Dextroamphetamine:* 5–60 mg/d PO
Contraindications:	Marked anxiety, agitation, Tourette's syndrome, MAOI usage
Drug Interactions:	↓ Efficacy of antihypertensives; β-blockers ↑ α-adrenergic stimulation; meperidine causes coma, convulsions, fever (NMS); MAOIs ↑ CV stimulation

METHYLPHENIDATE, DEXTROAMPHETAMINE *continued*

Key Points:	Carefully monitor hemodynamic variables due to potential interactions with adjunctive CV drugs during surgery

MODAFINIL

Trade Name:	**Provigil**
Indications:	Narcolepsy, shift work sleep disorder, postoperative fatigue
Pharmacokinetics:	Onset: 1 h; peak: 2–4 h; protein binding: 60%; duration: 24 h; $T_{1/2}$ β: 15 h (L-isomer × D-isomer); metabolized in liver, excreted in urine
Pharmacodynamics:	Promotes wakefulness analogous to sympathomimetics
CNS:	Headache, nervousness, dizziness, insomnia, ataxia, paresthesia, tremor, amblyopia, psychotic episodes
CV:	Arrhythmias, ↑ BP, orthostatic hypotension (↓ PVR), ischemia
GI:	Nausea, vomiting, dyspepsia, anorexia, diarrhea
GU:	Urine retention, abnormal ejaculation
Pulmonary:	Dyspnea, wheezing, rhinitis
Other:	Hyperglycemia, eosinophilia, "restless legs"
Dosage:	100–200 mg/d PO in the morning (max. 400 mg/d)
Contraindications:	Angina, tachyarrhythmias, LV failures, mitral valve prolapse
Drug Interactions:	Hepatic P_{450} inducers and inhibitors alter drug's level, ↓ effects of hormonal contraceptives; ↑ levels of TCAs, phenytoin, warfarin, and diazepam
Key Points:	↑ Anesthetic requirement and arrhythmias; recommend discontinuing prior to day of surgery; may ↓ postoperative fatigue when given after surgery

NICOTINE

Trade Names:	**Habitrol, Nicoderm, Nicotrol, Nicorette**
Indications:	Smoking cessation
Pharmacokinetics:	Onset: 15–30 min (oral), 5–6 h (TTS); peak: 1–2 h (oral), 3–9 h (TTS); protein binding: 5%; Vd: 2.5 L/kg; Cl: 1.2 L/min; $T_{1/2}$ β: 1–3 h; metabolized by liver, kidney, and lungs, excreted in urine
Pharmacodynamics:	Cholinergic nicotinic receptor antagonist
CNS:	Tremor, seizure, paresthesias

NICOTINE *continued*

CV:	↑ HR, ↑ BP (↑ PVR)
GI:	Nausea, vomiting
Pulmonary:	↑ Bronchial secretions, ↑ ventilation, dyspnea, pharyngitis
Other:	Myalgias, arthralgias
Dosage:	10 pieces of 2 mg gum/d; 2 sprays in each nostril 15–21 mg/d TTS
Contraindications:	Angina, arrhythmias, acute MI, pregnancy
Drug Interactions:	↑ Absorption of insulin; ↑ effects of sympathomimetic amines
Key Points:	Carefully monitor cardiovascular variables due to potential interactions with adjunctive drugs during perioperative period; remove TTS patch 6–12 h prior to surgery

PEMOLINE

Trade Names:	**Cylert, PemADD**
Indications:	Narcolepsy, ADHD
Pharmacokinetics:	Onset: <1 h; peak: 2–4 h; protein binding: 50%; duration: 12–24 h; $T_{1/2}$ β: 12 h; metabolized by liver, excreted 1° in urine
Pharmacodynamics:	CNS stimulant (analeptic)
CNS:	Insomnia, irritability, fatigue, seizures, dyskinesia, hallucinations
GI:	Anorexia, nausea, ↑ LFTs
Other:	Aplastic anemia, rash
Dosage:	18.75–75 mg/d (max. 112.5 mg/d); 50–200 mg/d (narcolepsy)
Contraindications:	Severe hepatorenal impairment
Drug Interactions:	Caffeine ↓ efficacy; ↑ anticonvulsants (due to ↓ seizure threshold)
Key Points:	Potential for intraoperative cardiovascular instability requires careful titration of volatile anesthetics

PERGOLIDE

Trade Name:	**Permax**
Indications:	Parkinson's disease
Pharmacokinetics:	Onset: <1 h; peak: 2–3 h; protein binding: 90%; $T_{1/2}$ β: 24 h; hepatic metabolism, excreted in urine

PERGOLIDE *continued*

Pharmacodynamics:	Ergot alkaloid, dopaminergic agonist at D_1 and D_2 sites
CNS:	Dyskinesia, dizziness, dystonia, confusion
CV:	Arrhythmias, angina, MI, edema
GI:	Nausea, constipation
Other:	UTI
Dosage:	0.05–3 mg/d PO
Contraindications:	Severe arrhythmias, sensitivity to ergot derivatives
Drug Interactions:	↓ Effects of dopamine antagonists (phenothiazines, butyrophenones, thioxanthines, metoclopramide); displaces highly protein bound drugs
Key Points:	Use of metoclopramide, droperidol, and physostigmine during anesthesia may worsen postoperative parkinsonian symptoms

PRAMIPEXOLE

Trade Name:	**Mirapex**
Indications:	Parkinson's disease
Pharmacokinetics:	Onset: <1 h; bioavailability: 90%; peak: 2 h; protein binding: <20%; duration: 8–12 h; Vd: 500 L; $T_{1/2}$ β: 8–12 h; minimal metabolism, excreted 1° in urine
Pharmacodynamics:	Dopamine agonist with intrinsic activity at the D_2 and D_3 receptors
CNS:	Hallucinations, drowsiness, insomnia, asthenia, dyskinesia
CV:	↓ BP, ↑ HR
GI:	Anorexia, nausea
Other:	Edema, fever, pneumonia
Dosage:	0.375–4.5 mg/d PO in divided doses
Contraindications:	Elderly with renal impairment
Drug Interactions:	Cimetidine, diltiagen, quinidine, ranitidine ↓ clearance; dopamine antagonist ↓ efficacy; ↑ L-dopa levels
Key Points:	↑ CNS depressant effects of anesthetic drugs

SELEGILINE

Trade Names:	**Atapryl, Carbex, Eldepryl, Selpak**
Indications:	Parkinson's disease (with levodopa)
Pharmacokinetics:	Onset: <0.5–2 h; bioavailability: 10%; peak: 1 h; protein binding: 94%; duration: 12 h; hepatic metabolism, excreted in urine

SELEGILINE *continued*

Pharmacodynamics:	Irreversible inhibition of MAOIs (type B), ↑ central dopamine levels
CNS:	Hallucinations, confusion, agitation, dyskinesia, mood changes, dizziness, drowsiness
CV:	Hypertensive crisis, angina, arrhythmias, ↓ HR, edema
GI:	Dry mouth, bleeding, abdominal pain
Other:	Urinary retention, BPH, wheezing, ↓ motor activity
Dosage:	5 mg PO bid (max. 10 mg/d)
Contraindications:	Peptic ulcer disease, use of meperidine
Drug Interactions:	Fluoxetine produces "serotonin syndrome" (i.e., confusion, myoclonus, hyperreflexia, fever, convulsions); meperidine and other MAOIs can cause NMS; TCAs and tyramine cause hypertensive crisis, ↑ side effects of levodopa; ↑ BP response to vasopressors
Key Points:	Use with high-dose opioid-based anesthesia techniques will ↑ complications during perioperative period

SUMATRIPTAN

Trade Name:	**Imitrex**
Indications:	Acute migraine headache
Pharmacokinetics:	Onset: <30 min; bioavailability: 15%; peak: 1–2 h; protein binding: 18%; $T_{1/2}$ β: 2 h; metabolized in liver, excreted in urine
Pharmacodynamics:	Selectively binds to 5-HT$_1$ receptor
CNS:	Dizziness, drowsiness, anxiety, weakness
CV:	Arrhythmias, angina, ↑ PVR
GI:	Nausea, vomiting, dysphagia, unusual taste
Other:	Tingling, burning sensations, flushing, muscle cramps
Dosage:	6 mg IM/SC bid; 25–100 mg PO bid (max. 200 mg/d); 0.1 mL nasal spray
Contraindications:	Use of MAOIs and ergotamines, uncontrolled hypertension, coronary artery disease (angina)
Drug Interactions:	Ergots ↑ vasospastic effects; MAOIs ↑ effects; SSRIs ↑ risk of weakness, hyperreflexia, and incoordination
Key Points:	Sympathomimetic drugs (e.g., phenylephrine) will accentuate ↑ peripheral vascular resistance and can cause life-threatening arrhythmias

THEOPHYLLINE

Trade Names: **Respbid, Quibron, Slo-Phyllin, Theox**

See Chapter 18, "Bronchodilators"

TRIHEXYPHENIDYL, BENZTROPINE, BIPERIDEN, ETHOPROPAZINE, PROCYCLIDINE

Trade Names: **Artane (trihexyphenidyl), Akineton (biperiden), Cogentin (benztropine), Kemadrin (procyclidine), Parsidol (ethopropazine)**

Indications: Idiopathic parkinsonism, drug-induced extrapyramidal reactions

Pharmacokinetics: Onset: 0.5–1 h; peak: 2–7 h; duration: 4–12 h; $T_{1/2}$ β: 6–10 h; hepatic metabolism, excreted 1° in urine

Pharmacodynamics: Blockade of central (striatal) cholinergic receptors
CNS: ↓ Tremor, blurred vision, ↑ IOP, confusion, delirium, dizziness
CV: ↑ HR, arrhythmia
GI: Dry mouth, constipation, nausea
Other: Urinary retention, ↓ airway secretions

Dosages: *Trihexyphenidyl:* 2–15 mg/d PO
Benztropine: 0.5–6 mg/d PO
Biperiden: 5 mg/mL, 2–8 mg/d PO
Ethopropazine: 50–600 mg/d PO
Procyclidine: 7.5–20 mg/d PO

Contraindications: Glaucoma, tardive dyskinesia, myasthenia gravis, cardiovascular instability, intestinal obstruction, urinary retention

Drug Interactions: Alcohol ↑ sedation; opioids, phenothiazines, TCA, antihistamines, produce central anticholinergic syndrome; antacids ↓ bioavailability

Key Points: Ensure adequate humidification of gases; use with anesthetics or hypnotics can ↑ CNS depressant effect and ↑ recovery

21

Cholinesterase Inhibitors

Cholinesterase Inhibitors

BETHANECHOL

Trade Names:	**Duvoid, Urecholine**
Indications:	Postoperative or postpartum period, nonobstructive urinary retention, neurogenic atony of bladder with retention
Pharmacokinetics:	Onset: 30–90 min; duration: 6 h PO, 2 h SC; unknown metabolism
Pharmacodynamics:	Stimulation of parasympathetic nervous system, ↑ release of acetylcholine at nerve endings
CNS:	Dizziness, headache, seizures
CV:	Hypotension with reflex tachycardia
GI:	Abdominal cramping, diarrhea, nausea, vomiting
Pulmonary:	Wheezing, bronchoconstriction
Other:	Flushing, sweating, body ache
Dosage:	5–50 mg PO q 6–12 h
Contraindications:	Hyperthyroidism, peptic ulcer disease, asthma, ↓ HR, coronary artery disease, parkinsonism, epilepsy, GI obstruction (mechanical)
Drug Interactions:	With ganglionic-blocking agents, combination may lead to precipitous fall in BP; procainamide or quinidine antagonizes anticholinergic activity; anticholinesterase drugs ↑ effect
Key Points:	Use of muscle relaxants and their reversal in patients receiving bethanechol should be based on use of nerve-muscle stimulator

CARBACHOLINE (CARBAMOYLCHOLINE)

Trade Names:	**Miostat Intraocular, Isopto Carbachol, Carbastat, Carboptic**
Indications:	Reduction of IOP in open-angle glaucoma and emergency treatment of angle-closure glaucoma prior to surgery
Pharmacokinetics:	After topical administration, miosis occurs within 10–20 min and persists 4–8 h; max. reduction in IOP within 2 h; after intraocular injection, peak effect for miosis is 2–5 min and lasts 24 h
Pharmacodynamics:	Stimulates motor end-plate of muscle cell and inhibits cholinesterase
CNS:	Seizures, headaches
CV:	↓ HR, ↓ BP
GI:	Nausea, vomiting, cramps
Pulmonary:	Bronchoconstriction, excessive secretions
Other:	Blurred vision, painful ciliary spasm, myalgias, weakness

CARBACHOLINE
(CARBAMOYLCHOLINE) *continued*

Dosage:	1–2 drops q 8 h 0.75–3%
Contraindications:	Risk of retinal detachment; hypersensitivity to miotics; acute iritis; caution in asthma, corneal abrasions, hyperthyroidism, urinary tract obstruction, severe coronary artery disease
Drug Interactions:	Additive effects in combination with topical epinephrine, timolol, or carbonic anhydrases
Key Points:	No interaction with anesthetic drugs reported

DEMECARIUM

Trade Name:	**Humorsol**
Indications:	Glaucoma and convergent strabismus
Pharmacokinetics:	Miosis: <30 min; max. miosis: 2–4 h; persists: 3–10 d; max. reduction in ↓ IOP: <24 h
Pharmacodynamics:	Inhibition of cholinesterase
CNS:	Headache, vertigo
CV:	↓ HR, ↓ BP
Pulmonary:	Bronchoconstriction, secretions, nasal congestion
Other:	Urinary frequency, nausea, diarrhea, cramping, muscle weakness
Dosages:	*Glaucoma:* 1–2 gtt 0.125–0.25% 2–10×/wk
	Strabismus: 1 gtt qd for 2–3 wk
Contraindications:	Risk of retinal detachment, hypersensitivity to miotics, marked vagotonia, asthma, hyperthyroidism, cardiac failure
Drug Interactions:	↑ Effects with ocular hypotensive agents, systemic cholinesterase inhibitors, general anesthetic agents; hyperactivity in patients with Down syndrome; ↓ effects of nondepolarizing muscle relaxants
Key Points:	Use with succinylcholine may produce a prolonged paralysis and requires careful neuromuscular blockade monitoring

DONEPEZIL

Trade Name:	**Aricept**
Indications:	Alzheimer's disease

DONEPEZIL *continued*

Pharmacokinetics:	Bioavailability: 100%; peak plasma concentrations: 3–4 h; $T_{1/2} \beta$: 70 h; plasma protein binding: 90%; Vd: 12 L/kg; metabolized by liver, excreted in urine
Pharmacodynamics:	↑ Acetylcholine via reversible inhibition of its hydrolysis by acetylcholinesterase
GI:	Upset, anorexia, nausea, diarrhea
Other:	Insomnia, muscle cramps
Dosage:	5–10 mg/d PO
Contraindications:	NK
Drug Interactions:	Inducers of CYP 2D6 and CYP 3A4 (e.g., phenytoin, carbamazepine, dexamethasone, rifampin, phenobarbital), ↑ elimination
Key Points:	Exaggerates succinylcholine-type muscle relaxation during anesthesia; careful neuromuscular blockade monitoring required

ECHOTHIOPHATE

Trade Name:	**Phospholine**
Indications:	Open-angle glaucoma and convergent strabismus
Pharmacokinetics:	Onset: 10 min–8 h; persists: >24 h; ↓ IOP: >4–8 h; max. reduction of IOP within 24 h; bound to serum and ocular tissues; oxidized and hydrolyzed by phosphoryl phosphatases
Pharmacodynamics:	Long-acting inhibition of cholinesterase
CNS:	Headache, vertigo, hyperactivity in Down syndrome
CV:	↓ HR, ↓ BP
Pulmonary:	Bronchoconstriction, secretions, nasal congestion
Other:	Urinary frequency, nausea, diarrhea, cramping, muscle weakness
Dosage:	1.5–12.5 mg (0.03–0.25%); 1 gtt q 12–48 h
Contraindications:	Risk of retinal detachment, hypersensitivity to miotics, marked vagotonia, asthma, hyperthyroidism, cardiac failure
Drug Interactions:	↑ Effect with ocular hypotensive agents, systemic cholinesterase inhibitors, general anesthetic agents; ↓ effects of nondepolarizing muscle relaxants
Key Points:	Use with succinylcholine requires neuromuscular blockade monitoring due to possibility of prolonged paralysis

EDROPHONIUM

Trade Names:	**Tensilon, Enlon, Reversol**
Indications:	Differential diagnosis of myasthenia gravis (MG), evaluation of emergency treatment of myasthenic crisis, reversal of neuromuscular blockade
Pharmacokinetics:	Onset: within 60 sec (IV); duration: 5–20 min (IV); Vd: 1.1 L/kg; CrCl: 9.6 mL/min/kg; $T_{1/2}$ β: 110 min
Pharmacodynamics:	↓ Acetylcholinesterase at sites of cholinergic transmission
CNS:	Convulsions, dysarthria, dysphonia, dysphasia
CV:	↓ HR, ↓ CO
GI:	↑ Salivary and gastric secretions, nausea, vomiting, ↑ peristalsis, cramping
Pulmonary:	↑ Secretions, laryngospasm, bronchiolar constriction
Other:	Muscle weakness, fasciculations
Dosages:	*MG:* 10–40 mg IV *Reversal:* 0.5–1.0 mg/kg IV (+ atropine)
Contraindications:	Asthma, urinary tract or intestinal obstruction, cardiac dysrhythmias
Drug Interactions:	Digitalis ↑ vagomimetic effects on heart; with succinylcholine causes prolonged phase 1 block of depolarizing muscle relaxants; mimics symptoms of anticholinesterase overdose with anticholinesterase drugs
Key Points:	Neuromuscular blockade monitoring required during anesthesia

GALANTAMINE

Trade Name:	**Reminyl**
Indications:	Alzheimer's disease
Pharmacokinetics:	Bioavailability: 90%; $T_{1/2}$ β: 7 h; Vd: 175 L; metabolized by liver isoenzymes, excreted in urine
Pharmacodynamics:	Competitive, reversible, centrally active cholinesterase inhibitor
GI:	Nausea, vomiting, anorexia, diarrhea
Dosage:	4–8 mg PO bid
Contraindications:	NK
Drug Interactions:	Ketoconazole, paroxetine ↑ galantamine level
Key Points:	↑ Blockade of depolarizing muscle relaxant (succinylcholine)

ISOFLUROPHATE

Trade Name:	**Floropryl**
Indications:	Glaucoma, convergent strabismus
Pharmacokinetics:	Miosis occurs after 5–10 min, max. miosis after 15–20 min; persists for 1–4 wk; max. reduction in IOP within 24 h; rapidly decomposes with moisture to hydrogen fluoride
Pharmacodynamics:	Long-acting inhibition of cholinesterase
CNS:	Headache, vertigo
CV:	↓ HR, ↓ BP
GI:	Nausea, diarrhea, cramping
Pulmonary:	Bronchoconstriction, secretions, nasal congestion
Renal:	Urinary frequency
Dosages:	*Glaucoma:* 0.5 cm 0.25% ointment every 8–72 h *Convergent strabismus:* 0.5 cm hs
Contraindications:	Risk of retinal detachment, hypersensitivity to miotics, marked vagotonia, asthma, hyperthyroidism, cardiac failure
Drug Interactions:	↑ Effects with ocular hypotensive agents, systemic cholinesterase inhibitors, some general anesthetic agents
Key Points:	Use with succinylcholine may produce prolonged paralysis

NEOSTIGMINE

Trade Name:	**Prostigmin**
Indications:	Myasthenia gravis (MG); reversal of effects of nondepolarizing neuromuscular blocking agents; postoperative distention and urinary retention (without mechanical obstruction)
Pharmacokinetics:	Onset: 50 min (PO), 4–8 min (IV); peak: 1–2 h; duration: 2–4 h; Vd: 1.0 L/kg; Cl: 9.6 mL/min/kg; $T_{1/2}$ β: 104 min; metabolized by liver, excreted in urine
Pharmacodynamics:	Inhibits hydrolysis of acetylcholine by acetylcholinesterase; ↑ cholinergic stimulation at myoneural junction
CNS:	Dizziness, convulsions, headache, miosis, visual changes
CV:	Arrhythmias (↑ HR, ↓ HR, AV block, nodal rhythm), ↓ BP, cardiac arrest
GI:	Nausea, emesis, flatulence, ↑ peristalsis
Pulmonary:	↑ Secretions, respiratory depression, bronchospasm
Other:	Rash, urticaria, urinary frequency, muscle cramps

NEOSTIGMINE *continued*

Dosages:	*MG:* 15 mg PO q 6–8 h (adults); 2 mg/kg/d (children) *Reversal of neuromuscular blockade:* 50–70 μg/kg IV (adults); 0.01–0.04 mg/kg IV/IM (children)
Contraindications:	Peritonitis or mechanical obstruction of GI tract
Drug Interactions:	↑ Nondepolarizing muscle relaxant dose for adequate paralysis; prolonged phase 1 block of depolarizing muscle relaxants ↑ effects of β-blockers
Key Points:	Adequate fluid replacement with concomitant use of vasodilating anesthetics; manipulation of the airway may precipitate bronchospasm; monitor adequacy of reversal

PHYSOSTIGMINE

Trade Names:	**Antilirium, Eserine**
Indications:	Glaucoma, atropine intoxication, TCA intoxication, postoperative somnolence, reversal of nondepolarizing muscle relaxation
Pharmacokinetics:	Onset: 3–5 min; duration: 0.5–5 h; $T_{1/2}$ α: 20–30 min; tertiary amine; crosses blood-brain barrier; destroyed by hydrolysis at ester linkage
Pharmacodynamics:	↑ Acetylcholine at site of cholinergic transmission
CNS:	Anxiety, delirium, hallucinations, seizures, blurred vision, miosis
CV:	↓ HR, ↓ BP
GI:	Emesis, diarrhea, nausea, hypersalivation
Pulmonary:	Bronchoconstriction
Other:	Urinary urgency, muscle fasciculation/weakness, diaphoresis
Dosages:	*Neuromuscular reversal:* 0.5–1 mg IM/IV (adults); 0.02 g/kg IM (children); *glaucoma:* 0.25% ointment tid
Contraindications:	Asthma, gangrene, diabetes, obstruction, corneal injury
Drug Interactions:	Echothiophate ↓ duration of action; belladonna alkaloids ↓ antiglaucoma, miotic action; succinylcholine prolongs phase 1 block of depolarizing muscle relaxants; atropine ↓ effects of nondepolarizing muscle relaxants
Key Points:	Avoid vasodilating anesthetics; patients with Parkinson's disease ↑ central cholinergic tone, exacerbating parkinsonian symptoms

PILOCARPINE

Trade Names:	**Salagen, Pilagan, Ocusert**
Indications:	Xerostomia, glaucoma
Pharmacokinetics:	Onset: 20 min; peak: 1 h; duration: 3–8 h; metabolized in neuronal synapses and in plasma, excreted in urine
Pharmacodynamics:	↑ Salivary gland secretions; ↑ cholinergic receptors in iris sphincter muscles (miosis), vasodilation of conjunctival vessels
CNS:	Dizziness, headache, tremor, asthenia, lacrimation, amblyopia
CV:	↑ BP, ↑ HR, edema
GI:	Nausea/vomiting, diarrhea, dysphagia
Other:	Myalgia, anaphylaxis, urinary frequency
Dosage:	5–10 mg tid PO; 0.25–8% solution, 1–2 gtt q 4–12 h
Contraindications:	Acute iritis, acute inflammatory disease of the anterior chamber, asthma, diabetes; obstruction of intestinal or urogenital tract; choline esters or depolarizing neuromuscular blockers
Drug Interactions:	Cholinergic drugs ↑ toxicity
Key Points:	Use with succinylcholine prolongs respiratory depression

PYRIDOSTIGMINE

Trade Names:	**Regonol, Mestinon**
Indications:	MG, postoperative urinary retention, antagonism of nondepolarizing muscle relaxants
Pharmacokinetics:	Duration of anticholinesterase activity may be prolonged in elderly; Vd: 1.1 L/kg; Cl: 8.6 mL/min/kg; $T_{1/2}$ β: 112 min
Pharmacodynamics:	Inhibits breakdown of acetylcholine by cholinesterase
CNS:	Confusion, seizures, nervousness, miosis
CV:	↓ HR, ↓ BP
GI:	Cramping, nausea, vomiting, diarrhea
Pulmonary:	Wheezing, ↑ secretions
Other:	Weakness, muscle cramping
Dosages:	*Antimyasthenic:* IV or IM, 10–20 mg/70 kg (adults); oral, 60–180 mg bid or qid (adults); IM, 0.05–0.15 mg/kg q 4–6 h (children) *Reversal:* 10–20 mg IV (with atropine 0.6–1.2 mg IV)
Contraindications:	Asthma, pneumonia, cardiac dysrhythmias, intestinal obstruction

PYRIDOSTIGMINE *continued*

Drug Interactions:	↓ Metabolism of ester-type local anesthetics; succinyl-choline prolongs phase 1 block; quinine, enflurane, halothane, aminoglycosides ↓ antimyasthenic effect on skeletal muscle; high doses of nondepolarizing muscle relaxants necessary for adequate paralysis
Key Points:	Adequate fluid replacement with concomitant use of vasodilating anesthetics; manipulation of airway may precipitate bronchospasm

TACRINE, RIVASTIGMINE

Trade Names:	**Cognex (tacrine), Exelon (rivastigmine)**
Indications:	Degenerative dementia (Alzheimer's type)
Pharmacokinetics:	*Tacrine:* Peak: 1–2 h; plasma protein binding: 55%; Vd: 349 L; $T_{1/2}$ β: 2–4 h; metabolized by liver *Rivastigmine:* Bioavailability: 36%; peak: 1 h; protein binding: 40%; duration: 12 h; $T_{1/2}$ β: 1.5 h; metabolized in liver, excreted in urine
Pharmacodynamics:	Centrally active, reversible, cholinesterase inhibitor, ↑ acetylcholine concentrations in cerebral cortex
CNS:	Headache, fatigue, agitation
GI:	Nausea, vomiting, diarrhea, anorexia, ↓ weight, ↑ LFTs
Other:	Rash, UTI
Dosages:	*Tacrine:* 10 mg qid for 4 wk, followed by 20 mg qid *Rivastigmine:* 1.5–3 mg bid
Contraindications:	Jaundice (bilirubin >3 mg/dL)
Drug Interactions:	↑ Symptoms of Parkinson's disease; ↑ effect other cholinergics; ↓ theophylline metabolism; fluvoxamine and cimetidine ↑ tacrine
Key Points:	Succinylcholine blockade may be prolonged

22

Dermatologic Drugs

ALUMINUM SALTS

Trade Names:	**Bluburo, Boropak, Burow's, Domeboro**
Indications:	Skin irritations/inflammation, contact dermatoses
Pharmacokinetics:	NK
Pharmacodynamics:	Astringent action ↓ friction
Dosage:	Apply to loose dressing q 15–30 min for 4–8 h
Contraindications:	Eyes, mucous membranes
Key Points:	Avoid use with occlusive dressings

ANTHRALIN

Trade Names:	**Drithocreme, Dritho-Scalp, Lasan**
Indications:	Psoriasis, alopecia areata
Pharmacokinetics:	Minimal absorption
Pharmacodynamics:	Antipsoriatic activity
Other:	Conjunctivitis
Dosage:	0.1–1%; apply 1–2×/d
Contraindications:	Acute eruptions, skin inflammation, facial application
Drug Interactions:	Photosensitizing effects, skin rash
Key Points:	No known interactions with anesthetic drugs

AZELAIC ACID

Trade Names:	**Azelex, Finacea**
Indications:	Acne, rosacea
Pharmacokinetics:	Systemic absorption: 4%; $T_{1/2}$ β: 12 h; excreted unchanged
Pharmacodynamics:	Inhibits microbial cellular protein synthesis
Pulmonary:	Wheezing
Other:	Hypopigmentation, pruritis, erythema, dry skin
Dosage:	3–5% topical cream
Contraindications:	Sensitivity to cream or lotion
Drug Interactions:	NK
Key Points:	No reported interactions with anesthetic drugs

BENZALKONIUM

Trade Names: **Benza, Mycocide NS, Ony-Clear, Zephiran**

Indications: Disinfection

Pharmacokinetics: NK

Pharmacodynamics: Cationic, bacteriostatic, or bactericidal effect

Dosage: 1:750 tincture or spray (unbroken skin); 1:5–10,000 solution (mucous membranes or denuded skin); 1:3–20,000 solution (irrigation)

Contraindications: Occlusive dressings or packs; skin inflammation (↓ concentration)

Key Points: Inactivated by anionic compounds (e.g., soap)

BENZOIN TINCTURE COMPOUND

Trade Name: **Same**

Indications: Demulcent and protectant (cutaneous ulcers, bedsores, cracked nipples, lip and anal fissures)

Pharmacokinetics: NK

Pharmacodynamics: Protects via coating actions

Dosage: Apply 1–2 times/d

Key Points: Useful in protecting skin from adhesive

BENZOYL PEROXIDE

Trade Names: **Desquam, Ben-Aqua, Benzac, PanOxyl, Clearasil, Noxzema**

Indications: Acne vulgaris, decubital (or stasis) ulcers

Pharmacokinetics: Absorption via skin, 5% excreted as benzoic acid in urine

Pharmacodynamics: Keratolytic activity
  Skin: Rash, feeling of warmth, drying effect

Dosage: 2.5–20%; apply to skin 1–4×/d

Contraindications: Acute skin inflammation, denuded skin

Drug Interactions: Skin irritation from peeling, desquamating, or abrasive agents

Key Points: No known adverse interaction with anesthetic drugs

CAPSAICIN

Trade Name:	**Zostrix**
Indications:	Reflex sympathetic dystrophy, herpes zoster, neuropathic pain
Pharmacokinetics:	NK
Pharmacodynamics:	↓ Painful impulses by depleting and preventing reaccumulation of substance P (neurokinin-1) in peripheral sensory C-fibers
CNS:	Analgesia (topical)
GI:	Antiemetic activity (at P_6 acupoint)
Dosage:	0.025–0.075%; apply 3–4×/d
Contraindications:	Intraocular use, open skin surface
Drug Interactions:	↑ Coughing with ACE inhibitors
Key Points:	Burning sensation on initial application

CHLOROXINE

Trade Name:	**Capitrol**
Indications:	Seborrheic dermatitis (dandruff)
Pharmacokinetics:	Absorption through scalp
Pharmacodynamics:	Antibacterial, antifungal, antiseborrheic activity
Dosage:	2% shampoo; apply to scalp twice/wk
Contraindications:	Acute inflammation, exudative scalp lesions
Drug Interactions:	NK
Key Points:	No known interaction with anesthetic drugs

CLOBETASOL

Trade Names:	**Olux (foam), Temovate (cream)**
Indications:	Dermatoses, psoriasis, atopic dermatitis (scalp)
Pharmacokinetics:	Metabolized in skin, small amounts excreted in urine and feces
Pharmacodynamics:	Analog of prednisolone, anti-inflammatory antipruritic actions
Skin:	Burning, pruritus, dryness, erythema, ↓ pigmentation
Other:	Folliculitis, hyperglycemia, Cushing's syndrome, ↓ hypothalamic-pituitary-adrenal (HPA) axis
Dosage:	0.05% solution/gel ointment; apply to affected area twice/d

CLOBETASOL *continued*

Contraindications:	Suppression, HPA axis, pregnancy, breast-feeding
Drug Interactions:	NK
Key Points:	Check perioperative glucose levels; consider corticosteroid supplementation

COAL TAR

Trade Names:	**Alphosyl, Aquatar, DHS Tar**
Indications:	Seborrheic dermatitis, atopic dermatitis, eczema, psoriasis
Pharmacokinetics:	NK
Pharmacodynamics:	Antipsoriatic and antiseborrheic activity
CV:	Vasoconstriction (topical)
Dosage:	1–25% solution; apply to skin 1–4×/d
Contraindications:	Acute inflammation, open wounds, skin infections
Drug Interactions:	↑ Photosensitizing effects of other drugs
Key Points:	No known adverse interactions with anesthetic drugs

DEXPANTHENOL

Trade Names:	**Ilopan, Panthoderm**
	See Chapter 24, "Gastrointestinals"

ECONAZOLE

Trade Name:	**Spectazole**
Indications:	Cutaneous candidiasis, tinea infections
Pharmacokinetics:	Rapid percutaneous absorption, minimal systemic effect
Pharmacodynamics:	Alters cellular membranes, interferes with intracellular enzymes
Skin:	Burning, pruritus, erythema, rash
Dosage:	1% cream; apply to affected areas twice/d
Contraindications:	NK
Drug Interactions:	Corticosteroids ↓ antifungal activity
Key Points:	No interactions with anesthetic drugs

ETRETINATE

Trade Name:	**Tegison**
Indications:	Psoriasis, lichen planus
Pharmacokinetics:	Absorption in small intestine; highly protein bound; $T_{1/2}$ β: >4 mo; 1st-pass metabolism to active form, excreted 1° in feces
Pharmacodynamics: *CNS:* *GI:* *Other:*	Retinoid with antiseborrheic activity Mood changes Nausea, ↑ LFTs, hepatic fibrosis, cirrhosis Hyperostosis, ↑ lipid level
Dosage:	0.75–1.0 mg/kg/d (10–25 mg) PO, then 0.5–0.75 mg/kg/d
Contraindications:	Diabetes, severe cardiovascular or hepatic disease, hypertriglyceridemia, sensitivity to vitamin A, pregnancy
Drug Interactions:	Alcohol ↑ hypertriglyceridemia; ↑ toxic effects by isotretinoin, tretinoin, vitamin A; tetracycline ↑ pseudotumor cerebri
Key Points:	Avoid anesthetics drugs, which can cause liver damage

FLUOCINONIDE

Trade Names:	**Lidemol, Lidex, Lyderm**
Indications:	Dermatoses
Pharmacokinetics:	Widely distributed, metabolized 1° in skin (small amount absorbed into systemic circulation), excreted in urine and feces
Pharmacodynamics: *Skin:* *Other:*	↓ Inflammatory response Burning, dryness, hypopigmentation, erythema, acne Hyperglycemia, Cushing's syndrome
Dosage:	0.05% cream; apply 2–3×/d
Contraindications:	NK
Drug Interactions:	NK
Key Points:	No interactions with anesthetic drugs

HEXACHLOROPHENE

Trade Names:	**pHisoHex, Septisol**
Indications:	Surgical scrub, skin cleanser
Pharmacokinetics:	NK

HEXACHLOROPHENE *continued*

Pharmacodynamics:	↓ Bacterial membrane–bound enzymes of gram-(+) bacteria
Dosage:	0.23–3% solution
Contraindications:	Eyes and mucous membranes, CNS irritability, infants
Key Points:	Avoid use on broken skin, on burns, under occlusive dressings

HYDROGEN PEROXIDE

Trade Name:	**Peroxyl**
Indications:	Cleaning wounds, necrotizing ulcerative gingivitis
Pharmacokinetics:	NK
Pharmacodynamics:	Oxidative antibacterial effect
Dosage:	1.5–3% solution/gel (wounds); 3% solution (ulcerative gingivitis)
Contraindications:	In closed body cavity or abscess
Key Points:	When instilled into closed body cavity, released gas cannot escape

HYDROXYPROPYL CELLULOSE

Trade Name:	**Lacrisert**
Indications:	Keratoconjunctivitis sicca, corneal erosions, exposure keratitis
Pharmacokinetics:	Not absorbed
Pharmacodynamics:	Ocular moisturizing effect
Dosage:	5 mg/mL; apply to conjunctiva once/d
Contraindications:	NK
Drug Interactions:	NK
Key Points:	No known interaction with anesthetic drugs

IODINE

Trade Names:	**Acu-dyne, Aerodine, Betadine, Betagen, Biodine, Etodine, Iodex, Operand, Polydine**
Indications:	Disinfection
Pharmacokinetics:	NK

IODINE *continued*

Pharmacodynamics: Broad-spectrum germicidal effects due to protein disruption

Dosage: 100% solution; apply prn

Contraindications: Povidone ↓ irritating effects of iodine

Key Points: Avoid ingestion; use thiosulfate as antidote

ISOTRETINOIN

Trade Name: **Accutane**

Indications: Acne vulgaris, rosacea, folliculitis, suppurative hidradenitis

Pharmacokinetics: Onset: 1–2 h; peak: 3 h; highly protein bound; $T_{1/2}$ β: 10–20 h; hepatic metabolism, excreted in urine and feces

Pharmacodynamics: Synthetic retinoid with keratolytic activity
  CNS: Mental depression (suicidal), mood changes, ocular changes
  GI: Inflammatory bowel disease, regional ileitis, bleeding gums
  GU: Proteinuria, hematuria, glomerulonephritis, abnormal menses
  Other: Hyperostosis, hypertriglyceridemia, hyperuricemia, palpitations

Dosage: 0.5–2 mg/kg/d PO in divided doses

Contraindications: Pregnancy, hypertriglyceridemia, diabetes; sensitivity to parabens

Drug Interactions: ↑ Skin irritation with alcohol-containing drugs; ↑ photosensitization of vitamin A derivatives; pseudotumor cerebri with tetracyclines

Key Points: No known interaction with anesthetic drugs

LINDANE

Trade Names: **Kwell, Bio-Well, Kildane, Kwildane, Scabene, Thionex**

Indications: Pediculosis capitis, pediculosis pubis, scabies

Pharmacokinetics: Absorption through skin. $T_{1/2}$ β: 18 h (in infants and children)

Pharmacodynamics: Scabicidal and pediculicidal activity
  CNS: Convulsions, dizziness

Dosage: 1% solution; apply to skin or scalp

LINDANE *continued*

Contraindications:	Convulsive disorders, irritated or broken skin
Drug Interactions:	↑ Absorption with other skin, scalp, or hair preparations
Key Points:	Proconvulsant, ↑ drugs with CNS-stimulating properties

MAGNESIUM

Other Name:	**Epsom Salt**
	See Chapter 7, "Anticonvulsants."

NITROFURAZONE

Trade Name:	**Furacin**
Indications:	Burns infected with gram-(+), gram-(−)organisms
Pharmacokinetics:	Minimal drug absorption with topical use
Pharmacodynamics:	Inhibits bacterial enzymes involved in carbohydrate metabolism
Skin:	Erythema, pruritus, contact dermatitis
Dosage:	0.2%; apply to affected area daily
Contraindications:	NK
Drug Interactions:	NK
Key Points:	No known interactions with anesthetic drugs

PERMETHRIN

Trade Names:	**Nix Cream Rinse, Elimite Cream**
Indications:	Pediculosis capitis, scabies
Pharmacokinetics:	Minimal absorption (2%); duration: 14 d; rapid ester hydrolysis to inactive metabolites, excreted in urine
Pharmacodynamics:	Pediculicidal activity
Skin:	Burning, itching, rash, redness, swelling, tingling of scalp
Dosage:	1–5%; apply in a single application to hair and scalp
Contraindications:	Acute scalp inflammation
Drug Interactions:	Sensitivity to chrysanthemums, pyrethrins, insecticides
Key Points:	No known adverse interactions with anesthetic drugs

PIMECROLIMUS

Trade Name:	**Elidel**
Indications:	Atopic dermatitis
Pharmacokinetics:	Minimal systemic absorption; protein binding: 80%; metabolized in liver, excreted in feces
Pharmacodynamics:	Inhibits T-cell activation by blocking cytokine transcription
CNS:	Headache, eye infection
GI:	Nausea, vomiting, diarrhea, gastroenteritis, abdominal pain
Pulmonary:	URI, cough, dyspnea, nasopharyngitis, bronchitis
Other:	Skin infections, urticaria, acne, dysmenorrhea, fever
Dosage:	1% cream; apply as thin layer to affected skin twice/d
Contraindications:	Acute cutaneous viral infections in immunocompromised patients
Drug Interactions:	Cytochrome P_{450} inhibitors ↓ metabolism (↑ levels)
Key Points:	No known interactions with anesthetic drugs

PODOPHYLLUM RESIN

Trade Names:	**Podocon, Podofin**
Indications:	Condylomata acuminatum (warts), superficial epitheliomatosis
Pharmacokinetics:	↑ Absorption via friable, bleeding, or recently biopsied warts
Pharmacodynamics:	Keratolytic activity, disruption of epithelial cell division
CNS:	Confusion, nervousness, excitement, autonomic neuropathy
GI:	Stomach pain, diarrhea, nausea, vomiting
Pulmonary:	Dyspnea
Other:	Muscle weakness, rash, pruritus
Dosage:	10–25% topical; apply to venereal warts (1/wk), epitheliomatosis and keratosis (1/d)
Contraindications:	Friable, bleeding, or recently biopsied warts; pregnancy
Drug Interactions:	NK
Key Points:	No known interactions with anesthetic drugs

PYRETHRINS, PIPERONYL BUTOXIDE

Trade Name:	**Pediculocide**
Indications:	Pediculosis corporis, capitis, pubis

PYRETHRINS, PIPERONYL BUTOXIDE *continued*

Pharmacokinetics:	Minimal absorption through intact skin
Pharmacodynamics: Other:	Pediculicidal activity Rash, sneezing, wheezing
Dosage:	0.18–0.33% (pyrethrins), 2.2–4% (piperonyl butoxide); apply to hair and scalp (repeat in 1–2 wk)
Contraindications:	Acute skin inflammation
Drug Interactions:	NK
Key Points:	No known interactions with anesthetic drugs

PYRITHIONE ZINC

Trade Names:	**Head & Shoulders, Danex, DHS Zinc**
Indications:	Seborrheic dermatitis (dandruff)
Pharmacokinetics:	Topical application
Pharmacodynamics:	Antiseborrheic, antibacterial, antifungal activity
Dosage:	1–2% cream/shampoo; apply to scalp twice/wk
Contraindications:	NK
Drug Interactions:	NK
Key Points:	No known interactions with anesthetic drugs

RESORCINOL

Trade Name:	**RA**
Indications:	Acne vulgaris, seborrheic dermatitis, eczema, psoriasis
Pharmacokinetics:	Absorption through skin or from ulcerated surfaces
Pharmacodynamics: CNS: GI: Other:	Keratolytic activity Dizziness, headache Diarrhea, nausea, abdominal pain, vomiting Methemoglobinemia, ↓ HR, dyspnea
Dosage:	2–3% (lotion) or 2–20% (ointment) and sulfur (5–8%); apply to skin
Contraindications:	NK
Drug Interactions:	Skin irritation with peeling, desquamating, or abrasive agents
Key Points:	Enhances CNS effects of β-blocking drugs in hypertensive patients

SALICYLIC ACID

Trade Names:	**Compound W, Duofilm, Freezone, Gordofilm, Hydrisalic, Keralyt, Occlusal-HP, Off-Ezy, Sal-Acid, Wart-Off**
Indications:	Scaling dermatoses, ↑ keratosis, calluses, warts
Pharmacokinetics:	NK
Pharmacodynamics:	Desquamation of cornified epithelium by ↑ hydration
Dosage:	Apply and cover with occlusive dressing qhs
Contraindications:	Aspirin-sensitive patients; contact with eye, face, genitals, mucous membranes; birthmarks, moles, hair follicle areas
Drug Interactions:	NK
Key Points:	No systemic effect; can cause topical mucosal damage

SELENIUM

Trade Names:	**Exsel, Glo-Sel, Head & Shoulders, Selsun Blue**
Indications:	Seborrheic dermatitis (dandruff), tinea versicolor
Pharmacokinetics:	Topical effect only (not absorbed)
Pharmacodynamics:	Antiseborrheic and antifungal activity
Dosage:	1–2.5% lotion; apply to scalp/body 1–2×/wk
Contraindications:	Acute dermatologic inflammation
Drug Interactions:	NK
Key Points:	No known interactions with anesthetics

SERTACONAZOLE

Trade Name:	**Ertaczo**
Indications:	Tinea pedis
Pharmacokinetics:	NK
Pharmacodynamics:	Imidazole antifungal ↓ synthesis of ergosterol in cellular membranes
Other:	Skin irritation (contact dermatitis), ↑ pigmentation
Dosage:	2% cream (0.5 g/100 cm); apply q 12 h
Contraindications:	Sensitivity to imidazoles
Drug Interactions:	NK
Key Points:	No interactions with anesthetic drugs

SULFAPYRIDINE

Trade Name:	**Dagenan**
Indications:	Dermatitis herpetiformis, pemphigoid, subcorneal pustular dermatitis, pyoderma gangrenosum
Pharmacokinetics:	Absorption incomplete; peak: 4–6 h; protein binding: ~ 50%; Vd: 0.8 L/kg; $T_{1/2}$ β: 6–14 h; hepatic metabolism, excreted in urine
Pharmacodynamics:	Inhibition of dermal cell protein synthesis
CNS:	Headache
GI:	Diarrhea, anorexia, nausea, vomiting, jaundice, ↑ LFTs
Other:	Bone marrow suppression, porphyria, fever, photosensitivity, Stevens-Johnson syndrome
Dosage:	0.25–1 g PO q 6–12 h (max. 6 g/d)
Contraindications:	Blood dyscrasias, G6PD deficiency, hepatic disorders, porphyria, renal function impairment, sulfa allergies
Drug Interactions:	Anticoagulants, anticonvulsants, antidiabetic agents, methotrexate, phenylbutazone ↑ effect (due to displacement from protein-binding sites); metabolism inhibited by sulfonamides; ↑ toxicity of hemolytics, methyldopa, methotrexate, phenytoin; cross-sensitivity with sulfonamides; ↑ sensitivity to sunlight
Key Points:	Avoid use with hepatotoxic anesthetics

SULFUR

Trade Names:	**Fostex, Finac, Fostril, Cuticura, Sulfacet**
Indications:	Acne vulgaris, seborrheic dermatitis, scabies, rosacea
Pharmacokinetics:	Topical effect
Pharmacodynamics:	Antiseborrheic, keratolytic, antibacterial activity
Dosage:	0.5–10% applied 1–3×/d
Contraindications:	Sensitivity to sulfur, renal impairment
Drug Interactions:	↑ Irritation of skin with alcohol-containing drugs; topical mercury compounds cause chemical reaction by releasing hydrogen sulfide
Key Points:	Renal function should be evaluated before surgery in chronic users

TRETINOIN

Trade Names:	**Retin-A, Renova**
Indications:	Acne, facial wrinkles, mottled hyperpigmentation
Pharmacokinetics:	Absorption minimal; $T_{1/2}$ β: 2 h; excreted in urine and feces
Pharmacodynamics:	Keratolytic effect, ↓ proliferation of primitive promyelocytes
Skin:	Erythema, blistering, hyper- or hypopigmentation, leukocytosis
Dosage:	0.025–0.1% (cream) or 0.01–0.025% (gel); apply daily
Contraindications:	Eczema, sunburn, pregnancy
Drug Interactions:	↑ Irritation of skin with alcohol-containing drugs; incompatible with benzoyl peroxide; ↑ absorption of topical minoxidil (↑ hypotension, arrhythmias, impotence); ↑ photosensitization with isotretinoin
Key Points:	St. John's wort ↑ skin photosensitivity

TRIOXSALEN

Trade Name:	**Trisoralen**
Indications:	Vitiligo, skin sensitivity to sunlight
Pharmacokinetics:	Absorbed from GI tract; activated by long wavelength ultraviolet light A (320–400 nm); metabolized in liver, excreted in urine
Pharmacodynamics:	Repigmentation of vitiliguous skin (requires functional melanocytes)
CNS:	Dizziness, headache, depression, cataracts
GI:	Nausea
Other:	Leg swelling, sunburn, ↑ risk of skin cancer
Dosage:	20–40 mg PO 3 h before UV light exposure, apply 2–3×/wk
Contraindications:	Photosensitization conditions (e.g., albinism), aphakia, cataracts, skin cancer, lupus, porphyria, leukoderma
Drug Interactions:	↑ Phototoxicity with sunlight, furocoumarin-containing foods (e.g., figs, limes, carrots), photosensitizing drugs
Key Points:	↑ Risk of perioperative bleeding in patients with defective coagulation systems (or receiving anticoagulants)

ZINC OXIDE (WITH CALAMINE AND GELATIN)

Trade Name:	**Dome-Paste**
Indications:	Protectant (lesions on extremities)
Pharmacokinetics:	NK
Pharmacodynamics:	Protects skin by forming occlusive barrier
Dosage:	3–4 in wet bandage; apply for 1 wk
Contraindications:	Constrictive bandage; remove previous application before reapplying
Key Points:	Apply with nap of hair to avoid folliculitis

23

Diuretics

ACETAZOLAMIDE

Trade Names:	**Dazamide, Diamox**
Indications:	Open-angle and acute angle-closure glaucoma, petit mal and myoclonic seizures, edema, acute mountain sickness, periodic paralysis
Pharmacokinetics:	Onset: 2 min (IV); 1 h (PO), 2 h (ER); peak: 15 min (IV), 1–3 h (PO) and 3–6 h (ER); protein binding: 90%; duration: 4–5 h (IV), 8–24 h; $T_{1/2}$ β: 2–6 h; excreted 1° unchanged in urine
Pharmacodynamics:	Noncompetitive reversible carbonic anhydrase inhibition, ↓ conversion of CO_2 and H_2O to HCO_3 and H+
CNS:	↓ CSF formation, ↓ ICP; drowsiness, paresthesias, confusion, tinnitus, ↓ aqueous humor formation, ↓ IOP
CV:	↓ BP
GI:	Nausea, vomiting, diarrhea, anorexia, bad taste, ↑ LFTs
GU:	Metabolic acidosis, polyuria, hematuria, renal calculi
Other:	Rash, photosensitivity, hyperglycemia, bone marrow depression
Dosage:	500 mg initially, then 125–250 mg PO qid, or 500 mg ER PO bid (max. 1 g/d); 8–30 mg/kg/d in divided doses (children)
Contraindications:	Severe hepatorenal insufficiency, electrolyte imbalance, adrenocortical insufficiency, sensitivity to sulfonamides
Drug Interactions:	Salicylates may induce coma; ↓ lithium, phenobarbital, salicylates levels; ↑ cyclosporin, amphetamine, quinidine, ephedrine, flecainide, protainamide levels
Key Points:	Perioperative hyperglycemia ↑ insulin requirement; use preoperatively with acute angle-closure glaucoma; avoid with chronic pulmonary insufficiency

AMILORIDE

Trade Name:	**Midamor**
Indications:	Hypertension, edema (due to CHF), adjunct to thiazide (or other K^+-wasting) diuretics
Pharmacokinetics:	Onset: 2 h; peak: 6–10 h; protein binding: 23%; duration: 24 h; $T_{1/2}$ β: 6–9 h; excreted unchanged in urine and feces
Pharmacodynamics:	Inhibits Na^+ reabsorption and K^+ excretion in distal renal tubules, ↓ K^+ loss in urine
CNS:	Dizziness, headache, paresthesias, confusion, weakness, fatigue
CV:	↓ BP, ↓ HR, CHF, angina, arrhythmias

AMILORIDE *continued*

GI:	Nausea, vomiting, abdominal pain, ↑ LFTs, anorexia
GU:	Electrolyte imbalance, polyuria, impotence
Other:	Dyspnea, rash, alopecia, aplastic anemia, muscle cramps
Dosage:	5–10 mg/d PO (max. 20 mg/d)
Contraindications:	Anuria, hepatorenal failure, hyperkalemia, diabetic nephropathy
Drug Interactions:	K⁺ supplements, K⁺-sparing diuretics, salt substitutes, K⁺-containing drugs (penicillin G), indomethacin, ACE inhibitors ↑ K⁺ levels; ↑ lithium and amantadine levels; NSAIDs ↓ diuretic effect; ↑ hypotensive effect of antihypertensives; ↓ clearance of digoxin
Key Points:	Monitor K⁺ levels during perioperative period due to ↑ risk of hyperkalemia; use with general anesthetics may enhance hypotensive effect

BUMETANIDE

Trade Name:	**Bumex**
Indications:	Edema, hypertension
Pharmacokinetics:	Onset: <20 min (IV), 30–60 min (PO); bioavailability: 80%; peak: 15–30 min (IV), 1–2 h (PO); protein binding: 95%; duration: 30–60 min (IV), 4–6 h (PO); Vd: 3–6 L; $T_{1/2}$ β: 1–2 h; metabolized in liver, excreted 1° in urine
Pharmacodynamics:	Inhibits Na⁺ and Cl⁻ reabsorption in proximal ascending loop of Henle; ↑ excretion of Na⁺, H_2O, Cl⁻, K⁺
CNS:	Ototoxicity (deafness, tinnitus), headache, dizziness
CV:	Hypovolemia, orthostatic hypotension, thromboembolism
GI:	Nausea, vomiting, abdominal pain, ↑ LFTs
GU:	Azotemia, premature ejaculation, oliguria
Other:	Hyperglycemia, electrolyte imbalance, hyperuricemia, myalgias, arthralgias, hypercholesterolemia, thrombocytopenia, pruritus
Dosage:	0.5–2 mg PO qid (max. 10 mg/d); 0.015 mg/kg/d (max. 0.1 mg/kg/d) (children), or 0.5–1 mg IV q 2–3 h
Contraindications:	Anuria, hepatic coma, electrolyte depletion, sensitivity to sulfonamides
Drug Interactions:	ACE inhibitors ↑ hypotension; ↑ digitalis toxicity; ↑ lithium level; ↑ ototoxicity with aminoglycosides; ↓ efficacy with indomethacin and probenecid; ↑ hypotensive effects of antihypertensives; K⁺-depleting drugs (e.g., amphotericin B and corticosteroids) ↑ K⁺ loss in urine

BUMETANIDE *continued*

Key Points: Preoperative assessment of electrolytes and volume
                       status is critical to avoid intraoperative CV complications

---

CHLOROTHIAZIDE

Trade Name: **Diuril**

Indications: Edema, hypertension

Pharmacokinetics: Onset: <15 min (IV), 1 h (PO); peak: <0.5 (IV),
                       2–3 h (PO); duration: 2 h (IV), 6–12 h (PO); $T_{1/2}$ β:
                       45–120 min; excreted unchanged in urine

Pharmacodynamics: Inhibits Na^+ reabsorption and K^+ excretion on the distal
                       renal tubules
  CNS: Lethargy, confusion, weakness, dizziness, blurred
                       vision
  CV: Hypovolemia, ↓ BP
  GI: Nausea, vomiting, constipation, jaundice, ↑ LFTs
  Other: Hyperglycemia, electrolyte imbalance, hyperuricemia,
                       ↑ lipid levels, photosensitivity, ↑ SLE symptoms, blood
                       dyscrasias, impotence

Dosage: 0.25–1 g PO bid; 20–30 mg/kg/d (children)

Contraindications: Anuria, hepatic coma, sensitivity to other
                       sulfonamides

Drug Interactions: NSAIDs ↓ efficacy; ↑ lithium level; ↑ hypokalemia
                       with ACTH and corticosteroids; ↑ digitalis toxicity

Key Points: Monitor glucose levels in diabetics (↑ insulin during
                       surgery and in postoperative period); use with
                       barbiturates and opioids ↑ hypotensive effect

---

CHLORTHALIDONE

Trade Names: **Hygroton, Thalitone**

Indications: Pedal edema, hypertension

Pharmacokinetics: Onset: 2–3 h; peak: 2–6 h; duration: 1–3 d; $T_{1/2}$ β: 54 h;
                       90% bound to erythrocytes; excreted 1° in urine as
                       unchanged drug

Pharmacodynamics: ↑ Excretion of Na^+ and H_2O by inhibiting Na^+
                       reabsorption in renal cortical diluting tubules
  CNS: Dizziness, headache, paresthesia, weakness,
                       restlessness
  CV: Hypovolemia, orthostatic hypotension
  GI: Anorexia, nausea, pancreatitis, vomiting, jaundice

CHLORTHALIDONE *continued*

GU:	Impotence, glycosuria
Other:	Hyperuricemia, hyperglycemia, metabolic alkalosis, rash
Dosage:	50–100 mg/d PO; 2 mg/kg q 2 d (children)
Contraindications:	Anuria, sensitivity to sulfonamides (e.g., thiazides)
Drug Interactions:	↑ Effect of amphetamine, quinidine, antihypertensives; cholestyramine and colestipol ↓ absorption; ↑ lithium level; methenamine ↓ efficacy; diazoxide ↑ side effects; NSAIDs ↓ renal function
Key Points:	↑ Hypotensive effects with inadequate fluid replacement during anesthesia; ↑ insulin requirements

ETHACRYNIC ACID

Trade Name:	**Edecrin**
Indications:	Edema, hypertension, ascites
Pharmacokinetics:	Onset: 5 min (IV), 30 min (PO); bioavailability: 100%; peak: 15–30 min (IV), 2 h (PO); protein binding: 90%; duration: 2 h (IV), 6–8 h (PO); hepatic metabolism, excreted 1° in urine
Pharmacodynamics:	Inhibits Na^+ and Cl^- reabsorption in proximal part of ascending loop of Henle, ↑ excretion of Na^+, H_2O, Cl^-, K^+
CNS:	Headache, blurred vision, confusion, ototoxicity
CV:	Hypovolemia, orthostatic hypotension, thromboembolism
GI:	Nausea, vomiting, diarrhea, anorexia, cramps, ↑ LFTs
GU:	Electrolyte imbalance, hematuria, oliguria, polyuria, azotemia
Other:	Hyperglycemia, hyperuricemia, ↑ lipid levels, photosensitivity, fever, bone marrow suppression, premature ejaculation
Dosage:	25–100 mg PO q 12–24 h (max. 200 mg/d); 0.5–1 mg/kg IM/IV (max. 100 mg)
Contraindications:	Anuria, electrolyte imbalance, severe diarrhea
Drug Interactions:	↑ Lithium level; ↓ efficacy with NSAIDs and probenecid; ↑ ototoxicity with aminoglycosides, cisplastin, and cephalosporins; ↑ warfarin anticoagulation effect; ↑ digitalis toxicity; ↑ GI bleeding with steroids
Key Points:	Use with cardiac glycosides, epinephrine, volatile anesthetics ↑ cardiovascular complications if electrolyte deficits are not corrected preoperatively; in diabetics, ↑ insulin requirement

FUROSEMIDE

Trade Name:	**Lasix**
Indications:	Edema, hypertension, hypercalcemia
Pharmacokinetics:	Onset: 5 min (IV), 30–60 min (PO); bioavailability: 62%; peak: 30 min (IV), 1–2 h (PO); protein binding: 95%; duration: 2 h (IV), 6–8 h (PO); $T_{1/2}$ β: 1–2 h; minimally metabolized by liver, excreted 1° unchanged in urine
Pharmacodynamics:	Inhibits Na^+ and Cl^- reabsorption in proximal part of ascending loop of Henle, excretion of Na^+, Cl^-, K^+, H_2O
CNS:	Headache, blurred vision, paresthesias, ototoxicity, ↓ ICP
CV:	Hypovolemia, orthostatic hypotension, thromboembolism
GI:	Nausea, vomiting, diarrhea, jaundice, anorexia, cramps
GU:	Electrolyte imbalance, azotemia, nocturia, polyuria
Other:	Hyperglycemia, hyperuricemia, ↓ bone marrow, photosensitivity, rash, pruritus, SLE
Dosage:	20–80 mg/d PO (max. 600 mg/d); 20–40 mg IM/IV q 1–2 h (max. 600 mg/d); 2 mg/d (max. 600 mg/kg/d) PO or 1 mg/kg/d IM/IV (children)
Contraindications:	Anuria, sensitivity to sulfonamides, hepatic coma
Drug Interactions:	↑ Lithium level; ↓ BP response to norepinephrine; ↓ effects with indomethacin; ↑ ototoxicity with aminoglycosides, cisplastin, ethacrynic acid; ↑ digitalis toxicity; ACE inhibitors ↑ hypotension; amphotericin B, corticosteroids, corticotropin, metolazone ↑ hypokalemia
Key Points:	Use with epinephrine, cardiac glycosides volatile anesthetics ↑ intraoperative arrhythmias; ↑ insulin requirement for diabetics during perioperative period; prolongs neuromuscular blockade

HYDROCHLOROTHIAZIDE (HCTZ)

Trade Names:	**Esidrix, Ezide, HydroDIURIL, Hydro-Par, Oretic**
Indications:	Edema, hypertension
Pharmacokinetics:	Onset: 2 h; peak: 4–5 h; duration: 6–12 h; $T_{1/2}$ β: 5–15 h; excreted 1° unchanged in urine
Pharmacodynamics:	↑ Excretion of Na^+ and H_2O by inhibiting Na^+ reabsorption in the renal cortical diluting tubules
CNS:	Dizziness, weakness, headache, paresthesia
CV:	Hypovolemia, orthostatic hypotension, myocarditis, angina

HYDROCHLOROTHIAZIDE
(HCTZ) *continued*

GI:	Nausea, vomiting, pancreatitis, diarrhea, hepatic failure
GU:	Electrolyte imbalance, polyuria, interstitial nephritis, renal failure
Other:	Hyperglycemia, hyperuricemia, ↑ lipid levels, agranulocytosis, photosensitivity, vasculitis, lymphadenopathy, thrombocytopenia

Dosage: 25–200 mg/d PO, then 25–100 mg/d; 2–3 mg/kg/d (children)

Contraindications: Anuria, hepatic coma, sensitivity to other sulfonamides

Drug Interactions: ↑ Lithium level; NSAIDs ↓ effect; ↓ response to vasopressors; ↑ hypotension with alcohol, antihypertensives, barbiturates, opioids; ↑ K$^+$ with corticosteroids and ACTH; ↑ digitalis toxicity; cholestyramine and colestipol ↓ absorption

Key Points: Preoperative signs of hypokalemia include muscle weakness and cramps, ↑ risk of intraoperative CV complications; ↑ insulin during surgery on diabetics

INDAPAMIDE

Trade Name: **Lozol**

Indications: Edema, hypertension

Pharmacokinetics: Onset: 1–2 h; peak: 2–5 h; protein binding: 75%; duration: 36 h; T$_{1/2}$ β: 14 h; metabolized in liver, excreted in urine

Pharmacodynamics: ↑ Excretion of Na$^+$ and H$_2$O by inhibiting Na$^+$ reabsorption in renal tubules

CNS:	Headache, dizziness, drowsiness, fatigue, paresthesias, insomnia
CV:	Orthostatic hypotension, hypovolemia, arrhythmia, flushing
GI:	Anorexia, nausea, vomiting, abdominal pain
Other:	Nocturia, impotence, hyperuricemia, ↓ Na$^+$, ↓ K$^+$, metabolic alkalosis, rash, pruritus, muscle cramps, weakness

Dosage: 1.25–2.5 mg/d PO

Contraindications: Anuria, sensitivity to sulfonamides

Drug Interactions: ↑ Effect of amphetamine, antihypertensives, quinidine; cholestyramine and colestipol ↓ absorption; ↑ lithium level; methenamine ↓ efficacy; diazoxide ↑ side effects

INDAPAMIDE *continued*

Key Points:	General anesthetics ↑ hypotensive effects of diuretics; adequate fluid and electrolyte replacement during anesthesia minimizes cardiovascular complications; ↑ insulin requirements in diabetics

MANNITOL

Trade Names:	Osmitrol, Resectisol
Indications:	Intracranial and intraocular hypertension, oliguria (due to ARF), toxic substances in urine, pedal edema (due to TURP solution)
Pharmacokinetics:	Onset: 1 h (diuresis); 15 min (↓ ICP and IOP); peak: 1–3 h; duration: 3–8 h; $T_{1/2}$ β: 100 min; minimally metabolized, excreted in urine
Pharmacodynamics:	↑ Osmotic pressure of glomerular filtrate, ↓ tubular reabsorption of H_2O and electrolytes
CNS:	↓ ICP (may ↑ ICP with disrupted blood-brain barrier), headache, blurred vision, dizziness, seizures
CV:	Pulmonary edema, hypovolemia, CHF, ↑ HR, angina
GI:	Nausea, vomiting, diarrhea
GU:	Electrolyte imbalance, difficulty urinating
Other:	Hyperosmolar hyperglycemia, rash, necrosis, fever, chills, urticaria, cough, wheezing, thrombophlebitis
Dosage:	12.5 g IV over 3–5 min, then 50–100 g over 90 min; or 1.5–2 g/kg IV over 30 min (to serum osmolality of 310–320 mOsm); 200 mg/kg IV over 3–5 min, then 2 g/kg IV over 30 min (children)
Contraindications:	Severe renal impairment, dehydration and electrolyte depletion, pulmonary edema, active intracranial bleeding
Drug Interactions:	If mixed with blood, can produce pseudoagglutination; ↑ digitalis toxicity; ↑ effect of carbonic anhydrase inhibitors; ↓ lithium level
Key Points:	After receiving mannitol, urethral catheter is necessary to monitor urine output and ensure adequate fluid replacement during surgery

METOLAZONE

Trade Names:	Zaroxolyn, Mykrox, Diulo
Indications:	Edema, hypertension, diuresis (unresponsive to furosemide)

METOLAZONE *continued*

Pharmacokinetics:	Onset: <1 h; bioavailability: 65%; peak: 2–8 h; 60% erythrocyte bound and 30% protein bound; duration: 12–24 h; $T_{1/2}$ β: 6–20 h; metabolized in liver, excreted in urine
Pharmacodynamics:	↑ Excretion of Na^+ and H_2O by ↓ Na^+ reabsorption in the renal tubules
CNS:	Dizziness, headache, fatigue, paresthesia, blurred vision
CV:	Hypovolemia, arrhythmias, orthostatic hypotension, angina
GI:	Nausea, vomiting, pancreatitis, dry mouth
GU:	Electrolyte imbalance, nocturia, impotence
Other:	Hyperglycemia, hyperuricemia, photosensitivity, muscle cramps
Dosage:	2.5–10 mg PO q 12–24 h
Contraindications:	Anuria, hepatic coma, sensitivity to sulfonamides
Drug Interactions:	↑ Lithium level; diuretic-induced hypokalemia ↑ digitalis toxicity; loop diuretics ↑ fluid or electrolyte losses; ↓ vascular response to pressor amines; ↑ effect of antihypertensives, opiates, barbiturates; cholestyramine, colestipol ↓ absorption; ↑ photosensitivity
Key Points:	Correction of K^+ and Mg^{++} preoperatively ↓ risk of arrhythmias with glycosides, vasopressor, volatile anesthetics; ↑ insulin requirement in diabetics

SPIRONOLACTONE

Trade Name:	**Aldactone**
Indications:	Primary aldosteronism, hypertension, diuretic-induced hypokalemia, CHF, precocious puberty, hirsutism, metrorrhagia
Pharmacokinetics:	Onset: <30 min; peak: 1–2 h; protein binding: 90%; duration: 2–3 d; $T_{1/2}$ β: 16.5 h (canrenone); metabolized to active metabolite (canrenone), excreted 1° in urine
Pharmacodynamics:	Competitively inhibits aldosterone effects at the distal renal tubules, ↑ Na^+ and H_2O excretion, ↓ K^+ excretion
CNS:	Drowsiness, confusion, headache, ataxia
CV:	↓ BP, ↓ HR
GI:	Nausea, vomiting, diarrhea, gastritis, bleeding, cramping
GU:	Electrolyte imbalance, ↓ penile erection, menstrual disturbances

SPIRONOLACTONE *continued*

Other:	Drug fever, gynecomastia, hirsutism, rash, muscle weakness
Dosage:	25–100 mg PO q 12–24 h; 1–3 mg/kg/d in 1–2 doses (children)
Contraindications:	Anuria, acute renal insufficiency, hyperkalemia
Drug Interactions:	K^+ supplements, K^+-sparing diuretics, salt substitutes, indomethacin, ACE inhibitors ↑ K^+ levels; ↓ effect of epinephrine and norepinephrine; ↑ digoxin level
Key Points:	Use with general anesthetics and antihypertensives ↑ risk of hypotension

TORSEMIDE

Trade Name:	**Demadex**
Indications:	Pedal edema, hypertension
Pharmacokinetics:	Onset: 10 min (IV), 1 h (PO); bioavailability: 95%; peak: 1 h (IV), 1–2 h (PO); protein binding: 99%; duration: 6–8 h; Vd: 12–15 L; $T_{1/2}$ β: 3.5 h; metabolized in liver, excreted 1° in urine
Pharmacodynamics:	Enhances excretion of Na^+, Cl^-, and H_2O by acting on ascending portion of loop of Henle
CNS:	Syncope, ototoxicity, dizziness, headache, insomnia
CV:	Hypovolemia, orthostatic hypotension, chest pain (angina)
GI:	Nausea, vomiting, dyspepsia, hepatic failure
Other:	Electrolyte disturbances, ↑ urination, weakness, cough
Dosage:	5–20 mg/d PO (max. 200 mg/d); 5–10 mg/d IM/IV
Contraindications:	Anuria, hepatic failure/ascites, sensitivity to sulfonylureas
Drug Interactions:	NSAIDs ↓ renal function; ↑ lithium levels; aminoglycosides ↑ ototoxicity; indomethacin and probenecid ↓ effects; antihypertensives ↑ hypotension
Key Points:	Adequate fluid replacement minimizes inadvertent hypovolemia and cardiovascular instability during perioperative period

TRIAMTERENE

Trade Name:	**Dyrenium**
Indications:	Pedal edema

TRIAMTERENE *continued*

Pharmacokinetics:	Onset: 2–4 h; peak: 6–8 h; protein binding: 67%; duration: 12–16 h; $T_{1/2}$ β: 3 h; hepatic metabolism (active metabolite), excreted 1° in feces
Pharmacodynamics:	Acts directly on distal renal tubules to inhibit Na^+ reabsorption and K^+ excretion
CNS:	Dizziness, headache, weakness
CV:	↓ BP, ↓ HR
GI:	Nausea, vomiting, diarrhea, jaundice, ↑ LFTs
GU:	Renal stones, azotemia, interstitial nephritis
Other:	Hyperglycemia, hyperuricemia, metabolic acidosis, photosensitivity, rash, thrombocytopenia, megaloblastic anemia
Dosage:	50–100 mg PO bid (max. 300 mg/d); 1–2 mg/kg bid (children)
Contraindications:	Anuria, acute or chronic renal failure, severe hepatic insufficiency
Drug Interactions:	K^+ supplements, K^+-sparing diuretics, salt substitutes, indomethacin, or ACE inhibitors ↑ K^+ levels; ↓ effect of norepinephrine; NSAIDs ↓ renal function; ↑ lithium levels; cimetidine ↑ bioavailability; ↑ photosensitivity
Key Points:	Use with vasodilators and general anesthetics ↑ hypotension; surgical blood loss and hemodynamic instability managed with fluid replacement; ↑ effects of nondepolarizing muscle relaxants

UREA (CARBAMIDE)

Trade Name:	**Ureaphil**
Indications:	Intracranial and intraocular hypertension, SIADH
Pharmacokinetics:	Onset: 20 min; peak: 1–2 h; duration: 5–6 h; $T_{1/2}$ β: 10 h; hydrolyzed in GI tract by bacterial urease, excreted in urine
Pharmacodynamics:	↑ Plasma osmolality, ↑ H_2O into extracellular fluid, ↑ osmolality at renal glomerulus, ↓ renal tubular reabsorption of H_2O
CNS:	↓ ICP (but ↑ ICP with disrupted blood-brain barrier), headache, syncope, confusion, nervousness, ↓ IOP, blurred vision
CV:	Venous thrombosis, ↑ HR
GI:	Nausea, vomiting, ↑ GI ammonia (with hepatic impairment)
Other:	Local tissue irritation, hyponatremia, hypokalemia
Dosage:	1–1.5 g/kg IV over 1–2.5 h (max. 120 g/d); 0.1–1.5 g/kg/d (children)

UREA (CARBAMIDE) *continued*

Contraindications: Severe hepatorenal disease, sickle cell anemia, active intracranial bleeding, severe dehydration and electrolyte depletion

Drug Interactions: ↓ Lithium level

Key Points: Ensure adequate perioperative assessment of blood volume, as urea masks effects of blood loss

24

Gastrointestinals

ACTIVATED CHARCOAL

Trade Names:	**Actidose-Aqua/Sorbitol, Charco-Aid, CharcoCaps, Liqui-Char**
Indications:	Chemical toxicity, intestinal gas, dyspepsia
Pharmacokinetics:	Onset immediate (not absorbed from GI tract), excreted in feces
Pharmacodynamics: GI:	Antidote with antiflatulent and antidiarrheal activity Diarrhea/constipation, vomiting, abdominal swelling, black stools
Dosage:	0.6–5 g/d PO (antidote) or 1–3 g PO tid (flatulence); 1 g/kg (children)
Contraindications:	Ileus, antidiarrheal use, dehydration, acute dysentery
Drug Interactions:	↓ Effectiveness of oral medications (e.g., acetylcysteine as antidote in acetaminophen overdose); milk ↓ effectiveness
Key Points:	Do not use if poisoning involves corrosive agents, cyanide, iron, mineral acids, or organic solvents

ALVIMOPAN

Trade Name:	**Entereg**
	See Chapter 35, "Opioid Agonists and Antagonists"

ATTAPULGITE

Trade Names:	**Diar-Aid, Diasorb, Kaopectate, Rheaban**
Indications:	Diarrhea
Pharmacokinetics:	Not absorbed
Pharmacodynamics: GI:	Antidiarrheal effect Constipation
Dosage:	1.2–1.5 g PO after each loose bowel movement (max. 9.0 g/d); 300–600 mg PO (max. 4.2 g/d) (children)
Contraindications:	Severe dehydration, acute dysentery, parasite diarrhea, bowel obstruction
Drug Interactions:	↓ Efficacy of anticholinergics; antidyskinetics, glycosides, lincomycins, loxapine, phenothiazines, thioxanthines, xanthines ↓ absorption
Key Points:	No interactions with anesthetic drugs reported

DEXPANTHENOL

Trade Names:	**Ilopan, Panthoderm**
Indications:	Adynamic ileus, eczema, decubitus ulcer
Pharmacokinetics:	Converts to pantothenic acid (coenzyme A), excreted in urine and feces
Pharmacodynamics:	Analog of pantothenic acid, a precursor of coenzyme A, a cofactor for acetylcholine synthesis, ↑ peristalsis and promotes wound healing
GI:	Vomiting, diarrhea, intestinal colic
Other:	Tingling, itching, dyspnea
Dosage:	250–500 mg IM, repeat q 6 h, or 500 mg IV infusion; 2% cream (topical)
Contraindications:	Obstructive ileus, hemophilia
Drug Interactions:	Antibiotics and barbiturates ↑ allergic responses
Key Points:	Prolongs succinylcholine-induced muscle relaxation

DIFENOXIN-ATROPINE

Trade Name:	**Motofen**
Indications:	Nonspecific diarrhea, acute exacerbations of chronic diarrhea
Pharmacokinetics:	Onset: <30 min; peak: 40–60 min; $T_{1/2}$ β: 12–24 h; hepatic metabolism, excreted in urine and feces
Pharmacodynamics:	Opioid with antidiarrheal effect (due to slowing intestinal motility)
CNS:	Drowsiness, confusion, blurred vision, dizziness, headache
GI:	Paralytic ileus, toxic megacolon, nausea, vomiting, cramps
Other:	Muscle cramps, difficult urination, ↓ respiration, diaphoresis
Dosage:	1–2 mg PO, then 1 mg q 3–4 h (max. 8 mg/d)
Contraindications:	Severe colitis, diarrhea (due to toxic *Escherichia coli*, *Shigella*, *Salmonella* sp. poisoning or dysentery), GI tract obstruction, hepatic dysfunction
Drug Interactions:	Alcohol ↑ CNS depressive effect; anticholinergics ↑ effects; MAOIs ↑ BP and ↓ detoxification; naltrexone ↑ withdrawal symptoms
Key Points:	Use with general anesthetics ↑ postoperative sedation and ↑ opioid-induced respiratory depression

DIPHENOXYLATE-ATROPINE

Trade Names:	**Logen, Lomanate, Lomotil, Lonox, Lofene**
Indications:	Acute nonspecific diarrhea
Pharmacokinetics:	Onset: 45–60 min; peak: 3 h; duration: 3–4 h; $T_{1/2}$ β: 2.5 h; excreted into breast milk; hepatic metabolism, excreted 1° in feces
Pharmacodynamics:	Meperidine analog that inhibits GI motility
CNS:	Nervousness, restlessness, irritability, paresthesia, depression, headache, mydriasis, blurred vision, dizziness
GI:	Paralytic ileus, toxic megacolon, pancreatitis, cramps
Other:	Dry mouth, flushing, hyperthermia, pruritus, urticaria, angioedema, ↑ HR, urinary retention, ↓ respiration
Dosage:	2.5 mg PO diphenoxylate (0.025–0.05 mg atropine), then 2.5 mg PO 2–3×/d; 0.3–0.4 mg/kg/d (children)
Contraindications:	Severe colitis, diarrhea (due to broad-spectrum antibiotics or organisms that penetrate intestinal mucosa), acute dysentery (in children), GI tract obstruction, ↓ hepatic function, breast-feeding
Drug Interactions:	Alcohol ↑ CNS depression; anticholinergics ↑ effects; MAOIs ↑ hypertension ↓ detoxification; naltrexone ↑ withdrawal symptoms
Key Points:	Adequate fluid and electrolyte replacement preoperatively ↓ intraoperative hypotension; use with general anesthetics and opioid analgesics ↑ CNS depressant effects

ESOMEPRAZOLE

Trade Name:	**Nexium**
	See Chapter 3, "Antacids and Antisecretories"

KAOLIN-PECTIN

Trade Names:	**Kapectolin, Kaodene Donnagel**
Indications:	Acute diarrhea (mild)
Pharmacokinetics:	Not absorbed (pectin decomposed in GI tract)
Pharmacodynamics:	Antidiarrheal absorbent with gut protectant effects
GI:	Constipation
Dosage:	5.8 g kaolin and 130 mg pectin in 180 mL; 60–120 mL after each loose bowel movement; 15–30 mL (children)

KAOLIN-PECTIN *continued*

Contraindications:	Severe dehydration, acute dysentery, parasite-associated diarrhea
Drug Interactions:	Anticholinergics, antidyskinetics, erythromycin, glycosides, lincomycin, loxapine, phenothiazines, thioxanthines, xanthines ↓ effect
Key Points:	No adverse interactions with anesthetic drugs reported

LANSOPRAZOLE

Trade Name:	**Prevacid**
	See Chapter 3, "Antacids and Antisecretories"

LAXATIVES

Other Names:	**Bulk-forming agent, stool softener, hyperosmotic lubricant (or emollient), bowel stimulants**
Indications:	Constipation, laxative dependency, hyperacidity, hyperammonemia, biliary tract disorders, irritable bowel syndrome
Pharmacokinetics:	Local absorption, elimination in feces
Pharmacodynamics:	Absorbs water in the gut, ↑ stool bulk, ↑ peristaltic activity and bowel evacuation
GI:	Rectal irritation, esophageal blockage, impaction (bulk-forming), discoloration of feces
Renal:	Discoloration of urine, ↑ magnesium
Other:	Skin irritation, electrolyte imbalance
Dosages:	*Bulk-forming:* Psyllium, 2.5–8 g, 1–3×/d; methylcellulose, 0.5–2 g, 1–3×/d; children >6 y; calcium polycarbophil, 0.5–1 g 1–4×/d *Stool softener:* Docusate sodium, 50–250 mg/d, 20–60 mg/d (children) *Hyperosmotics:* Glycerin, magnesium citrate, lactulose, 10–20 g/d (Fleet's Enema) *Lubricant/emollient:* Mineral oil, 2.1–8.4 g/d *Stimulant:* Phenolphthalein, castor oil, 15–60 mL/d
Contraindications:	Appendicitis, acute abdomen, rectal bleeding *Bulk-forming:* dysphagia *Hyperosmotic:* severe dehydration, renal impairment *Lubricant:* dysphagia, at risk of aspiration, diabetes (lactulose)

LAXATIVES *continued*

Drug Interactions:	*Bulk-forming agent:* ↓ effects of anticoagulants, cardiac glycosides, salicylates; ↓ effects of tetracycline and calcium *Magnesium-containing agent:* ↓ effectiveness of anticoagulants, digitalis, phenothiazines; polystyrene sulfonate ↑ alkalosis, forms nonabsorbable complexes with tetracycline *Lubricant:* ↓ effectiveness of anticoagulants, contraceptives, glycosides, fat-soluble vitamins *Stimulant:* Antacids, H_2-receptor antagonists and milk ↑ gastric irritation *Stool softener:* ↑ absorption of dantheon, mineral oil, phenolphthalein
Key Points:	Adequate preoperative fluid replacement (hydration) ↓ hypotension after induction of anesthesia; opioid-sparing analgesic techniques ↓ constipation/ileus

LOPERAMIDE

Trade Names:	**Imodium, Kaopectate, Maalox Antidiarrheal**
Indications:	Diarrhea
Pharmacokinetics:	Peak: 2.5–5 h; protein binding: 97%; duration: 12–24 h; $T_{1/2}$ β: 9–14 h; poorly absorbed (<40%); metabolized by liver, excreted primarily in feces
Pharmacodynamics:	↓ Intestinal motility by acting directly on intestinal mucosal nerve endings, inhibits fluid and electrolyte secretion
CNS:	Drowsiness, dizziness, fatigue
GI:	Toxic megacolon, dry mouth, abdominal pain, constipation
Dosage:	2–4 mg PO, then 2 mg bid (max. 16 mg/d); 80–240 µg/kg/d (1–2 mg) in divided doses (children)
Contraindications:	Ulcerative colitis, bloody diarrhea, hyperthermia, hepatic dysfunction
Drug Interactions:	Opioid analgesics ↑ constipation; rash; naloxone does not antagonize "overdose"
Key Points:	Minimize perioperative use of opioid analgesics because of risk of postoperative constipation; use with general anesthetics can produce ↑ CNS depression

MESALAMINE
(5-AMINOSALICYLIC ACID)

Trade Names:	**Asacol, Canasa, Pentasa, Rowasa**
Indications:	Ulcerative colitis, proctosigmoiditis, proctitis
Pharmacokinetics:	Poorly absorbed (25%); $T_{1/2}$ β: 1 h (5–10 h for metabolite); metabolized to active metabolite, excreted in urine and in feces
Pharmacodynamics:	↓ Inflammation by blocking cyclooxygenase (COX) isoenzymes, and ↓ prostaglandin production in colon
CNS:	Headache, malaise, paresthesia, fever, fatigue
CV:	Chest pain, ↑ HR
GI:	Cramps, bloody diarrhea, pancreatitis, dyspepsia, flatulence, ↑ LFTs
Other:	Myalgia, arthralgia, pruritus, rash, alopecia, rhinitis, dysuria
Dosage:	0.8–1 g PO tid; 500 mg PR (1 sup bid)
Contraindications:	Allergic to sulfite (rectal suppository)
Drug Interactions:	NK
Key Points:	No known interaction with anesthetic drugs

MISOPROSTOL

Trade Name:	**Cytotec**
	See Chapter 3, "Antacids and Antisecretories"

NITAZOXANIDE

Trade Name:	**Alinia**
	See Chapter 12, "Antimicrobials"

OCTREOTIDE

Trade Name:	**Sandostatin**
Indications:	Carcinoid tumors, acromegaly, AIDS-associated diarrhea, diarrhea due to vasoactive intestinal peptide-secreting (VIP) tumors
Pharmacokinetics:	Onset: <10 min; peak: 0.5–1 h; protein binding: 65%; duration: <12 h; $T_{1/2}$ β: 1.5 h; rapidly absorbed, excreted in urine

OCTREOTIDE *continued*

Pharmacodynamics:	Somatostatin-like ↓ secretion of gastroenterohepatic peptides
CNS:	Dizziness, headache, fatigue, blurred vision
CV:	↓ HR, arrhythmias
GI:	Nausea, diarrhea, abdominal pain, vomiting, fat malabsorption
GU:	Urinary frequency, UTI
Other:	Hypothyroidism, Δ glucose level, ↓ GH, gastrin and insulin secretion, gallstones, pain at injection site, myalgias
Dosage:	Parenteral: 0.05, 0.1, 0.2, 0.5 mg/mL; 10, 20, 30 mg/5 mL (PR); 50 μg IM (max. 750 μg/d); 1–10 μg/kg/d (children)
Contraindications:	Gallbladder disease, diabetes mellitus, severe renal impairment
Drug Interactions:	↓ Cyclosporin level
Key Points:	To prevent carcinoid crisis during surgery, administer 250–500 μg SC 1–2 h before induction of anesthesia; unstable glucose levels during perioperative period

OLSALAZINE

Trade Name:	**Dipentum**
Indications:	Inflammatory bowel disease (intolerant of sulfasalazine)
Pharmacokinetics:	Onset: 0.5 h; peak: 1 h; protein binding: >99%; $T_{1/2}$ β: 0.9 h (active metabolite 7 d); converted to 5-aminosalicylic acid (5-ASA); metabolized 1° in colon, excreted 1° in feces
Pharmacodynamics:	↓ Inflammation by blocking cyclooxygenase (COX) isoenzymes and inhibiting prostaglandin production in the colon
CNS:	Drowsiness, dizziness, headache, anxiety, insomnia
GI:	↑ Ulcerative colitis, pancreatitis, bloating, diarrhea, nausea, ↑ LFTs
Other:	Muscle pain, arthralgia, fever, rash, itching, acne
Dosage:	250–500 mg PO bid
Contraindications:	Sensitive to salicylates, renal impairment
Drug Interactions:	↑ PT with warfarin
Key Points:	Salicylate-like activity ↑ risk of perioperative GI bleeding

PANCREATIN

Trade Names:	**Creon, Digepepsin, Pancrezyme**
Indications:	Digestive disorders (to replace deficient digestive enzymes)
Pharmacokinetics:	Acts locally in GI tract, excreted in feces
Pharmacodynamics:	Proteolytic, amylolytic and lipolytic enzymes
GI:	Perianal irritation, nausea
Other:	Rash
Dosage:	0.5–8 g of pancreatin, lipase, protease, and amylase with meals
Contraindications:	Sensitive to pork protein, pancreatitis, pregnancy, breast-feeding
Drug Interactions:	Antacids (Ca^{2+}, Mg^{++}) $\downarrow$ activity; $\downarrow$ iron absorption
Key Points:	No known interaction with anesthetic drugs

PANCRELIPASE

Trade Names:	**Cotazym, Creon, Ilozyme, Ku-Zyme, Lipram, Pancrease, Protilase, Ultrase, Viokase, Zymase**
Indications:	Pancreatic insufficiency or duct obstruction, malabsorption, steatorrhea
Pharmacokinetics:	Acts locally in GI tract and excreted in feces
Pharmacodynamics:	Proteolytic, amylolytic, lipolytic enzymes, $\uparrow$ digestion of proteins, starches, fats
GI:	Mouth irritation, nausea, cramping, diarrhea
Pulmonary:	Respiratory difficulty, wheezing (if inhale powder)
Other:	Hyperuricemia, hyperuricosuria, rash
Dosage:	8000 lipase; 30,000 protease; 30,000 amylase and 16,000 lipase; 70,000 protease; 70,000 amylase in capsules; 1–3 with meals
Contraindications:	Acute pancreatitis, sensitivity to pork protein
Drug Interactions:	Antacids $\downarrow$ pancrelipase activity; $\downarrow$ iron absorption
Key Points:	No known interactions with anesthetic drugs

PANTOPRAZOLE

Trade Name:	**Protonix**
	See Chapter 3, "Antacids and Antisecretories"

POLYETHYLENE GLYCOL-ELECTROLYTES SOLUTION (PEG-ES)

Trade Names:	**CoLyte, GoLytely, NuLytely**
Indications:	Preprocedural bowel evacuation, acute iron overdose
Pharmacokinetics:	Onset: 30 min; peak: 60 min; duration: 4 h; negligible absorption, excreted in feces
Pharmacodynamics:	Acts as osmotic product
GI:	Bloating, nausea, vomiting, abdominal cramps, anal irritation
Other:	Rhinorrhea, urticaria, rash
Dosage:	240 mL q 10 min (up to 4 L); 25–40 mL/kg/h (children)
Contraindications:	Intestinal obstruction, paralytic ileus, perforated bowel, severe ulcerative colitis, toxic colitis (megacolon)
Drug Interactions:	↓ Absorption of oral medications
Key Points:	Assess volume status and electrolyte levels prior to induction of anesthesia to prevent hypotension when treatment <4 h prior to surgery

RABEPRAZOLE

Trade Name:	**Aciphex**
	See Chapter 3, "Antacids and Antisecretories"

SIMETHICONE

Trade Names:	**Gas-X, Mylicon, Phazyme**
Indications:	Excess GI gas, adjunct in gastroscopy, bowel radiography
Pharmacokinetics:	Elimination unchanged in feces
Pharmacodynamics:	Defoaming agent, ↓ formation of mucous-coated gas bubbles
GI:	Belching, rectal flatus
Dosage:	40–125 mg PO after meals and hs (max. 500 mg/d)
Contraindications:	NK
Drug Interactions:	NK
Key Points:	No known interaction with anesthetic drugs

SUCRALFATE

Trade Name:	**Carafate**
Indications:	Duodenal ulcer, aspirin-induced gastric erosion
Pharmacokinetics:	Onset: <1 h; acts locally; peak: 2–3 h; duration: 6 h
Pharmacodynamics:	Adheres to proteins at ulcer site forming a protective coating against gastric acid, pepsin, bile salts; ↓ pepsin secretion
CNS:	Dizziness, drowsiness, headache
GI:	Nausea, dyspepsia, bezoar formation, dry mouth, flatulence
Other:	Rash, pruritus, myalgia
Dosage:	1 g PO q 6–12 h
Contraindications:	NK
Drug Interactions:	Antacids ↓ binding to gastroduodenal mucosa; ↓ PT with anticoagulants; ↓ absorption of cimetidine, digoxin, fat-soluble vitamins, ketoconazole, phenytoin, quinidine, quinolones, ranitidine, tetracycline, theophylline
Key Points:	↑ Doses of chronic oral medications prior to surgery due to ↓ GI absorption; consider H$_2$-blockers and gastrokinetic drugs for prophylaxis

25

Herbal Medicines and Dietary Supplements

ANDROSTENEDIONE

Trade Name:	**Primobolan**
Other Names:	**Androstenedione, androstenediol, norandrostenedione**

See Chapter 26, "Hormones"

AZELAIC ACID

Trade Names:	**Azelex, Finacea**

See Chapter 22, "Dermatologic Drugs"

BLUE COHOSH

Other Names:	**Papoose root, squaw root, *Caulophyllum thalictroides***
Indications:	Uterine cramps, uterine stimulant (labor)
Pharmacokinetics:	NK
Pharmacodynamics:	Smooth muscle stimulant
CV:	Chest pain, ↑ HR, ↑ BP, coronary vasoconstriction
GI:	Cramping, diarrhea, ↑ gastric motility
GU:	Abortifacient (termination of pregnancy), uterine bleeding
Other:	Hyperglycemia
Dosage:	Liquid extract (NK)
Contraindications:	Diarrhea, diabetes, cancer, preterm parturients
Drug Interactions:	↑ Effect of vasoactive drugs; nicotine ↑ toxicity
Key Points:	Avoid hypertension and vasoconstrictive drugs to ↓ risk of myocardial ischemia; monitor glucose levels to avoid hyperglycemia

CARNITINE, LEVOCARNITINE

Trade Names:	**Carnitor, VitaCarn**
Indications:	L-carnitine deficiency, valproic acid overdose, lactic acidosis
Pharmacokinetics:	Rapid absorption, metabolized in liver, excreted in urine and feces
Pharmacodynamics:	Essential cofactor for fatty acid metabolism
CNS:	Lethargy, weakness
GI:	Nausea, vomiting, diarrhea
Other:	Body odor

CARNITINE, LEVOCARNITINE *continued*

Dosage:	0.5–1.0 g in divided doses; 50–100 mg/kg/d, max. 3 g/d (children)
Contraindications:	NK
Drug Interactions:	NK
Key Points:	Continue medication to avoid acute hypoglycemia and lactic acidosis due to primary carnitine deficiency; use dextrose-containing fluid to ↓ hypoglycemia

CHITOSAN

Other Name:	**None**
Indications:	Periodontitis, weight loss, ↓ cholesterol levels
Pharmacokinetics:	NK
Pharmacodynamics:	Cationic polysaccharide component of crustacean skeletons interacts with erythrocyte cellular membranes
GI:	Abdominal pain, flatulence, bulky stool, nausea
Other:	↓ Cholesterol, ↑ hemoglobin level, ↓ BUN/Cr
Dosage:	NK
Contraindications:	Allergy to shellfish
Drug Interactions:	NK
Key Points:	No scientific evidence to support indications

CHOLESTIN

Other Name:	**None**
Indications:	↓ Cholesterol biosynthesis
Pharmacokinetics:	NK
Pharmacodynamics:	Inhibits HMG CoA reductase
GI:	Cholestatic jaundice, ↑ LFTs
Other:	Depression, myositis, ↓ lipid levels, rash, pruritus
Dosage:	2.4 g PO bid
Contraindications:	Hepatic impairment, muscle diseases
Key Points:	No known adverse interaction with anesthetic drugs

CHONDROITIN, GLUCOSAMINE

Other Name:	**None**
Indications:	Osteoarthritis, degenerative joint disease

CHONDROITIN, GLUCOSAMINE *continued*

Pharmacokinetics:	Onset: 1 mo; high bioavailability; peak: 8 wk; duration: 1–2 mo (after discontinuing therapy); excreted in urine
Pharmacodynamics:	↑ Proteoglycan synthesis in articular cartilage, anti-inflammatory (due to local inhibition of interleukin-1β)
GI:	Nausea, vomiting, gastric irritation
Other:	↓ Platelet adhesion (glucosamine)
Dosages:	*Chrondroitin:* 1–2 g/d PO
	Glucosamine: 1.5–2.5 g/d PO
Contraindications:	Sensitivity to shark cartilage
Drug Interactions:	NK
Key Points:	No known adverse interactions with anesthetic drugs

CHROMIUM

Other Name:	**None**
	See Chapter 32, "Minerals"

CRANBERRY

Other Name:	**None**
Indications:	Periodontal gum disease, UTI
Pharmacokinetics:	NK
Pharmacodynamics:	↑ Hippuric acid, ↓ urinary pH, ↓ bacterial adherence to mucosal surfaces
GU:	↑ Stone formation (urolithiasis), urinary frequency/urgency
Other:	↓ Dental plaque formation, ↓ gingivitis
Dosage:	300–400 mL/d
Contraindication:	Urolithiasis
Key Points:	No known interactions with anesthetic drugs

CREATINE

Other Names:	**None**
Indications:	↑ Muscle size and strength, creatine deficiency
Pharmacokinetics:	Metabolized to creatinine, excreted in urine
Pharmacodynamics:	High-energy phosphate ↑ muscle activity (via phosphagen energy system), ↑ phosphocreatine levels in skeletal muscle

CREATINE *continued*

CV:	Hypovolemia, ↓ BP
Other:	↓ Cholesterol level
Dosage:	20–25 g/d × 1 wk, then 5–10 g/d for 10–12 wk
Contraindications:	CHF, severe hypertension, dehydration
Drug Interactions:	↑ Hypotension with antihypertensives, diuretics, H₂-blockers
Key Points:	Assess volume status before induction of general anesthesia

DANDELION

Other Name:	***Taraxacum officinale***
Indications:	Fluid retention, hepatitis, bile duct inflammation and gallstones, liver congestion, cystitis, dietary supplement
Pharmacokinetics:	NK
Pharmacodynamics:	Stimulates bile release, diuretic action
CV:	Hypovolemia, orthostatic hypotension, ↑ HR
GI:	↑ Gastric secretion, diarrhea, polydipsia
Other:	Polyuria, hypoglycemia, skin rash
Dosage:	250–500 mg (or 4–8 mL extract) PO tid; 2–8 g tid (dried root)
Contraindications:	Pregnancy, breast-feeding, acute cholecystitis
Drug Interactions:	Atopic (e.g., plant pollens)
Key Points:	Careful assessment of volume status prior to induction of anesthesia; ↑ CV depressant effects of general anesthetics

ECHINACEA

Other Names:	**None**
Indications:	Immune system stimulant, URI
Pharmacokinetics:	NK
Pharmacodynamics:	Anti-inflammatory, ↑ release of tumor necrosis factor from lymphocytes, inhibits bacterial hyaluronidase, ↑ phagocytosis
Dosage:	1–3 g PO tid, 3–5 mL/d (tincture)
Contraindications:	AIDS, tuberculosis, autoimmune disorders

ECHINACEA *continued*

Drug Interactions:	↑ Hepatotoxicity with methotrexate, ketoconazole, cyclosporine, phenytoin, amiodarone
Key Points:	No known adverse interaction with anesthetic drugs

EPHEDRA

Other Name:	**Ma Huang**
Indications:	Obesity, low energy state, asthma, URI
Pharmacokinetics:	Onset: <30 min; peak: 1–2 h; $T_{1/2}$ β: 6 h; crosses blood-brain barrier; excreted in urine
Pharmacodynamics:	Contains ephedrine and pseudophedrine, ↑ release of norepinephrine, ↑ sympathetic stimulation of α- and β-adrenoceptors
CNS:	Headache, confusion, hemorrhage (CVA), seizure
CV:	↑ BP, angina, MI, arrhythmias, sudden death, myocarditis
Other:	Heat stroke, uterine stimulant, ↑ LFTs
Dosage:	25 mg/d PO (max. 100 mg/d)
Contraindications:	Pregnancy, breast-feeding, impaired cerebral circulation, glaucoma, HTN, pheochromocytoma, thyrotoxicosis, CV disease
Drug Interactions:	Tachyphylaxis to ephedrine; ↑ insulin requirements in diabetics; TCAs, antihistamines, antihypertensives, thyroid hormone ↑ side effects; MAOIs ↑ risk of high fever
Key Points:	Sympathomimetics, cardiac glycosides, volatile anesthetics ↑ arrhythmias; ketamine or enflurane ↑ seizures; direct-acting adrenergic agonist (e.g., phenylephrine) should be used to control hypotension; discontinue use ≥ 24 h prior to surgery

EVENING PRIMROSE OIL (EPO)

Other Names:	**Fever plant, huile d'onagre, night willow herb, scabish, Ozark sundrops**
Indications:	Menopausal symptoms, asthma, atopic eczema, autoimmune disorders, whooping cough, mastalgia, GI disorders, wound healing
Pharmacokinetics:	Onset: 3–4 mo; essential fatty acid γ-linolenic acid (GLA) is metabolized to a precursor of prostaglandins

EVENING PRIMROSE OIL (EPO) *continued*

Pharmacodynamics:	Essential fatty acids for prostaglandin biosynthesis, antiarteriosclerotic, ↓ cholesterol level, antihypertensive, anti-inflammatory, immunomodulator properties
CNS:	↓ Headache; "hot flashes" (due to menopause)
GU:	Prolonged rupture of membranes, arrest of descent during delivery
Other:	↓ Cholesterol level, ↓ platelet aggregation, antioxidant, ↓ arthralgias
Dosage:	8% GLA 3–8 g/d PO; 1–4 g/d (children)
Contraindications:	Seizure disorders, pregnancy, estrogen-induced breast cancer
Drug Interactions:	↑ Seizures in schizophrenics treated with epileptogenic drugs (e.g., phenothiazines); ↑ effect of oxytocin; ↑ effect of antihypertensives
Key Points:	Use with general anesthesia and central neuroaxis blockade ↑ hypotension

FISH OIL (OMEGA-3 FATTY ACIDS)

Other Names:	**Eicosapentaenoic acid (EPA), docosahexaenoic acid (DHA)**
Trade Names:	**Cardi-Omega 3, Promega, Proto-Chol, Sea-Omega**
Indications:	Hypercholesterolemia, CAD, CVA, collagen vascular diseases, IgA and diabetic nephropathies, severe depression
Pharmacokinetics:	NK
Pharmacodynamics:	Antihypercholesterolemic, ↓ triglycerides, ↓ VLDL, ↓ chylomicrons, ↑ RBC deformability, antithrombogenic and anti-inflammatory
CV:	↑ BP, vasoconstriction
GI:	Abdominal distention, belching, dyspepsia, flatulence, diarrhea
Other:	Rash, hypoglycemia, ↓ platelet aggregation, ↑ bleeding time
Dosage:	1 g/d or bid (includes eicosapentaenoic acid [180 mg] and docosahexaenoic acid [120 mg])
Contraindications:	Coagulation disorders, concomitant use of anticoagulants
Drug Interactions:	↑ Bleeding with aspirin, ticlopidine, heparin, warfarin, dipyridamole, sulfinpyrazone, ASA, NSAIDs
Key Points:	Can ↑ operative site bleeding; may ↑ hemorrhage with peripheral nerve blocks

GARLIC

Other Name:	***Allium sativum***
Indications:	Hypercholesterolemia, CAD, hypertension, diabetes; antibacterial, antiviral, antifungal, and antiparasitic activity
Pharmacokinetics:	NK
Pharmacodynamics:	↑ Activity of allinase, converting alliin to allicin, a potent antibacterial agent, a byproduct of allicin (ajoenes) possesses antithrombotic activity
GI:	Dyspepsia, eructation, flatulence, halitosis
Other:	↓ Cholesterol, hypoglycemia, ↓ platelet aggregation, ↑ bleeding
Dosage:	1–4 g/d over 3–6 mo, 2–5 mg/d allicin extract
Contraindications:	Coagulation disorders, gastritis, pregnancy
Drug Interactions:	↑ Bleeding with ASA, NSAIDs, platelet inhibitors, thrombolytic drugs; ↑ effects of antidiabetic drugs, ginger, ginkgo biloba, ginseng
Key Points:	Assess coagulation to ↓ hemorrhagic complications and intraoperative hypotension; monitor blood glucose levels; discontinue usage 7–10 d prior to surgery

GINGER

Other Name:	***Zingiber officinale***
Indications:	Loss of appetite, motion sickness, flatulence
Pharmacokinetics:	Onset: <30 min; peak: 1–2 h; duration: 4 h
Pharmacodynamics:	Inhibits thromboxane synthetase, stimulates prostacyclin
CNS:	Depression, anticonvulsant
CV:	(+) inotropic effect, ↓ BP, ↓ HR, arrhythmias
GI:	↓ Nausea, ↑ gastric/intestinal motility, ↑ salivary/gastric secretion
Other:	↑ Bleeding time, pungent constituents
Dosage:	2–4 g/d PO; 1.5–3 mL qid; <100 mg (2 h before travel)
Contraindications:	Gallstones
Drug Interactions:	↑ Bleeding with heparin, warfarin, antiplatelet drugs
Key Points:	↑ CNS depressant effects of anesthetic drugs; ↑ surgical bleeding

GINKGO BILOBA

Other Names:	**Ginkgo nut, Bioginkgo, Gincosan**
Indications:	Improving memory, dementia, intermittent claudication, Alzheimer's disease, Parkinson's disease
Pharmacokinetics:	Onset: <4 h; peak: 2–3 h; crosses blood-brain and placental barriers
Pharmacodynamics:	Ca-membrane stabilizer, ↑ uptake of oxygen and glucose, antioxidant activity
CNS:	Seizures, headache, ↑ CBF
GI:	Nausea, vomiting, ↑ salivation
Other:	↓ Blood viscosity, ↓ platelet aggregation, ↑ bleeding, hyphemas
Dosage:	40–80 mg PO tid (25% flavonoids and 6% terpenes)
Contraindications:	Coagulopathy or bleeding disorders; pregnancy; use with meperidine, SSRIs, MAOIs, OTC cold/flu products
Drug Interactions:	↑ Bleeding with antiplatelet, antithrombotic, anticoagulant drugs; ↑ effect of β-blockers and opioid analgesics
Key Points:	↑ CNS depressant and hypotensive effects of anesthetic and analgesic drugs; hypertension may occur with local anesthetics containing epinephrine; due to ↓ platelet function, discontinue 1–2 wk before surgery

GINSENG

Other Names:	*Panax ginseng, Panax quinquefolius,* Siberian ginseng (*Eleutherococcus senticosus*)
Indications:	Fatigue, impotence, ↑ performance, ↑ immune response
Pharmacokinetics:	Rapidly absorbed from GI tract, eliminated in urine
Pharmacodynamics:	↑ Vascular endothelium nitric oxide production in lung, heart, kidney, corpus cavernosum
CNS:	Agitation, restlessness
CV:	↑ BP, ↑ HR
Other:	Hypoglycemia, mastalgia, postmenopausal bleeding, ↓ platelet aggregation
Dosage:	200–400 mg/d PO
Contraindications:	Hypertension, bleeding disorders, use of estrogens, corticosteroids, or phenelzine; pregnancy, breast-feeding, schizophrenia, mania
Drug Interactions:	↑ Bleeding with anticoagulants, antiplatelets, antithrombotics; ↑ effect of antidiabetic drugs, MAOIs, digoxin; ↓ analgesic effects of opioid analgesics; ↓ anticoagulant effect of warfarin

GINSENG *continued*

Key Points: Ginseng should be discontinued 7–10 d before surgery due to ↑ risk of bleeding during perioperative period

GLYCINE

Other Name:	**None**
Indications:	Hyperaldosteronism, BPH, irrigant during TURP, psychiatric disorders, gastric ulcer, acute stroke
Pharmacokinetics:	NK
Pharmacodynamics:	↑ Influx of Na^+ and Ca^{2+} via NMDA receptor stimulation
CNS:	Headache, visual changes, drowsiness, seizures (↑ cerebral edema)
CV:	↓ HR (via Cushing's reflex), ↓ BP, pulmonary edema
GI:	Nausea, ↓ gastric acid
Other:	TURP syndrome, hyponatremia
Dosage:	0.1 g/d PO initially, then 0.4–0.8 mg/kg/d
Contraindications:	NK
Drug Interactions:	↓ Toxicity of anticonvulsant, neuroleptic, antidepressant drugs; ↑ efficacy of haloperidol; ↓ clozapine efficacy
Key Points:	Monitor for glycine toxicity during TURP procedures (e.g., hyponatremia); glycine-receptor antagonist (felbamate) ↑ seizure threshold and ↓ stroke infarct size; volatile anesthetics and alcohol ↑ glycine activity

GOLDEN SEAL

Other Names:	**Orange root, yellow root, turmeric root, *Hydrastis canadensis***
Indications:	Diarrhea, ulcerative colitis, irritable bowel syndrome, peptic ulcers, influenza and sinus infections, diuretic, hemostatic
Pharmacokinetics:	NK
Pharmacodynamics:	Isoquinoline, alkaloids, hydrastine, berberine (intraluminally)
CNS:	Agitation, hallucinations, seizures
CV:	↑ BP, (+) inotropic, ↓ HR, vasoconstriction
GI:	Diarrhea, jaundice, gastric irritation
Pulmonary:	Bronchospasm, dyspnea
Other:	Hypoglycemia, muscle spasm, diuresis, uterine stimulation

GOLDEN SEAL *continued*

Dosage:	Berberine: 5–10 mg/kg/d (×6); 1 mL tincture tid (×1 wk)
Contraindications:	Epilepsy, hypercoagulable states, pregnancy, breast-feeding
Drug Interactions:	↑ Insulin-like activity, ↓ heparin and warfarin anticoagulants
Key Points:	Monitor perioperative glucose levels and coagulation status; can ↑ volatile anesthetic requirement due to CNS stimulant properties

GRAPEFRUIT JUICE

Other Name:	**None**
Indications:	Dietary supplement
Pharmacodynamics:	Inhibits hepatic cytochrome P_{450}–dependent drug metabolism
Key Points:	↑ Clinical effects (and duration of activity) of anesthetic drugs dependent on hepatic metabolism for clearance; ↓ efficacy of prodrugs dependent on P_{450} metabolism for generation of active metabolites

GREEN TEA

Other Name:	**None**
Indications:	Depression, atherosclerosis, vascular headaches
Pharmacokinetics:	NK
Pharmacodynamics:	CNS stimulant properties
CNS:	Restlessness, insomnia
CV:	Palpitations
GI:	Vomiting, abdominal pain, constipation
Dosage:	3 cups/d (max. 5 cups/d); polyphenol (80%), epigallocatechin gallate (55%), caffeine (60 mg)
Contraindications:	CHF, recent MI
Key Points:	Potential for CNS stimulation and emetic side effects

LICORICE

Other Name:	*Glycyrrhiza glabra*
Indications:	Chronic fatigue syndrome, ↓ immune function, gastric and duodenal ulcer, bronchitis, Addison's disease, atherosclerosis

LICORICE *continued*

Pharmacokinetics:	Metabolized by liver, excreted in urine and feces
Pharmacodynamics:	Glycyrrhizin/glycrrhetinic acid inhibits 11-β-hydroxysteroid dehydrogenase (↓ cortisol), prostaglandin dehydrogenase and reductase (↓ prostaglandin E)
CNS:	Headache (vascular), paresthesia, visual changes
CV:	↑ BP, arrhythmias, fluid retention, pedal edema
GI:	Diarrhea, dark stool
Other:	↓ Blood clotting, ↑ glucose level, ↓ platelet aggregation, pseudohyperaldosteronism, hypernatremia, hypokalemia
Dosage:	1–5 g PO tid; 380–760 mg before meals; 1–5 mL PO tid (as extract)
Contraindications:	Cholestatic hepatitis, CHF, hepatorenal impairment
Drug Interactions:	↑ Effects of diuretics and steroids; interferes with oral hypoglycemics and BCP; ↑ arrhythmias with digoxin
Key Points:	Potential for glucose and electrolyte disturbances and fluid retention; discontinue 1–2 wk before elective surgery; may alter response to nondepolarizing muscle relaxants

MELATONIN

Other Names:	*N*-Acetyl-5-methoxytryptamine, Melatonex
	See Chapter 26, "Hormones"

S-ADENOSYL-ʟ-METHIONINE

Trade Name:	SAMe
Indications:	Depression, dementia, Alzheimer's and Parkinson's diseases, migraine headache, fibromyalgia, hepatic disorders
Pharmacokinetics:	Onset: 1–2 h; peak: 3–5 h; $T_{1/2}$ β: 100 min; rapidly crosses blood-brain barrier; metabolized to homocysteine (1st-pass effect), excreted in urine and feces
Pharmacodynamics:	↑ Hormones and neurotransmitters; ↑ efficiency of receptor-effector coupling, stimulates articular cartilage growth
CNS:	Anxiety, confusion
GI:	Nausea, vomiting, diarrhea, flatulence
Dosage:	400–1600 mg/d PO, or 200–400 mg/d IV
Contraindications:	Concurrent use of MAOIs

S-ADENOSYL-L-METHIONINE *continued*

Drug Interactions:	↑ Efficacy of antidepressants; ↑ side effects of MAOIs; ↓ hepatotoxic effect of alcohol, acetaminophen, steroids, phenobarbital
Key Points:	Adverse effects on CNS neurotransmitter function

SAW PALMETTO

Other Names:	***Serenoa repens**, sabal berry, *Sabal fructus**
Indications:	BPH, sexual stimulation
Pharmacokinetics:	Variable absorption; peak: 1–2 h; $T_{1/2}$ β: 1.9 h
Pharmacodynamics:	Inhibits 5α-reductase; ↓ cytokines, leukotriene B_4, thromboxane B_2
GI:	Nausea, abdominal pain
GU:	↓ Nocturia, ↓ dysuria
Other:	Gynecomastia, ↑ testosterone level
Dosage:	1–2 g (sabal berry) or 32 mg (*N*-hexane extract)
Contraindications:	Pregnancy
Drug Interactions:	↑ Urinary retention with anticholinergics
Key Points:	No known perioperative complications

β-SITOSTEROL

Other Name:	None
Indications:	↑ Immune system, BPH, ↑ cholesterol, gallstones, migraine headache, chronic fatigue syndrome, bronchitis, SLE, alopecia, colon cancer prophylaxis, ↓ sexual activity
Pharmacokinetics:	NK
Pharmacodynamics:	Constituent in rye germ oil with ability to emulsify fats, ↑ activity of T-cells, ↓ prostaglandin synthesis (in prostate gland)
CV:	Chest pain (angina)
GI:	Nausea, vomiting, flatus
Pulmonary:	Bronchospasm (wheezing)
Dosage:	60–800 mg PO tid
Contraindications:	Inherited lipid storage disease (sitosterolemia)
Drug Interactions:	↓ Absorption of vitamin E and β-carotene; antihyperlipidemic drugs have additive effects in ↓ cholesterol; pravastatin ↓ level

β-SITOSTEROL *continued*

Key Points:	No known interactions with anesthetic drugs

SOY

Other Name:	**None**
Indications:	Dietary supplement, enuresis, BPH, common cold
Pharmacokinetics:	NK
Pharmacodynamics:	Isoflavones with potent antioxidant and weak estrogen, ↓ tyrosine kinase
GU:	↑ Vaginal secretions, ↓ hot flashes
Other:	↓ Lipid levels, ↓ insulin dosage, venous thromboembolism, ↑ folate level
Dosage:	50–100 mg PO bid
Contraindications:	Soy allergic, hormone replacement therapy, pregnancy, breast-feeding
Drug Interactions:	NK
Key Points:	Propofol emulsion also contains soybean oil

ST. JOHN'S WORT

Other Name:	*Hypericum perforatum*
Indications:	Depression, anxiety, menstrual cramps
Pharmacokinetics:	Onset: <30 min; $T_{1/2}$ β: 43 h; hepatic metabolism, excreted in urine
Pharmacodynamics:	Inhibitor of serotonin, norepinephrine, dopamine reuptake
CNS:	Fatigue, restlessness
CV:	↑ HR, ↑ BP (rare)
Other:	Photosensitivity, rash, nausea
Dosage:	300–500 mg PO tid
Contraindications:	Sensitivity to light, lactation, pregnancy
Drug Interactions:	↑ Photosensitivity with tetracyclines and vitamin A; SSRIs and MAOIs ↑ risk of serotonin-like syndrome; ↓ effects of warfarin, benzodiazepines, β-blockers, steroids, Ca^{2+}-channel blockers, cyclosporin; ↓ digoxin level
Key Points:	↑ CNS depressant effects of opioid analgesics; ↑ clearance of drugs metabolized by cytochrome P_{450}; discontinue intake at least 1 wk before surgery

VALERIAN

Other Name:	***Valeriana officinalis***
Indications:	Insomnia, anxiety, muscle spasms, benzodiazepine withdrawal
Pharmacokinetics:	NK
Pharmacodynamics:	Binds to CNS barbiturate and benzodiazepine receptors
CNS:	Drowsiness, blurred vision, restlessness
CV:	Arrhythmias
Dosage:	2–3 g/d, 2–6 mL/d (liquid extract) or 5–15 mL/d (tincture)
Contraindications:	Pregnancy, breast-feeding, severe hepatic disease
Drug Interactions:	↑ Sedation with MAOIs, opioid analgesics, benzodiazepines
Key Points:	↑ CNS depressant effects of anesthetic drugs, prolongs emergence from general anesthesia; benzodiazepine-like withdrawal syndrome when discontinued; ↑ effects of muscle relaxants; recommend slow withdrawal over 1–2 wk prior to surgery

26

Hormones

ABARELIX

Trade Name:	**Plenaxis**
	See Chapter 13, "Antineoplastics"

CALCITONIN

Trade Names:	**Calcimar, Miacalcin, Salmonine**
Indications:	Paget's disease, osteogenesis imperfecta, osteoporosis, hypercalcemia
Pharmacokinetics:	Onset: <3 min; peak: 0.5 h (topical), 4 h; duration: 1 h (topical), 8–24 h; rapid metabolism in kidney, excreted in urine
Pharmacodynamics:	Inhibits bone resorption of Ca^{2+}, $\uparrow$ cAMP level in bone cells $\downarrow$ renal tubular resorption of Ca^{2+}
CNS:	Headache, weakness, dizziness, paresthesia, eye pain
CV:	Angina, pedal edema
GI:	Diarrhea, anorexia, nausea, vomiting, abdominal pain, bad taste
GU:	Urinary frequency, nocturia, $\uparrow$ excretion of Ca^{2+}, PO_4^{2-}, Na^+
Other:	Facial flushing, rash, rhinitis, $\downarrow$ bone pain
Dosage:	200 IU/d (one spray); 100 IU/d IM, for maintenance; 50–100 q2d, 4–8 IU/kg/d IM (hypercalcemia)
Contraindications:	Sensitivity to salmon calcitonin
Drug Interactions:	Ca^{2+}-containing preparations and vitamin D $\downarrow$ effects of calcitonin
Key Points:	Check electrolytes (Ca^{2+}, PO_4^{2-}, Na^+) prior to surgery

CLOMIPHENE

Trade Names:	**Clomid, Milophene, Serophene**
Indications:	Anovulation (or oligo-ovulation), male infertility
Pharmacokinetics:	Onset: <1 h; duration: 6–12 h; $T_{1/2}$ β: 5 d; metabolized by liver, excreted in feces
Pharmacodynamics:	$\uparrow$ Release of pituitary gonadotropin, FSH, LU, leads to development and maturation of ovarian follicle
CNS:	Headache, blurred vision, nervousness, insomnia
GI:	Abdominal discomfort, nausea, vomiting, flatulence
GU:	$\uparrow$ Urine output, ovarian hyperstimulation syndrome, menorrhagia
Pulmonary:	Cough, dyspnea
Other:	$\uparrow$ Secretion of LH and FSH, "hot flashes"
Dosage:	50–100 mg/d PO

CLOMIPHENE *continued*

Contraindications:	Pregnancy, uncontrolled thyroid (or adrenal) dysfunction, hepatic dysfunction, intracranial lesion, ovarian cyst, genital bleeding
Drug Interactions:	NK
Key Points:	No known interactions with anesthetic drugs

CORTICOTROPIN (ADRENOCORTICOTROPIC HORMONE [ACTH])

Trade Name:	**Acthar**
Indications:	Infantile spasms, multiple sclerosis, hormone replacement, test of adrenocortical function
Pharmacokinetics:	Onset: <10 min; peak: 1 h; duration: 2–4 h; $T_{1/2}$ β: 15 min; excreted by kidney
Pharmacodynamics:	Stimulates synthesis of adrenal steroids
CNS:	Seizures, ↑ ICP, dizziness, pseudotumor cerebri, cataract, glaucoma
CV:	↑ BP, CHF, necrotizing vasculitis, shock
GI:	Peptic ulceration, nausea, vomiting, pancreatitis (↑ amylase)
Other:	Muscle weakness, electrolyte disturbances, ecchymoses, impaired wound healing, acne, diaphoresis, hyperglycemia
Dosage:	10–20 U IM qid (80 U); 20–40 U/d or 80 U IM q 2 d (children)
Contraindications:	Peptic ulcer, scleroderma, osteoporosis, fungal infections, CHF, hypertension, sensitivity to pork products, Cushing's syndrome
Drug Interactions:	Amphotericin B, carbonic anhydrase inhibitors and diuretics ↑ electrolyte losses; ↑ digitalis toxicity; cortisone, estrogens, hydrocortisone ↑ cortisol level; indomethacin, NSAIDs, salicylates ↑ GI bleeding; ↑ oral hypoglycemic and insulin requirement
Key Points:	Consider supplemental glucocorticoids preoperatively due to atrophy of the ACTH-producing cells in anterior pituitary

COSYNTROPIN

Trade Name:	**Cortrosyn**
Indications:	Evaluation of adrenocortical function
Pharmacokinetics:	Onset: <10 min; peak: 45–60 min; duration: 4–8 h

COSYNTROPIN *continued*

Pharmacodynamics:	Anterior pituitary hormone binds specific receptors in adrenal cell
CNS:	Seizures, anxiety, dizziness, pseudotumor cerebri, glaucoma
GI:	Peptic ulcer, pancreatitis, abdominal distention, nausea, vomiting
Other:	Menstrual irregularities, myopathy, petechiae, diaphoresis, acne
Dosage:	0.25–0.75 mg IV/IM; 0.125 mg IV/IM (children)
Contraindications:	NK
Drug Interactions:	Blood and plasma products inactivate; cortisone, estrogens, hydrocortisone ↑ cortisol level
Key Points:	Less likely to cause allergic reactions than ACTH (corticotropin)

DARBEPOETIN ALFA

Trade Name:	**Aranesp**
Indications:	Anemia (due to chemotherapy), CRF
Pharmacokinetics:	Peak: 34 h (SC); duration: 49 h (SC), 21 h (IV); $T_{1/2}$ β: 21 h (IV), 49 h (SC); steady-state levels within 4 wk
Pharmacodynamics:	Glycoprotein which stimulates erythropoiesis
CNS:	Headache, dizziness, fatigue, asthenia, fever, seizures
CV:	↑ BP, thrombosis, arrhythmia, acute MI, angina
GI:	Nausea, vomiting, diarrhea, constipation
Pulmonary:	Dyspnea, cough, pulmonary embolus
Other:	Myalgia, dehydration, pruritus, rash
Dosage:	2.25 µg/kg/wk (max. 4.5 µg/kg) SC/IV
Contraindications:	Uncontrolled hypertension; hemolytic and sickle cell anemia, thalassemia, porphyria
Drug Interactions:	NK
Key Points:	Use with ketamine, etomidate, enflurane may ↑ risk of seizure-like activity

DESMOPRESSIN (DEAMINO-D-ARGININE VASOPRESSIN [DDAVP])

Trade Name:	**Stimate**
Indications:	Diabetes insipidus (neurogenic), polydipsia, uria, hemophilia A, von Willebrand's disease, Factor VIII deficiency, nocturnal enuresis

DESMOPRESSIN *continued*

Pharmacokinetics:	Onset: <30 min (IV), 1 h (topical); peak: 1–5 h; duration: 4–12 h; $T_{1/2}$ β: 75 min (↑ in von Willebrand's factor over 3 h, Factor VIII over 24 h)
Pharmacodynamics:	*Antidiuretic:* ↑ Water permeability at renal tubules and collecting ducts
	Antihemorrhagic: ↑ Release endogenous Factor VIII
CNS:	Headache, confusion, seizures, coma
CV:	Cardiovascular instability, flushing
GI:	Abdominal cramps, nausea
GU:	↑ Water reabsorption (↓ urine output, ↑ urine osmolality, ↓ serum osmolality), vulvar pain
Pulmonary:	Rhinitis, epistaxis, nasal congestion, sore throat, cough
Other:	Hyponatremia, water intoxication, ↑ clotting Factor VIII, ↑ von Willebrand's factor activity, ↓ platelet aggregation, local erythema
Dosage:	2-4 μg/d IV over 15 min; 0.05–0.6 mg PO bid; 0.1–0.4 mL/d
Contraindications:	Factor VIII concentrations ≤5%; Factor VIII antibodies, severe coronary artery disease; renal failure; seizures, cystic fibrosis
Drug Interactions:	↑ Antidiuretic effect with carbamazepine, chlorpropamide, clofibrate; ↓ antidiuretic effect with demeclocycline, lithium, norepinephrine, heparin, epinephrine; alcohol ↑ side effects
Key Points:	Administration of glucocorticoids preoperatively ↑ antidiuretic potency; avoid hyponatremia during urologic procedures

DEXTROTHYROXINE (D-THYROXINE)

Trade Name:	**Choloxin**
Indications:	Primary hypercholesterolemia (type II hyperlipidemia)
Pharmacokinetics:	Onset: 1–2 h; bioavailability: 25%; peak: 1–2 mo; protein binding: 100%; duration 12–24 h; $T_{1/2}$ β: 18 h; metabolized in liver, excreted in urine
Pharmacodynamics:	Generalized ↑ metabolic activity, ↓ cholesterol levels
CV:	Arrhythmias
Hepatic:	↑ Catabolism of LDL
Other:	Weak thyroid effects (due to levothyroxine), gallstones
Dosage:	1–8 mg/d PO; 0.05–0.4 mg/kg/d (max. 4 mg/d) (children)

DEXTROTHYROXINE
(D-THYROXINE) *continued*

Contraindications:	Coronary artery disease, hepatorenal impairment, hypertension
Drug Interactions:	↓ Effect of β-blockers; ↓ effect of digoxin; TCAs ↑ CNS stimulation (irritability) and arrhythmias, ↑ effects of anticoagulants; cholestyramine, ursodiol, colestipol ↓ effects
Key Points:	Use with volatile anesthetics, epinephrine, or α-adrenergic agonists ↑ arrhythmias during perioperative period

EPOETIN ALFA
(ERYTHROPOIETIN)

Trade Names:	**Epogen, Procrit**
Indications:	Anemia
Pharmacokinetics:	Onset: <1 h; peak: 1–2 h (IV), 6–24 h (SC); duration: 2 wk; $T_{1/2}\,\beta$: 4–13 h
Pharmacodynamics:	Glycoprotein that stimulates erythropoiesis, ↑ RBC production
CNS:	Seizures, headache, paresthesia
CV:	↑ BP, edema, angina, ↑ HR
GU:	Renal impairment, electrolyte imbalance, hyperuricemia
Other:	↑ Thrombosis, rash, urticaria, cough, arthralgia, polycythemia, dyspnea
Dosage:	25–100 U/kg IV/SC (3×/wk)
Contraindications:	Sensitivity to mammalian cell–derived products or albumin, hypertension, hypercoagulable disorders, myelodysplastic syndromes
Drug Interactions:	NK
Key Points:	Anesthetics with proconvulsant activities (e.g., ketamine, etomidate, enflurane) should be carefully titrated to avoid CNS stimulation

GLUCAGON

Trade Name:	GlucaGen
Indications:	Severe hypoglycemia (due to oral antidiabetics or insulin), relaxation of smooth musculature for GI radiology and endoscopy procedures, relief of foreign body obstruction in esophagus

GLUCAGON *continued*

Pharmacokinetics:	Onset: 5–20 min; peak: 30 min; duration: 60–90 min; Vd: 0.25 L/kg; Cl: 13.5 mL/kg/min; $T_{1/2}$ β: 3–6 min; metabolized in liver, excreted in urine
Pharmacodynamics:	↑ Plasma glucose levels, causes smooth muscle relaxation and (+) inotropic on myocardium
CNS:	Dizziness
CV:	Arrhythmias, ↑ BP
GI:	↓ Peristalsis activity, nausea, vomiting
Other:	Hypokalemia, rash, muscle weakness (cramps)
Dosage:	1 mg IV, repeat dose after 15 min; 20–30 µg/kg IV (children)
Contraindications:	Diabetes mellitus, insulinoma, pheochromocytoma
Drug Interactions:	↑ Effect of anticoagulants; epinephrine ↑ hyperglycemia
Key Points:	α-Adrenergic agonists ↑ risk of arrhythmia during surgery

HUMAN CHORIONIC GONADOTROPIN (hCG)

Trade Names:	**Chorex, Chorigon, Follutein, Gonic, Glukor, Profasi**
Indications:	Cryptorchidism, infertility, hypogonadotropic hypogonadism
Pharmacokinetics:	Onset: 2 h; peak: 6 h; duration: 36 h; $T_{1/2}$ β: 11–23 h; excreted in urine unchanged
Pharmacodynamics:	Mimics action of LH, stimulates testicular Leydig's cells
CNS:	Headache, irritability, depression, fatigue
CV:	↑ Vascular permeability, thromboembolism
GI:	Abdominal pain, dyspepsia, nausea, vomiting, diarrhea
GU:	Early puberty, ovarian cysts, gynecomastia
Other:	↑ Androgen production (by testes); ↑ ovarian progesterone and estrogen production, pelvic pain, weight gain, pedal edema
Dosage:	500–1000 U/d IM
Contraindications:	Pituitary tumor, precocious puberty, fibroid uterine tumors, ovarian cyst, thrombophlebitis, androgen-dependent neoplasms
Drug Interactions:	NK
Key Points:	No adverse interactions with anesthetics reported

INSULIN

Other Names:	**Humulin, Lantus, Lente Insulin, NPH Insulin, Regular Insulin, Semilente Insulin, Ultralente U, Novalog**
Indications:	Diabetes mellitus, chronic pancreatitis
Pharmacokinetics:	*Regular (Humulin):* Onset: 0.5–1 h; peak: 2–3 h; duration: 5–7 h *Intermediate (NPH, Lente):* Onset: 1–2 h; peak: 4–15 h; duration: 12–24 h *Long-acting (Ultralente):* Onset: 4–8 h; peak: 20 h; duration: 36 h
Pharmacodynamics:	Facilitates glucose uptake by skeletal muscle, fat, storage as glycogen in liver; inhibition of hepatic glucose production
CNS:	Somnolence, confusion, seizure activity
Other:	Hypoglycemia, hyperglycemia (due to Somogyi effect); ↑ muscle uptake of glucose and amino acids, ↑ protein biosynthesis, hypokalemia, lipohypertrophy (due to ↑ storage of fat in adipose cells); ↓ lipolysis, weight gain, pedal edema
Dosage:	0.1–1 U/kg/d in divided doses; 0.1–1 U/kg/d IV/SC (children); 5–10 U over 5 min (K^+)
Contraindications:	Sensitivity to insulin formation (porcine insulin is less antigenic than bovine products); K^+-lowering drugs (e.g., diuretics)
Drug Interactions:	Furosemide, epinephrine, corticosteroids, thyroxine, glucagons, estrogens ↓ effect; alcohol, MAOIs, guanethidine ↑ hypoglycemia; α-agonists, β-blockers, somatostatin, diazoxide, thiazide diuretics, volatile anesthetics ↓ effect
Key Points:	$β_1$-Blockers can inhibit clinical signs of hypoglycemia under anesthesia; diabetics with underlying CV disease are sensitive to hemodynamic depressant effects of IV and volatile anesthetics

LEVOTHYROXINE (L-THYROXINE) [T_4])

Trade Names:	**Cytomel, Levoid, Levothroid, Levoxine, Synthroid, Thyrolar**
Indications:	Thyroid hormone deficiency (hypothyroidism), chronic lymphocytic thyroiditis, myxedema coma

LEVOTHYROXINE
(L-THYROXINE) [T$_4$] *continued*

Pharmacokinetics:
Onset: 24 h (oral); peak: 1–3 wk after oral therapy begins; protein binding: 99%; T$_{1/2}$ β: 6–7 d; deiodinated in peripheral tissues to T$_3$; metabolized in liver (deiodinated), excreted in feces

Pharmacodynamics:
Promotes gluconeogenesis, ↑ glycogen stores, ↑ protein synthesis

CNS: Tremors, headache, nervousness, insomnia

CV: ↑ HR, arrhythmias, angina, cardiac arrest

GI: ↑ Appetite, ↑ GI motility, ↑ hepatic blood flow

GU: ↑ Renal blood flow, ↑ GFR, menstrual irregularity

Other: Catabolic (calorigenic) and anabolic effects, hyperglycemia, ↑ free fatty acids, ↑ basal metabolism, ↑ erythropoiesis, ↑ RBC turnover, muscle cramps and weakness, rash, urticaria, alopecia

Dosage:
50 μg/d PO, ↑ by 25–50 μg/d (max. 200 μg/d); 3–8 μg/kg/d (children)

Contraindications:
Adrenocortical/pituitary insufficiency, acute MI, hyperthyroidism

Drug Interactions:
↓ Clearance of adrenocorticoids with ↓ levels; ↑ anticoagulant effect; TCAs ↑ therapeutic and toxic effects; ↑ requirement for antidiabetic drugs; β-blockers ↓ conversion of T$_4$ and T$_3$; cholestyramine ↓ absorption; estrogens, phenytoin ↑ dose requirements

Key Points:
Anesthetics, β-stimulant properties (e.g., ketamine) predispose to tachycardia and possible myocardial ischemia

LIOTHYRONINE (T$_3$), LIOTRIX (T$_3$ AND T$_4$)

Trade Names:
Cytomel, Triostat (liothyronine), Thyrolar (liotrix)

Indications:
Hypothyroidism, myxedema, thyroid goiter

Pharmacokinetics:
Onset: <1 h; peak: 2–5 d; duration: 3 d; T$_{1/2}$ β: 1–2 d; metabolized in liver, kidney, intestines; excreted in feces

Pharmacodynamics:
Promotes gluconeogenesis, ↑ metabolic rate of tissue, stimulates protein synthesis, ↑ mobilization of glycogen

CNS: Nervousness, insomnia, tremor, headache

CV: ↑ HR, angina

GI: Diarrhea, vomiting, constipation

Other: Diaphoresis, heat intolerance, menstrual irregularities, dyspnea

LIOTHYRONINE (T₃),
LIOTRIX (T₃ AND T₄) *continued*

Dosage:	5–25 µg/d up to 100 µg/d PO; 25–50 µg IV
Contraindications:	Acute MI, thyrotoxicosis, adrenal insufficiency
Drug Interactions:	↑ Effects of TCAs, sympathomimetics; estrogens ↑ requirements; ↑ effects of anticoagulants; ↑ requirement for antidiabetic drugs
Key Points:	Concomitant administration of β-blockers ↓ conversion of T_4 to T_3

MELATONIN

Other Name:	**N-Acetyl-5-methoxytryptamine**
Trade Name:	**Melatonex**
Indication:	Regulation of sleep-wake cycle (jet lag, shift work), autism (Rett's syndrome)
Pharmacokinetics:	Bioavailability: 40%; $T_{1/2}$ β: 45 min; crosses blood-brain barrier; extensively metabolized in liver (1st-pass effect), excreted in urine
Pharmacodynamics:	Resets the body to the environmental clock to normalize physiologic and behavioral sleep patterns
CNS:	Drowsiness, somnolence
Other:	Dyspnea, palpitations
Dosage:	2.5–10 mg PO hs (×3–5 d)
Drug Interactions:	↑ Benzodiazepine-induced sedation; alcohol ↑ side effects
Key Points:	↑ CNS depressant effects of anesthetic and analgesic drugs

MENOTROPINS

Trade Names:	**Humegon, Pergonal**
Indications:	Infertility (↑ ovarian follicle development and spermatogenesis); ovulation and implantation; ↑ testosterone due to pituitary hypofunction
Pharmacokinetics:	Onset: 9–12 d; $T_{1/2}$ β: 70 h; excreted in urine
Pharmacodynamics:	↑ Growth and maturation of ovarian follicles by mimicking endogenous LH and FSH; ↑ spermatogenesis with hCG
CNS:	Headache, malaise, dizziness, fever
CV:	↑ HR
GI:	Nausea, vomiting, diarrhea, cramps, bloating

MENOTROPINS *continued*

GU:	Ovarian enlargement, ectopic pregnancy, electrolyte imbalance
Other:	ARDS, pulmonary embolism, rash, erythrocytosis, gynecomastia
Dosage:	75–150 IU FSH and 75–150 IU LH IV (women > men)
Contraindications:	Pituitary tumor, fibroma, pregnancy, abnormal vaginal bleeding, ovarian cyst, 1° ovarian and testicular failure, hypoadrenalism
Drug Interactions:	NK
Key Points:	Check pregnancy test and electrolyte status preoperatively

OXYTOCIN

Trade Names:	**Pitocin, Syntocinon**
Indications:	Induction of labor, postpartum bleeding, induce abortion
Pharmacokinetics:	Onset: 3–5 min; peak: 10–30 min; protein binding: 30%; duration: 1–3 h; $T_{1/2} \beta$: 3–5 min; metabolized in kidney and liver, excreted in urine
Pharmacodynamics:	$\uparrow Na^+$ permeability of uterine myofibrils, $\uparrow$ contractions of uterine smooth muscle
CNS:	Subarachnoid hemorrhage, seizures/coma (due to water intoxication)
CV:	$\uparrow$ BP, $\uparrow$ HR, $\uparrow$ CVP
GI:	Nausea, vomiting
GU:	Abruptio placentae, $\downarrow$ uterine blood flow, uterine tetany
Other:	Water retention, afibrinogenemia, rhinorrhea
Dosage:	1–10 U/min (max. 100 U)
Contraindications:	Toxemia, hypertonic uterus, placenta previa; cephalopelvic disproportion
Drug Interactions:	Sympathomimetics $\uparrow$ vasopressor effects
Key Points:	Thiopental may cause delayed induction of anesthesia, $\uparrow$ sympathomimetic activity with desflurane

PEGVISOMANT

Trade Name:	**Somavert**
Indications:	Acromegaly
Pharmacokinetics:	Onset: slow; bioavailability: 57%; peak: 33–77 h; Vd: 7 L; Cl: 28–36 mL/h; $T_{1/2} \beta$: 6 d; less than 1% in urine

PEGVISOMANT *continued*

Pharmacodynamics:	Synthetic analog of human growth hormone (GH) that interferes with GH signal transduction
CNS:	Dizziness
GI:	↑ LFTs
Other:	Infection, peripheral edema, sinusitis, hypoglycemia
Dosage:	10–20 mg/d SC (max. 30 mg/d)
Contraindications:	Latex allergy
Drug Interactions:	Opioid analgesics ↑ dosage requirement; ↓ insulin, oral hypoglycemic agents
Key Points:	Monitor glucose levels during perioperative period

SOMATROPIN

Trade Names:	**Genotropin, Humatrope, Nutropin, Serostim**
Indications:	Growth failure, GH deficiency, Turner's syndrome, cachexia
Pharmacokinetics:	Onset: 1 h; peak: 2–4 h; duration: 12–48 h; $T_{1/2}$ β: 22 min; metabolized in liver, excreted in urine
Pharmacodynamics:	Purified (synthetic) GH, stimulates organ growth
CNS:	Headache, otitis media, ↑ ICP
Other:	↑ Erythropoietin, ↑ hematocrit, ↑ bone growth, ↑ muscle, muscle pain/weakness, edema, ↑ protein synthesis, hypothyroidism, leukemia, nausea, vomiting, pancreatitis, hypoglycemia
Dosage:	0.01–0.25 mg/kg/d SC
Contraindications:	Hypothyroidism, patients with closed epiphyses
Drug Interactions:	ACTH and adrenocorticoid hormones ↓ GH response; thyroid hormone accelerates epiphyseal closure
Key Points:	Perioperative glucocorticoid coverage with coexistent deficiency

TERIPARATIDE

Trade Name:	**Forteo**
Indications:	Osteoporosis in postmenopausal women and ↑ bone mass in men with hypogonadal osteoporosis
Pharmacokinetics:	Onset: rapid; bioavailability: 95%; peak: 0.5 h; Vd: 0.12 L/kg; Cl: 60–90 L/h; $T_{1/2}$ β: 1–2 h; metabolized in the liver and excreted in urine
Pharmacodynamics:	Synthetic parathyroid hormone (PTH) stimulates osteoblasts, GI and renal Ca^{2+} absorption

TERIPARATIDE *continued*

CNS:	Headache, asthenia, insomnia, dizziness, depression
CV:	Hypertension, angina, orthostatic hypotension
GI:	Nausea, constipation, dyspepsia, vomiting
Pulmonary:	Rhinitis, cough, pharyngitis, dyspnea, pneumonia
Other:	Arthralgia, leg cramps, rash, sweating
Dosage:	20 μg/d SC (3 mL prefilled disposable pen) for up to 24 mo
Contraindications:	Paget's disease of the bone, prior radiation therapy ↑ risk of osteosarcoma; bone metastases or history of skeletal malignancies; pregnancy and/or breast-feeding; children
Drug Interactions:	Furosemide may ↑ Ca^{2+} level
Key Points:	Hypercalcemia may predispose patients to digitalis toxicity and alter response to CCB drugs

VASOPRESSIN (ANTIDIURETIC HORMONE [ADH])

Trade Name:	**Pitressin**
Indications:	Diabetes insipidus, upper GI tract hemorrhage, postoperative abdominal distention (to expel gas)
Pharmacokinetics:	Onset: <30 min; no protein binding; duration: 2–8 h; $T_{1/2}$ β: 10–20 min; metabolized in liver and kidney, excreted in urine
Pharmacodynamics:	Antidiuretic hormone (ADH) effect at the renal tubules, ↑ GI, peristalsis, vasoconstriction of capillaries and small arterioles
CNS:	Tremor, headache, vertigo, seizures, lightheadedness
CV:	↑ BP, arrhythmia, vasoconstriction, ↓ CO, acute MI
GI:	Abdominal cramps, diarrhea, nausea, vomiting
Other:	Water intoxication, necrosis, gangrene, diaphoresis
Dosage:	0.2–0.4 U/min (GI hemorrhage); 5–15 U (expel gas)
Contraindications:	Renal disease, seizure disorder, CAD, hypertension
Drug Interactions:	↑ ADH effect with carbamazepine, chlorpropamide, TCAs, fludrocortisone, clofibrate; ↓ ADH effect with demeclocycline, epinephrine, alcohol, heparin, lithium, norepinephrine
Key Points:	Fluid retention due to antidiuretic effect in patients with borderline cardiac function may precipitate CHF during perioperative period

27

Immunomodulators

ADALIMUMAB

Trade Name:	**Humira**
Indications:	Severe rheumatoid arthritis
Pharmacokinetics:	Onset: slow; bioavailability: 64%; peak: 131 h; Vd: 4.7–6.0 L; Cl:12 mL/h; $T_{1/2}$ β: 2 wk
Pharmacodynamics:	Recombinant IgG monoclonal antibody that inactivates tumor necrosis factor (TNF)-alpha cytokine
CNS:	Headache, confusion, paresthesia, tremor, dizziness
CV:	Hypercholesterolemia, hyperlipidemia, hematuria
GI:	Nausea, abdominal pain, ↑ alkaline phosphatase
GU:	UTI
Pulmonary:	Respiratory infection, sinusitis
Other:	Erythema, pruritus, back pain, lupus-like rash
Dosage:	40 mg qo wk SC
Contraindications:	Active tuberculosis (TB)
Drug Interactions:	Methotrexate ↓ clearance
Key Points:	May lead to activation of latent TB

ALEFACEPT

Trade Name:	**Amevive**
Indications:	Psoriasis
Pharmacokinetics:	Onset: slow; bioavailability: 63%; Vd: 94 mL/kg; Cl: 0.25 mL/h/kg; $T_{1/2}$ β: 270 h
Pharmacodynamics:	Reduces stimulation and production of T-lymphocytes
CNS:	Dizziness
GI:	Nausea, ↑ LFTs
Other:	Pharyngitis, pruritus, myalgia, chills, cancer, lymphopenia
Dosage:	7.5 mg IV (or 15 mg IM) q wk for 12 wk
Contraindications:	Pregnancy
Drug Interactions:	NK
Key Points:	No known interactions with anesthetic drugs

AURANOFIN

Trade Name:	**Ridaura**
Indications:	Rheumatoid and psoriatic arthritis, SLE, Felty's syndrome

AURANOFIN *continued*

Pharmacokinetics:	Onset: 1 h; peak: 2 h; protein binding: 60%; duration: 24 h; $T_{1/2}$ β: 26 d; eliminated in urine (60%) and feces (40%)
Pharmacodynamics:	Reduces inflammation by altering immune system
CNS:	Confusion, seizures
GI:	Nausea, stomatitis, diarrhea, dyspepsia, ulcerative colitis
GU:	Proteinuria, hematuria, nephrotic syndrome, ARF
Other:	Rash, pruritus, exfoliative dermatitis, ↓ bone marrow, interstitial pneumonitis
Dosage:	6 mg/d PO (max. 9 mg/d)
Contraindications:	Gold toxicity, necrotizing enterocolitis, pulmonary fibrosis, hematologic disorder, exfoliative dermatitis
Drug Interactions:	Drugs that may cause blood dyscrasias ↑ hematologic toxicity
Key Points:	N_2O should be avoided due to potential bone marrow suppression; coagulation profile needs to be checked before major regional blocks

AZATHIOPRINE

Trade Name:	**Imuran**
Indications:	Renal transplantation, rheumatoid arthritis (severe)
Pharmacokinetics:	Onset: <1 h; peak: 2 h; protein binding: 30%; duration: 24 h; $T_{1/2}$ β: 5 h; metabolized to mercaptopurine (6-MP); both compounds cross placental barrier and are rapidly eliminated from blood erythrocytes and liver, 2° to metabolites excreted in urine
Pharmacodynamics:	Inhibition of mitosis and interference with coenzyme formation
GI:	Anorexia, nausea, vomiting, ↑ LFTs, pancreatitis, steatorrhea
Other:	Bone marrow suppression, hyperuricemia, rash, ecchymoses, myalgias, arthralgia, alopecia, pneumonitis
Dosage:	3–5 mg/kg/d PO initially; then 1–2 mg/kg/d
Contraindications:	Pregnancy, breast-feeding
Drug Interactions:	ACE inhibitor ↓ bone marrow; allopurinol ↑ level; ↓ cyclosporine levels

AZATHIOPRINE *continued*

Key Points: Antagonizes neuromuscular blockade produced by nondepolarizing muscle relaxants, enhances effect of succinylcholine

BASILIXIMAB

Trade Name:	**Simulect**
Indications:	Prophylaxis prior to kidney transplantation
Pharmacokinetics:	Onset/peak/duration: NK; $T_{1/2}$ β: 7 d (adults), 12 d (children)
Pharmacodynamics:	Binds to and blocks IL-2 receptor on the surface of T-lymphocytes, inhibits IL-2
CNS:	Headache, dizziness, tremor, agitation, hypoesthesia, insomnia, blurred vision, paresthesia, tremor, asthenia
CV:	Arrhythmias, angina, CHF, ↑ HR, edema
GI:	Candidiasis, abdominal pain, constipation, nausea
GU:	Dysuria, hematuria, UTI, renal tubular necrosis, urinary frequency
Pulmonary:	Bronchospasm, bronchitis, dyspnea, pulmonary edema, pharyngitis
Other:	Acne, herpes, diabetes, hypertrichosis, rash, acidosis dehydration, hypercholesterolemia, hyperuricemia, electrolyte disturbance
Dosage:	10–20 mg IV <2 h before surgery and for 4 d after surgery
Contraindications:	Anaphylactoid reactions to foreign protein
Drug Interactions:	NK
Key Points:	Check electrolytes prior to surgery to avoid untoward anesthetic interactions

BOTULISM IMMUNE GLOBULIN

Trade Names:	**Baby BIG, BIG-IV**
Indications:	Infant botulism
Pharmacokinetics:	Duration: 6 mo; $T_{1/2}$ β: 28 d
Pharmacodynamics: *Other:*	IgG against botulinum neurotoxins type A and B Rash/erythema, renal dysfunction, dysphagia
Dosage:	50 mg/kg IV
Contraindications:	Age >1 yr, anaphylaxic reaction to IgG products, IgA deficiency
Drug Interactions:	NK
Key Points:	No known interaction with anesthetic drugs

CYCLOSPORINE

Trade Names:	**Neoral, Sandimmune, Gengraf**
Indications:	Prevention of organ transplant rejection, severe rheumatoid arthritis, psoriasis
Pharmacokinetics:	Onset: 1 h; peak: 3 h; protein binding: 90%; duration: >24 h; Vd: distributed largely outside the blood volume; $T_{1/2}$ β: 7–19 h; crosses placental barrier; extensively metabolized in liver, excreted via bile in feces
Pharmacodynamics:	Inhibition of IL-2 response
CNS:	Headaches, tremor, paresthesias, seizures
CV:	↑ BP, flushing
GI:	Nausea, vomiting, diarrhea, anorexia, gastritis, oral candidiasis, ↑ LFTs
Other:	Hemolytic-uremic syndrome (microangiopathic hemolytic anemia, renal failure, thrombocytopenia), myalgias, gynecomastia, hirsutism, gingivitis, acne, ↑ K^+, hyperuricemia, hypomagnesemia, hyperlipidemia, fever, chills
Dosage:	10–15 mg/kg/d PO IV prior to and for 1–2 wk after transplantation, tapering to 5–10 mg/kg/d; 2.5 mg/kg PO bid (max. 4 mg/kg/d; RA, psoriasis)
Contraindications:	Sensitivity to castor oil, renal impairment, severe hypertension
Drug Interactions:	Cimetidine, erythromycin, ketoconazole, miconazole, CCBs, grapefruit, aminoglycosides, NSAIDs, loop diuretics ↑ levels; carbamazepine, phenytoin, rifampin, rafcillin ↓ levels; ↓ Cl prednisolone, digoxin, lovastatin
Key Points:	Anesthetic drugs that depend on renal excretion (e.g., pancuronium) and ↓ seizure threshold (e.g., lidocaine, ketamine, enflurane) should be avoided; use prophylactic antiemetics to ↓ PONV

CYTOMEGALOVIRUS IMMUNE GLOBULIN (CMV-IGIV)

Trade Name:	**CytoGam**
Indications:	CMV disease (prophylaxis and attenuation)
Pharmacokinetics:	NK
Pharmacodynamics:	Antibody against CMV
	CMV disease
CV:	↓ BP, flushing
GI:	Nausea, vomiting

CYTOMEGALOVIRUS IMMUNE
GLOBULIN (CMV-IGIV) *continued*

Pulmonary:	Bronchospam (wheezing)
Other:	Anaphylaxis, fever, chills, myalgias, arthralgias
Dosage:	150 mg/kg by infusion within 72 h of transplant, then 50–100 mg/kg/wk
Contraindications:	IgΛ deficiency
Drug Interactions:	↓ Immune response to live virus vaccines
Key Points:	Defer vaccination for at least 3 mo after CMV Ig is administered

DIPHTHERIA, TETANUS TOXOIDS, ACELLULAR PERTUSSIS, HEPATITIS B (RECOMBINANT) AND INACTIVATED POLIOVIRUS VACCINES

Trade Name:	**Pediarix**
Indications:	Immunization against diphtheria, tetanus, pertussis (whooping cough), hepatitis B virus, poliomyelitis
Pharmacokinetics:	NK
Pharmacodynamics:	Active immunization against infectious organisms
CNS:	Convulsions, encephalopathy, headache, hypotonia, somnolence, malaise, irritability, asthenia
GI:	Abdominal pain, anorexia, diarrhea, intussusception, nausea, vomiting, jaundice, ↑ LFTs
Pulmonary:	Cyanosis, edema, pallor
Other:	Fever, sudden infant death syndrome (SIDS), arthralgias
Dosage:	0.5 mL IM (3 doses at 6–8 wk intervals)
Contraindications:	Hypersensitivity to yeast, neomycin, polymyxin B, encephalopathy <7 d of pertussis-containing vaccine; progressive neurologic disorder (infantile spasms, uncontrolled epilepsy, or progressive encephalopathy)
Drug Interactions:	Anaphylactic reactions; Arthus-type (local) reaction; Guillain-Barré syndrome
Key Points:	Caution in the use of succinylcholine in the presence of neurologic symptoms

EFALIZUMAB

Trade Name:	**Raptiva**
Indications:	Severe placque psoriasis

Pharmacokinetics:	NK
Pharmacodynamics:	Recombinant IgG kappa monoclonal antibody binds to CD11a inhibiting adhesion of leukocytes to other cells
CNS:	Headache, fever
GI:	Nausea
Other:	Thrombocytopenia, myalgia, flu syndrome, cancer
Dosage:	0.7–1 mg/kg SC q wk (×10 wk)
Contraindications:	Use of other immunosuppressive drugs; phototherapy
Drug Interactions:	NK
Key Points:	Check platelet count prior to "blood loss" procedures

ETANERCEPT

Trade Name:	**Enbrel**
Indications:	Rheumatoid and psoriatic arthritis
Pharmacokinetics:	Onset: >24 h (SC); peak: 72 h; $T_{1/2}$ β: 115 h
Pharmacodynamics:	Antagonizes tumor necrosis factor (TNF), ↓ inflammatory response
CNS:	Asthenia, headache, dizziness, fever, chills
CV:	Peripheral edema, hemodynamic instability
GI:	Vomiting, abdominal pain
Other:	Rash, muscle stiffness, ↓ bone marrow, URI, cough
Dosage:	25 mg SC 3×/wk, 0.4 mg/kg 2×/wk (children)
Contraindications:	Sepsis, administration of live vaccines
Drug Interactions:	NK
Key Points:	No known interaction with anesthetic drugs

FILGRASTIM (GRANULOCYTE COLONY–STIMULATING FACTOR [G-CSF])

Trade Name:	**Neupogen**
Indications:	Nonmyeloid malignancies, AIDS-associated neutropenia
Pharmacokinetics:	Onset: 5–60 min; peak: 2 h (IV), 2–8 h (SC); duration: 1–7 d; Cl: 0.5–0.7 mL/min/kg; Vd: 150 mg/kg; $T_{1/2}$ β: 3.5 h
Pharmacodynamics:	Cytokine glycoprotein, stimulate progenitor cells, ↑ WBC, ↑ human granulocyte colony–stimulating factor (G-CSF)

FILGRASTIM (GRANULOCYTE COLONY–STIMULATING FACTOR [G-CSF]) *continued*

CNS:	Fatigue, headache
CV:	Arrhythmias (e.g., SVT), vasculitis
GI:	Nausea, vomiting, diarrhea, mucositis, anorexia
Other:	Leukocytosis, splenomegaly, alopecia, cough, bone pain

Dosage:	5 µg/kg/d SC/IV
Contraindications:	Sensitivity to *Escherichia coli*–derived protein
Drug Interactions:	↑ Release of neutrophils; lithium ↑ effect
Key Points:	No known interactions with anesthetic drugs

HEPATITIS A VACCINE

Trade Names:	**Havrix, Vagta**
Indications:	Immunization against hepatitis A virus
Pharmacokinetics:	Onset: 1–15 d; duration: 6 mo
Pharmacodynamics:	Inactivated vaccine, ↑ immunity to hepatitis A virus
CNS:	Fatigue, headache, insomnia, vertigo, fever
GI:	Anorexia, nausea, abdominal pain, diarrhea, jaundice, ↑ LFTs
Other:	Arthralgia, myalgia, rash, pruritus, urticaria, URI
Dosage:	1440 ELISA (EL) units IM, then a booster dose at 6–12 mo; 720 EL units IM, then a booster dose at 6–12 y (children)
Contraindications:	NK
Drug Interactions:	NK
Key Points:	Delay vaccination in patients with acute febrile illnesses

HEPATITIS B IMMUNE GLOBULIN (HBIG)

Trade Names:	**BayHep, Nabi-HB**
Indications:	Hepatitis B exposure
Pharmacokinetics:	Onset: 1–6 d; peak: 3–9 d; duration: 2 mo
Pharmacodynamics:	Passive immunity to hepatitis B
Other:	Urticaria, angioedema, pain at injection site
Dosage:	0.06 mL/kg IM at <7–14 d after exposure

HEPATITIS B IMMUNE
GLOBULIN (HBIG) *continued*

Contraindications:	Anaphylactic reactions to immunoglobulin (Ig) serum
Drug Interactions:	↓ Immune response to other virus vaccines (e.g., measles, mumps, rubella)
Key Points:	No known interactions with anesthetic drugs

HEPATITIS B VACCINE

Trade Names:	**Engerix-B, Recombivax HB**
Indications:	Immunization against hepatitis B, pre- and post-exposure prophylaxis
Pharmacokinetics:	Onset: 2 wk after last dose; peak: >6 mo; duration: >3 y
Pharmacodynamics:	Promotes active immunity to hepatitis B
CNS:	Headache, dizziness, insomnia, paresthesia, blurred vision, fatigue
GI:	Nausea, vomiting, anorexia, diarrhea
Other:	Arthralgia, myalgia, local inflammation, anaphylaxis
Dosage:	20 μg *Engerix-B* or 10 μg *Recombivax HB* IM, 2nd dose at 30 d and 3rd at 6 mo; 10 μg *Engerix-B* or 5 μg *Recombivax HB* IM, 2nd dose at 30 d and 3rd at 6 mo (children)
Contraindications:	Sensitivity to yeast
Drug Interactions:	Corticosteroids and immunosuppressants ↓ immune response
Key Points:	No known interactions with anesthetic drugs

IMIQUIMOD

Trade Name:	**Aldara TM**
Indications:	Genital and perianal warts, condyloma acuminata
Pharmacokinetics:	Absorption minimal; excreted in urine and feces
Pharmacodynamics:	Induces cytokines
Skin:	Erythema, erosion, excoriation, edema, itching, burning
Dosage:	5% cream applied 3×/wk
Contraindications:	NK
Drug Interactions:	NK
Key Points:	No known interactions with anesthetic drugs

IMMUNE GLOBULIN, IMMUNE SERUM GLOBULIN (ISG), IMMUNE GLOBULIN IV (IGIV)

Trade Names:	**BayGam, Gamimune N, Venoglobulin 1, Gamma-P**
Other Names:	**Gamma globulin**
Indications:	Agamma- and hypogamma-globulinemia, immune deficiency, ITP, bone marrow transplantation
Pharmacokinetics:	Onset: <30 min (IV); peak: 2 d (IM)
Pharmacodynamics:	Passive immunity ($\uparrow$ antibody titer)
CNS:	Headache, faintness, malaise, fever, chills
CV:	Chest pain, MI, palpitations, $\uparrow$ HR
GI:	Nausea, vomiting, abdominal cramps
Pulmonary:	Dyspnea, pulmonary edema
Other:	Arthralgias, erythema, urticaria, $\uparrow$ BUN, diaphoresis
Dosage:	100–200 mg/kg (or 2–4 mL/kg) infusion over 30 min (immunodeficiency); 1–2 mg/kg IM (exposure prophylaxis)
Contraindications:	NK
Drug Interactions:	$\downarrow$ Immune response to live vaccines (e.g., measles, mumps, rubella)
Key Points:	Possible association between IGIV and thrombotic events

INFLIXIMAB

Trade Name:	**Remicade**
Indications:	Crohn's disease, rheumatoid arthritis
Pharmacokinetics:	$T_{1/2} \beta$: 9–10 d
Pharmacodynamics:	Monoclonal antibody binds to TNF-α, $\downarrow$ inflammation in intestine and joint
CNS:	Headache, fatigue, dizziness, fever, conjunctivitis
CV:	$\downarrow$ BP, $\uparrow$ HR, edema, flushing
GI:	Nausea, vomiting, dyspepsia, constipation, ulcerative stomatitis
Pulmonary:	URI, cough, dyspnea, rhinitis
Other:	Anemia, myalgia, rash, pruritus, chills, diaphoresis, dysuria
Dosage:	5 mg/kg IV over 2 h, repeat at 2 and 6 wk (max. 10 mg/kg)
Contraindications:	NK
Drug Interactions:	NK
Key Points:	No known interactions with anesthetic drugs

INFLUENZA VIRUS VACCINE

Trade Names:	**Fluvarin, FluMist (live)**
Indications:	Influenza A and B (flu) prophylaxis
Pharmacokinetics:	Duration of immunity approximately 1 y
Pharmacodynamics:	Active immunity by inducing antibody production
CNS:	Malaise, dizziness, headache, chills, fever
GI:	Nausea, vomiting, diarrhea
Pulmonary:	Runny nose, nasal congestion, pharyngitis, cough (live)
Other:	Myalgias, anaphylaxis, erythema, pain at injection site, edema
Dosage:	0.5 mL IM; 0.25 mL SC, repeat in 4 wk; 0.5 mL nasal spray ("live")
Contraindications:	Allergy to chicken and egg products; defer vaccination in patients with active infections and neurologic disorders (Guillain-Barré syndrome)
Drug Interactions:	↓ Phenytoin level, ↑ theophylline level; corticosteroids and immunosuppressants ↓ immune response; ↑ PT with warfarin
Key Points:	No known interactions with anesthetic drugs

INTERFERON ALPHA

Trade Names:	**Roferon-A, Intron-A**
Indications:	Chronic hepatitis C and B, hairy cell leukemia, HIV-related Kaposi's sarcoma, CML, malignant melanoma, condylomata acuminata
Pharmacokinetics:	Vd: 0.4 L/kg; $T_{1/2}$ β: 5 h; hepatic metabolism, excreted in urine
Pharmacodynamics:	Recombinant antibody, ↓ viral replication and antiproliferation action
CNS:	Fatigue, confusion, anxiety, paresthesia, dizziness
CV:	Orthostatic hypotension, edema, angina, arrythmias
GI:	Anorexia, nausea, vomiting, abdominal pain, ↑ LFTs
Pulmonary:	Dyspnea, cough
Other:	Myalgia, fever, ↑ proteinuria, hypothyroidism
Dosage:	30–35 million IU/wk SC/IM (hepatitis B); 3 million IU 3×/wk (hepatitis C); 36 million IU/d (Kaposi's sarcoma); 3–9 million IU/d (leukemia)
Contraindications:	Sensitivity to benzyl alcohol (preservative), hepatorenal dysfunction

INTERFERON ALPHA *continued*

Drug Interactions:	↓ Barbiturate and theophylline metabolism; RT and immunosuppressant effects on bone marrow; ↑ side effects of liver vaccines
Key Points:	Potential prolongation of residual CNS depression of anesthetics

INTERFERON BETA

Trade Names:	**Avonex, Rebif, Betaseron**
Indications:	MS
Pharmacokinetics:	Peak: 3–8 h; $T_{1/2}$ β: 10 h
Pharmacodynamics:	Interacts with surface receptors to ↓ exacerbations of MS
CNS:	Depression, depersonalization, seizures, myasthenia gravis
CV:	↑ BP, ↑ HR
GI:	Nausea, vomiting
Other:	Cushing's syndrome, diabetes insipidus, hypothyroidism, leukopenia, anemia, flulike syndrome, asthesia, ataxia, menorrhagia, pelvic pain
Dosage:	8 million IU SC (0.25 mg) q 2 d
Contraindications:	Sensitivity to human albumin, pregnancy
Drug Interactions:	NK
Key Points:	Avoid anesthetics with stimulant properties (e.g., methohexital, ketamine, etomidate) due to ↓ seizure threshold

INTERFERON GAMMA

Trade Name:	**Actimmune**
Indications:	Chronic granulomatous disease, malignant osteopetrosis
Pharmacokinetics:	Well-absorbed (90%); peak: 4–7 h; $T_{1/2}$ β: 6 h
Pharmacodynamics:	Phagocytic activity, interacts with interleukins
CNS:	Fatigue, dizziness
GI:	Nausea, vomiting, diarrhea, anorexia
GU:	Proteinuria
Other:	Bone marrow suppression, weight loss, rash, erythemia
Dosage:	50 μg/m^2 SC 3×/wk
Contraindications:	Sensitivity to genetically engineered products from *E. coli*

INTERFERON GAMMA *continued*

Drug Interactions: ↓ Hepatic metabolism of drugs via cytochrome P_{450} system, myelosuppressants ↑ side effects

Key Points: ↑ Recovery of drugs with high hepatic clearance rates (e.g., propofol)

LEFLUNOMIDE

Trade Name: **Arava**

Indications: RA

Pharmacokinetics: Onset: 6–12 h; bioavailability: 80%; peak: 2 mo; protein binding: 99%; $T_{1/2}$ β: 2 wk; metabolized to active metabolite, excreted in urine and feces

Pharmacodynamics: Inhibits dihydroorotate dehydrogenase in pyrimidine synthesis pathway, antiproliferative and anti-inflammatory activity

CNS: Headache, dizziness, paresthesia, migraine, insomnia, blurred vision

CV: ↑ HR, vasodilation, edema, chest pain (angina)

GI: Stomatitis, gingivitis, gastroenteritis, colitis, ↑ LFTs, anorexia, nausea, vomiting, diarrhea

GU: UTI, albuminuria, menstrual disorder

Pulmonary: Cough, URI, asthma, pneumonia

Other: Myalgia, muscle cramps, tenosynovitis, alopecia, rash, hyperglycemia, hypokalemia, hyperthyroidism, weight loss

Dosage: 100 mg/d PO for 3 d, then 20 mg/d

Contraindications: Pregnancy, breast-feeding, hepatic insufficiency

Drug Interactions: Activated charcoal and cholestyramine ↓ level; hepatotoxic drugs (e.g., methotrexate) ↑ hepatotoxicity; rifampin ↑ level

Key Points: Avoid inhaled anesthetics with risk of hepatotoxicity and potential for bone marrow suppression

LEVAMISOLE

Trade Name: **Ergamisol**

Indications: Colorectal carcinoma, malignant melanoma

Pharmacokinetics: Rapidly absorbed; peak: 1–2 h; $T_{1/2}$ β: 4 h; hepatic metabolism, excreted 1° in urine and feces

Pharmacodynamics: Stimulates T-cell, monocytes, macrophage, neutrophil activity

CNS:	Ataxia, blurred vision, confusion, paresthesias, tardive dyskinesia
GI:	Nausea, vomiting, stomatitis, anorexia, jaundice
Other:	Bone marrow suppression, flulike syndrome
Dosage:	50 mg PO q 8 h alone, or in combination with fluorouracil
Contraindications:	NK
Drug Interactions:	$\uparrow$ Coumarin effect ($\uparrow$ PT); a disulfiram-like syndrome develops with alcohol; $\uparrow$ phenytoin levels
Key Points:	Prolonged exposure to N_2O may $\uparrow$ bone marrow suppression

LYMPHOCYTE IMMUNE GLOBULIN (ANTI-THYMOCYTE GLOBULIN [ATG])

Trade Name:	**Atgam**
Indications:	Prevention of renal allograph rejection; aplastic anemia
Pharmacokinetics:	Onset: <10 min; peak: 5 d; duration: <24 h; $T_{1/2}$ β: 6 d; crosses placenta (in last 4 wk); excreted in urine
Pharmacodynamics:	Antilymphocytic effect on T-cell function
CNS:	Headache, dizziness, seizures, fatigue
CV:	$\downarrow$ BP, $\uparrow$ HR, angina, clotted AV fistula, iliac vein obstruction, renal artery thrombosis, thrombophlebitis
GI:	Nausea, vomiting, dyspepsia, diarrhea, stomatitis
Pulmonary:	Dyspnea, pulmonary edema, laryngospasm, hiccups
Other:	Leukopenia, thrombocytopenia, myalgias, arthralgia, hyperglycemia, rash, fever, chills
Dosage:	5–30 mg/kg/d PO
Contraindications:	Systemic reaction to equine gamma globulin, late pregnancy
Drug Interactions:	Immunosuppressor drugs $\uparrow$ infection and $\uparrow$ risk of lymphoma
Key Points:	Give folinic acid (or vitamin B_{12}) with $\uparrow$ use of N_2O

MYCOPHENOLATE

Trade Names:	**CellCept, Myfortic**
Indications:	Prophylaxis against organ rejection (in combination with cyclosporine and steroids)

MYCOPHENOLATE *continued*

Pharmacokinetics:	Onset: 0.5 h; bioavailability: 94%; peak: 2 h; protein binding: >98%; duration: 8–18 h; Vd: 1–2 L/kg; Cl: 140 mL/min; $T_{1/2}$ β: 8–16 h; 93% renally excreted; excreted 1° in urine
Pharmacodynamics:	Inhibits IMP dehydrogenase, ↓ guanosine nucleotide synthesis and both T- and B-lymphocyte responses, cytostatic effect on lymphocytes
GI:	Nausea, diarrhea, constipation
Other:	Nasopharyngitis, anemia, leukopenia, UTI, insomnia
Dosage:	360–720 mg PO bid
Contraindications:	Hypersensitivity to drug or 1° metabolite (mycophenolic acid); live vaccines; pregnancy
Drug Interactions:	Antacids and food ↓ absorption; cholestyramine ↓ enterohepatic recirculation
Key Points:	No known interactions with anesthetic drugs

PEGFILGRASTIM

Trade Name:	**Neulasta**
Indications:	Nonmyeloid malignancies
Pharmacokinetics:	$T_{1/2}$ β: 15–80 h (SC)
Pharmacodynamics:	Neutrophil growth stimulator; ↑ proliferation and differentiation of neutrophils
CNS:	Dizziness, headache, insomnia, fatigue
GI:	Nausea, vomiting, stomatitis, dyspepsia
Pulmonary:	ARDS
Other:	Hyperuremia, arthralgia, myalgia, alopecia, neutropenia, granulocytopenia
Dosage:	6 mg SC (per cycle)
Contraindications:	Sensitivity to *E. coli*–derived proteins; avoid before and after therapy
Drug Interactions:	NK
Key Points:	Prolonged exposure to N_2O may ↑ bone marrow suppression

PEGINTERFERON ALFA/2a

Trade Names:	**PEG-Intron, Pegasys**
Indications:	Chronic hepatitis C infection

PEGINTERFERON ALFA/2a *continued*

Pharmacokinetics:	Peak: 72–96 h; duration: 7 d; $T_{1/2}$ β: 40 h; excreted 1° by kidneys
Pharmacodynamics:	Antiviral action, ↑ oligoadenylate synthetase, ↓ proliferation of infected cells
CNS:	Dizziness, hypertonia, depression, insomnia, headache, anxiety
GI:	Nausea, vomiting, anorexia, dyspepsia, diarrhea
Other:	Myalgias, cough, flulike symptoms (rigors), flushing
Dosage:	50–180 μg SC (1 μg/kg/wk) for 48 wk
Contraindications:	Autoimmune hepatitis, hepatic failure, pregnancy, suicidal tendency, severe infections
Drug Interactions:	Didanosine (fatal reactions); ↓ effect of stavudine and zidorudine; ↑ theophylline levels; ↓ dosages of high-clearance anesthetic drugs (e.g., propolol)
Key Points:	Check thyroid function if evidence of hypo- or hyperthyroidism

PNEUMOCOCCAL VACCINE

Trade Names:	**Pneumovax, Pnu-Immune**
Indications:	Pneumococcal immunization
Pharmacokinetics:	Onset: 2–3 wk; duration: 5 y
Pharmacodynamics:	Promotes active immunity against 23 pneumococcal subtypes
CNS:	Headache, fever
GI:	Nausea, vomiting
Other:	Myalgia, arthralgia, local inflammation, anaphylaxis
Dosage:	25 μg (0.5 m) IM/SC
Contraindications:	Hodgkin's disease, sensitivity to phenols
Drug Interactions:	Steroids and immunosuppressants ↓ immune response
Key Points:	No known interactions with anesthetic drugs

POLIOVIRUS VACCINE

Trade Names:	**Orimune, Sabin (live [TOPV]), IPOL (inactivated [IPV])**
Indications:	Poliovirus immunization
Pharmacokinetics:	Onset: 7–10 d; peak: 21 d; duration: >10 y, lasts for years

POLIOVIRUS VACCINE *continued*

Pharmacodynamics:	Promotes immunity to poliomyelitis by ↑ humoral and secretory antibodies
CNS:	Drowsiness, fever
GI:	↓ Appetite (anorexia)
Other:	Local inflammation, poliomyelitis
Dosage:	Two 0.5-mL doses 8 wk apart, 3rd dose at 6–12 mo
Contraindications:	Oral (live) immunosuppressed patients; inactivated IPV; allergy to neomycin, streptomycin, or polymyxin B
Drug Interactions:	Steroids and immunosuppressants ↓ immune response to vaccine
Key Points:	Defer vaccination in patients receiving blood transfusion, immune serum globulin, or blood products (<3 mo)

RABIES IMMUNE GLOBULIN (RIG) AND VACCINE, HUMAN DIPLOID CELL (HDCV)

Trade Names:	**BayRab, Imogam Rabies-HT (RIG); Imovax (HDCV)**
Indications:	Preexposure prophylaxis for high-risk patients, postexposure rabies prophylaxis exposure only (RIG)
Pharmacokinetics:	Onset: 24 h (RIG); peak: 2 wk after 3 doses (RIG), 1–2 mo (HDCV); duration: >2 yr (HDCV)
Pharmacodynamics:	Promote active (HDCV) and passive immunity (RIG)
CNS:	Fever, fatigue, headache, dizziness
GU:	Nephrotic syndrome (RIG)
Other:	Myalgia, local inflammation, abdominal pain, nausea
Dosage:	1 mL IM at 1, 7, 21, 28 d (preexposure); 1 mL IM HDCV at 1, 3, 7, 14, 28 d after exposure and 20 IU/kg RIG at 1st postexposure dose
Contraindications:	NK
Drug Interactions:	Corticosteroids and immunosuppressants ↓ immune response
Key Points:	Avoid live-virus vaccines (HDCV) <3 mo after giving RIG vaccine

RHo(D) IMMUNE GLOBULIN (HUMAN)

Trade Name:	**Rhophylac**
Indications:	Suppression of Rh isoimmunization in nonsensitized Rh(−) women, Rhesus prophylaxis for obstetrical complications

RHo(D) IMMUNE GLOBULIN
(HUMAN) *continued*

Pharmacokinetics:	Onset: rapid (RBC elimination); bioavailability: 69%; peak: 2–7 d; duration: 9 wk; Cl: 0.2 mL/min; $T_{1/2}$ β: 16 d
Pharmacodynamics:	Mechanism of action unknown
CNS:	Malaise, headache
Other:	Anaphylactic reactions, local pain, fever
Dosage:	1500 IU (300 µg) IM/IV
Contraindications:	Hypersensitivity to human globulin
Drug Interactions:	↓ Efficacy live virus vaccines (<3 mo)
Key Points:	Consider premedication with H_1 antagonist

SARGRAMOSTIM (GRANULOCYTE-MACROPHAGE COLONY–STIMULATING FACTOR)

Trade Name:	**Leukine**
Indications:	Acute myelogenous leukemia, aplastic anemia, myelodysplastic syndromes, bone marrow transplant (prophylaxis)
Pharmacokinetics:	Onset: 15 min; peak: 2–4 h; metabolism and excretion unknown
Pharmacodynamics:	↑ Cellular responses by binding to receptors on target cell surfaces
CNS:	Malaise, asthenia
CV:	Pericardial effusion, peripheral edema, arrhythmias
GI:	Nausea, vomiting, diarrhea, anorexia, stomatitis, ↑ LFTs
Other:	Hemorrhage, rash, alopecia, pleural effusion, ↑ BUN, fever
Dosage:	250 µg/m^2/d infusion over 2–4 h for 21 d
Contraindications:	Leukemic myeloid blast cells, <24 h of chemo- or radiation therapy
Drug Interactions:	Corticosteroids and lithium ↑ myeloproliferative effects
Key Points:	No known interactions with anesthetic drugs

SIROLIMUS

Trade Name:	**Rapamune**
Indications:	Prevention of renal transplant rejection

SIROLIMUS *continued*

Pharmacokinetics:	Onset: <1 h; bioavailability: 14%; peak: 1–3 h; protein binding: 92%; duration: 24 h; extensively metabolized by cytochrome P_{450} system, excreted 1° in feces
Pharmacodynamics:	Inhibits T-lymphocyte activation, proliferation, antibody formation
CNS:	Headache, insomnia, tremor, anxiety, depression, asthenia, malaise, neuropathy, paresthesia, blurred vision, tinnitus, fever
CV:	Vasodilation, ↓ BP, ↑ HR, pedal edema, arrhythmias, angina, CHF
GI:	Nausea, vomiting, anorexia, flatulence, ascites, dysphagia, dyspepsia, gastroenteritis, gingivitis, stomatitis, constipation/diarrhea
GU:	Dysuria, hematuria, tubular necrosis, UTI, impotence, nephrotoxicity, urinary frequency/retention/incontinence
Pulmonary:	Cough, dyspnea, URI, pleural effusion, pharyngitis, epistaxis
Other:	Pancytopenia, rash, pruritus, myalgias, acne, hypercholesterolemia, electrolyte disturbances
Dosage:	6 mg/d PO initially, then 2 mg/d; 3 mg/m^2 (children)
Contraindications:	Severe hyperlipidemia, impaired hepatorenal function
Drug Interactions:	Aminoglycosides, amphotericin, cyclosporin ↑ nephrotoxicity; cytochrome P_{450} inhibitors and grapefruit ↑ levels; ↓ effectiveness of vaccines
Key Points:	Check electrolytes and blood glucose levels preoperatively

TACROLIMUS

Trade Name:	**Prograf**
Indications:	Prevention of organ transplant rejection
Pharmacokinetics:	Onset: <10 min; bioavailability: 15%; peak: 1–4 h; protein binding: 99%; duration: 12 h; elimination $T_{1/2}$ β: 32 h; metabolized by cytochrome P_{450} (SYP3A), excreted 1° in feces
Pharmacodynamics:	Macrolide that inhibits T-lymphocyte activation by ↓ phosphatase activity of calcineurin
CNS:	Asthenia, headache, tremor, insomnia, paresthesias, fever
CV:	↑ BP, pedal edema
GI:	Nausea/vomiting, dysphagia, ascites, diarrhea/constipation, ↑ LFTs

TACROLIMUS *continued*

GU:	Nephrotoxicity, UTI, oliguria
Pulmonary:	Pleural effusion, dyspnea, atelectasis
Other:	Pancytopenia, myalgia, rash, purpura, electrolyte disturbances, hyperglycemia
Dosage:	0.05–0.1 mg/kg IV initially, then 0.15–0.3 mg/kg PO bid (adult); 0.1 mg/kg IV or 0.3 mg/kg PO (children)
Contraindications:	Hyperlipidemia, hepatorenal impairment, sensitivity to castor oil
Drug Interactions:	Barbiturates, phenytoin, carbamazepine, rifampin ↓ levels; diltiazem, antifungals, cimetidine, corticosteroids, other cytochrome P_{450} inhibitors ↑ levels
Key Points:	Check electrolytes and glucose levels during perioperative period

TETANUS TOXOID, TETANUS IMMUNE GLOBULIN (TIG)

Other Name:	**BayTet**
Indications:	Tetanus prophylaxis/treatment (TIG); 1° immunization (tetanus toxoid)
Pharmacokinetics:	Onset: 8–10 wk; duration: >10 y
Pharmacodynamics:	Promotes passive and active immunity by inducing tetanus antitoxin
CNS:	Malaise, headache, seizure (toxoid)
CV:	↓ BP, ↑ HR (toxoid)
GU:	Nephrotic syndrome (TIG)
Other:	Anaphylaxis, fever
Dosage:	(TIG) 250 U IM (prophylaxis), 3000–6000 U IM (treatment); 0.5 mL IM at 4–8 wk (×2), 3rd dose at 6–12 mo (tetanus toxoid)
Contraindications:	Thrombocytopenia, immunosuppressed patients
Drug Interactions:	Chloramphenicol, steroids, immunosuppressants ↓ immune response
Key Points:	Delay vaccination in patients with acute febrile illnesses

THALIDOMIDE

Trade Name:	**Thalomid**
Indications:	ENL, aphthous stomatitis, graft versus host disease (GVHD)
Pharmacokinetics:	Slowly absorbed from GI tract; peak: 3–6 h; $T_{1/2}$ β: 5–7 h
Pharmacodynamics:	Immunomodulatory action
CNS:	Drowsiness, dizziness, peripheral neuropathy, amblyopia
CV:	↓ HR, ↓ BP, orthostatic hypotension, edema
GI:	Dry mouth, oral candidiasis, anorexia, ↑ LFTs, nausea, dyspepsia
GU:	Albuminuria, hematuria, impotence
Other:	Bone marrow suppression, lymphadenopathy, rash, fever, acne
Dosage:	100–400 mg/d PO (ENL); 800–1600 mg/d (GVHD)
Contraindications:	Pregnancy
Drug Interactions:	↑ Sedation with barbiturates, alcohol, chlorpromazine, reserpine
Key Points:	Use prior to general anesthetics can ↑ recovery and hypotension; perform neurologic exam prior to peripheral nerve block

28

Inhalation Anesthetics

DESFLURANE

Trade Name:	**Suprane**
Indications:	Maintenance of general anesthesia
Pharmacokinetics:	Volatile, nonflammable liquid; blood:gas solubility: 0.42; extremely rapid onset and recovery; MAC: 5%–8% (depending on age); minimally metabolized (<0.02% excreted in urine)
Pharmacodynamics:	Halogenated anesthetic that ↑ release of inhibitory neurotransmitter, ↓ excitatory synaptic transmission
CNS:	CNS depression, rapid emergence from anesthesia, ↑ ICP, headache
CV:	↓ PVR, ↓ BP, ↑ HR (concentration-dependent)
GI:	Nausea, vomiting
Musculoskeletal:	Muscle relaxation
Pulmonary:	↓ TV, ↑ respiratory rate, ↑ end-tidal CO_2 airway irritant (at high concentrations), highly pungent odor, breath-holding, laryngospasm
Dosage:	Usual inspired concentration 4–6% (depending on adjuvants used)
Contraindications:	Malignant hyperpyrexia (MH); inhalation induction (due to airway irritation)
Drug Interactions:	↑ Effects of muscle relaxants; sympatholytic drugs, opioids, N_2O, benzodiazepines, ↓ anesthetic requirement
Key Points:	Provides for rapid emergence and precise control of anesthetic depth; associated with agitation in presence of inadequate analgesia; facilitates fast-tracking process; pressurized, electrically heated vaporizer required for delivery

ENFLURANE

Trade Name:	**Ethrane**
Indications:	Maintenance of general anesthesia
Pharmacokinetics:	Volatile, nonflammable liquid; blood:gas solubility: 1.9; rapid onset and recovery; MAC: 0.5–0.8% (depending on age), slight metabolism in liver (2%)
Pharmacodynamics:	Halogenated anesthetic that ↑ release of inhibitory neurotransmitters
CNS:	Generalized CNS depression, epileptiform paroxysmal spike activity (at high concentrations), ↑ ICP (similar to isoflurane)
CV:	Myocardial depressant, ↓ PVP, ↓ BP, ↑ HR, arrhythmias
GI:	Nausea, vomiting

ENFLURANE *continued*

Pulmonary:	Moderate airway irritation, respiratory depression
Other:	Shivering, muscle relaxation, nephrotoxicity (rare)
Dosage:	Usual inspired concentration is 0.4%–1.6%; max. vaporizer setting of 5% inadequate for induction of anesthesia
Contraindications:	Epilepsy, MH, renal impairment
Drug Interactions:	↑ Effects of muscle relaxants; sympatholytics, opioids, N_2O, benzodiazepines ↓ anesthetic requirement
Key Points:	↑ CNS stimulant activity in patients with ↓ seizure threshold

HALOTHANE

Trade Name:	**Fluothane**
Indications:	Induction and maintenance of general anesthesia
Pharmacokinetics:	Volatile, nonflammable liquid; blood:gas solubility: 2.5; moderate onset, but slow recovery times; MAC: 0.5–0.8% (depending on age); only 70% eliminated unchanged through lungs in 1st 24 h
Pharmacodynamics:	Halogenated anesthetic that ↑ release of both inhibitory and excretory neurotransmitters
CNS:	Generalized CNS depressant activity, cerebral vasodilation (↑ ICP)
CV:	↓ HR (vagal stimulation), ↓ BP, ↓ CO, arrhythmias
GI:	↓ Bowel motility, nausea, vomiting, ↑ LFTs (halothane hepatitis)
Pulmonary:	↓ TV, ↑ RR, bronchodilator, nonirritant, ↓ secretions
Other:	Shivering, skeletal muscle and uterine relaxant
Dosage:	Usual inspired concentration 2–3% (induction); 0.5–1% during the maintenance period
Contraindications:	Predisposition to MH; hepatic impairment; hepatitis
Drug Interactions:	↑ Effects of muscle relaxants; sympatholytics, opioids, N_2O, benzodiazepines; N_2O ↓ anesthetic requirement
Key Points:	Repeated administration to adult in combination with hepatotoxic drugs, obesity, advanced age, use of cytochrome P_{450}–inducing drugs ↑ risk of postanesthetic hepatitis

ISOFLURANE

Trade Name:	**Forane**
Indications:	Maintenance of general anesthesia

ISOFLURANE *continued*

Pharmacokinetics:	Volatile, nonflammable liquid; blood:gas solubility: 1.4; moderate induction and recovery times; MAC: 1–1.5% (depending on age); minimal metabolism, <2% excreted in urine as metabolites
Pharmacodynamics:	Halogenated anesthetic that inhibits neurotransmission in the CNS
CNS:	CNS depressant activity, ↑ ICP, headache, emergence excitement
CV:	↓ BP, ↑ HR, ↓ CO, ↓ PVR
GI:	Nausea, vomiting
Pulmonary:	Airway irritant, respiratory depression (↑ end-tidal CO_2)
Other:	Shivering, muscle relaxation
Dosage:	Usual inspired concentration: 0.5–1.5%
Contraindications:	Predisposition to MH
Drug Interactions:	↑ Effects of muscle relaxants, sympatholytics, opioids, N_2O, benzodiazepines; N_2O ↓ end-tidal anesthetic requirement
Key Points:	Widely used maintenance anesthetic that is being replaced by less-soluble agents desflurane (adults) and sevoflurane (children)

NITROUS OXIDE

Other Name:	**N_2O**
Indications:	Intraoperative amnesia and analgesia, adjuvant to volatile anesthetic
Pharmacokinetics:	Gaseous, nonflammable drug; blood:gas solubility: 0.47; extremely rapid onset and recovery times; MAC: ≈105%; not metabolized
Pharmacodynamics:	Inhaled anesthetic with prominent amnestic and weak analgesic properties
CNS:	Sedation, amnesia and analgesia, excitement, disorientation
CV:	↑ HR, ↑ PVR, ↓ CO (in presence of cardiac impairment)
GI:	Nausea, vomiting (when combined with opioid analgesics)
Pulmonary:	Nonirritant, respiratory depressant (mild), diffusion hypoxia
Other:	Megaloblastic anemia and agranulocytosis (with prolonged exposure)
Dosage:	Usual inspired concentration 40–70% in oxygen (or combined with volatile anesthetic)

NITROUS OXIDE *continued*

Contraindications:	Tension pneumothorax, pneumoencephalography, middle ear surgery, mechanical bowel obstruction
Drug Interactions:	↓ Volatile anesthetic requirement in concentration-dependent fashion; opioids ↑ PONV
Key Points:	Facilitates recovery when administered in combination with more highly soluble volatile agents; anesthetic- and analgesic-sparing effect

SEVOFLURANE

Trade Names:	**Ultane, Sevorane**
Indications:	Induction and maintenance of general anesthesia
Pharmacokinetics:	Volatile, nonflammable; blood:gas solubility: 0.69; rapid onset and recovery times; MAC: 1.5%–2.2% (depending on age); metabolized in liver to hexafluoro-isopropanol (nontoxic) and CO_2; 3%–5% eliminated in urine as metabolites (compound A is potentially nephrotoxic)
Pharmacodynamics:	Halogenated (volatile) anesthetic that inhibits CNS excitatory neurotransmitter systems
CNS:	Generalized depression of CNS activity, excitement (on emergence), ↑ ICP
CS:	↓ PVR, ↓ BP
GI:	Nausea, vomiting
Musculoskeletal:	Muscle relaxation
Pulmonary:	Respiratory depression, pungency, airway irritation (mild)
Dosage:	Usual inspired concentration: 0.8–1.5 with 4–8% for induction and 0.5–2% for maintenance of anesthesia
Contraindications:	Trigger to MH, prolonged exposure using closed-circuit anesthesia; ↑ risk of nephrotoxicity
Drug Interactions:	↑ Effects of muscle relaxants; opioids, N_2O, benzodiazepines ↓ end-tidal anesthetic concentration
Key Points:	Ideally suited for inhalation induction in patients with difficult airways (e.g., ENT surgery), lacking IV access (e.g., children), or with reactive airway and coronary artery disease

XENON

Trade Name:	**None**
Indications:	Induction and maintenance of anesthesia, inhalation analgesia

XENON *continued*

Pharmacokinetics:	Nonexplosive, nonflammable, colorless, odorless, tasteless gas; blood:gas partition: 0.14; extremely rapid induction and recovery; MAC: 63% (more potent than N_2O); eliminated through lungs (100%)
Pharmacodynamics:	Gaseous anesthetic that inhibits NMDA (aspartate) receptors in the CNS
CNS:	Concentration-dependent CNS depression, ↑ frontal theta-band and posterior delta-band EEG activity, ↑ cerebral flow, potent analgesic
CV:	↓ BP (mild)
GI:	Nausea, vomiting
Pulmonary:	↓ RR, ↑ tidal volume, ↑ airway resistance
Dosage:	Usual inspired concentration 40–70% in oxygen
Contraindications:	Acute bronchospasm (active wheezing)
Drug Interactions:	↑ Myocardial depression when combined with volatile anesthetics
Key Points:	When administered as part of balanced anesthetic technique, ↓ opioid analgesic requirement; useful in patients with coronary artery disease

29

Intravenous Anesthetics and Sedatives

AMOBARBITAL, SECOBARBITAL

Trade Names:	**Tuinal (amobarbital), Seconal (secobarbital)**
Indications:	Preoperative sedation, insomnia
Pharmacokinetics:	Onset: <15–30 min; bioavailability: 90%; peak: 30 min; protein binding: 40%; duration: 3–6 h; $T_{1/2}$ β: 20–30 h; metabolized in liver, excreted in urine
Pharmacodynamics:	↓ Presynaptic and postsynaptic membrane excitability by ↑ GABA activity
CNS:	Drowsiness, confusion, ataxia, dizziness, "hangover" feeling, paradoxical excitement (in elderly)
GI:	Nausea, vomiting, constipation
Pulmonary:	Respiratory depression, dyspnea
Other:	↑ Porphyria, rash, angioedema, fever, bleeding
Dosages:	*Secobarbital:* 100–200 mg PO hs (insomnia); 200–300 mg (premedication); 2–6 mg/kg, max. 100 mg (children) *Amobarbital:* 30–60 mg PO tid (insomnia); 200 mg (premedication); 2 mg/kg/d (children)
Contraindications:	Porphyria, diabetes, COPD
Drug Interactions:	Antidepressants, antihistamines, opioids, sedative-hypnotics, alcohol ↑ CNS and respiratory depression; ↑ metabolism of corticosteroids, digitoxin, doxycycline, estrogens (OCPs), theophylline, anticoagulants; disulfiram, MAOIs, valproic acid ↓ metabolism; rifampin ↓ level
Key Points:	Preoperative use with anesthetics and other sedative-hypnotics, ↑ CNS and respiratory depressive effects, prolonging recovery from general anesthesia

BUTALBITAL

Trade Names:	**Fioricet, Fiorinal, Phrenilin**
Indications:	Tension headache, muscle relaxation
Pharmacodynamics:	Barbiturate with central depressant effect, spinal-mediated muscle relaxant
CNS:	Drowsiness, confusion, dizziness, paradoxical excitement (elderly)
GI:	Nausea, vomiting, abdominal cramps, bloating
Pulmonary:	Dyspnea
Dosage:	50 mg PO (in combination with acetaminophen [or aspirin] and caffeine)
Contraindications:	Porphyria, hyperthyroidism, aspirin sensitivity, pregnancy, breast-feeding

BUTALBITAL *continued*

Drug Interactions:	↑ Sedation in presence of CNS depressant drugs
Key Points:	May ↓ IV anesthetic requirements with short-term use and ↑ anesthetic requirement with chronic use

CHLORAL HYDRATE

Trade Name:	**Aquachloral**
Indications:	Preoperative sedation, insomnia, hypnosis, alcohol withdrawal
Pharmacokinetics:	Onset: 0.5 h; peak: 1–2 h; protein binding: 40%; duration: 4–8 h; $T_{1/2}$ β: 8–10 h (trichloroethanol); metabolized by liver and erythrocytes to active metabolite (trichloroethanol), excreted in urine
Pharmacodynamics:	Sedative-hypnotic which depresses reticular activating system
CNS:	Drowsiness, hypnosis, delirium, ataxia
GI:	Nausea, vomiting, diarrhea, flatulence
Other:	Leukopenia
Dosage:	0.5–1 g PO initially, then 250 mg PO tid (adult); 50 mg/kg, then 8 mg/kg tid, or 325–650 mg pr (children)
Contraindications:	Hepatorenal impairment, severe cardiac disease
Drug Interactions:	CNS depressants ↑ sedative effect; with oral anticoagulants ↑ PT
Key Points:	Use with anesthetics and sedative-hypnotics ↑ CNS depressive effects and delays early recovery from general anesthesia

ETOMIDATE

Trade Name:	**Amidate**
Indications:	Induction of anesthesia, procedural sedation
Pharmacokinetics:	Onset: <2 min; peak: 3–5 min; protein binding: 76%; duration: 5–15 min; Vd: 3–4 l/kg; Cl: 20 mL/kg/min; $T_{1/2}$ β: 4 h; metabolized in liver, excreted in urine
Pharmacodynamics:	↑ CNS action of GABA at $GABA_A$ receptor
CNS:	Sedation-hypnosis, ↓ CBF, myoclonic activity, ↓ IOP
CV:	↓ SVR, ↓ BP (minimal)
GI:	Nausea, vomiting

ETOMIDATE *continued*

Pulmonary:	↓ Tidal volume, ↓ respiratory rate, transient apnea
Other:	↓ Adrenosteroidogenesis (↓ cortisol), pain on injection, hiccups
Dosages:	*Induction (hypnosis):* 0.15–0.3 mg/kg (age-dependent) *Maintenance (sedation):* 25–100 µg/kg/min
Contraindications:	Prolonged sedation, seizure disorders, adrenocortical impairment
Drug Interactions:	Concurrent use of potent opioid analgesics ↓ myoclonic activity; sedative-hypnotic and opioids ↓ anesthetic requirement
Key Points:	IV induction in presence of coronary artery or cerebrovascular disease, unstable cardiovascular status or depleted intravascular volume

GAMMA HYDROXYBUTYRATE (GHB)

Other Names:	**Fantasy, soap, liquid ecstasy, "date rape" drug, nature's quaalude, blue nitro, gamma G, vita-G, wolfies**
Indications:	ICU sedation, total IV anesthesia, brain injury, narcolepsy, alcohol, opioid withdrawal (investigational)
Pharmacokinetics:	Onset: 5–7 min (IV), <30 min (oral); peak: 20–60 min; duration: 1–7 h; $T_{1/2}$ β: 20 min; extensively metabolized in liver to CO_2 and H_2O
Pharmacodynamics:	Endogenous byproduct of GABA synthesis that causes ↑ serotonin and acetylcholine level, ↓ CNS release of dopamine
CNS:	Sedation-hypnosis, euphoria, dizziness, disorientation (hallucinations), aggressive behavior, myoclonic activity, psychological dependence
CV:	↓ HR, orthostatic hypotension
GI:	Vomiting
GU:	↑ Libido, ↑ erection
Pulmonary:	Respiratory depression, Cheyne-Stokes pattern
Other:	Hyperglycemia, hypokalemia, ↓ cholesterol level, hypothermia
Dosage:	70–120 mg/kg IV loading dose, then 40 mg/kg/h infusion; 120–150 mg/kg IM, or 100–200 mg/kg pr (children)
Contraindications:	Hypokalemia, myasthenia gravis, alcohol overdose

GAMMA HYDROXYBUTYRATE
(GHB) *continued*

Drug Interactions:	NK
Key Points:	↑ CNS depressant effects of anesthetic and analgesic drugs, withdrawal syndrome occurs after prolonged use; reversal of sedative effects using physostigmine

KETAMINE

Trade Names:	**Ketalar, Ketaject**
Indications:	Induction of general anesthesia, sedation analgesia
Pharmacokinetics:	Onset: 30 sec (IV), 3–4 min (IM); peak: 3–5 min (IV), 10–25 min (IM); duration 8–15 min (IV), 30–60 min (IM); Vd: 2–4 L/kg; Cl: 16–18 mL/kg/min; $T_{1/2}$ α: 10–15 m, β: 1–2 h; metabolized in liver, excreted in urine
Pharmacodynamics:	Activates limbic system, producing dissociative anesthetic state, S (+) isomer is more potent hypnotic-analgesic than racemic mixture
CNS:	Sedation, hypnosis, cerebral vasodilation (↑ CBF); nystagmus, emergence delirium, seizures, tremor, hallucinations, analgesia
CV:	↑ BP, ↑ HR, ↑ CO (unless depleted catecholamine stores), ↑ myocardial oxygen consumption, arrhythmias
GI:	↑ Salivary gland secretion, nausea
Pulmonary:	↓ Respiratory rate, apnea, ↑ airway secretions, bronchodilation
Other:	Hypertonus, purposeful skeletal movements, rash
Dosages:	*Induction:* 0.5–2.5 mg/kg IV (adults); 2–4 mg/kg IV or 6–10 mg/kg IM (children) *Maintenance:* 75–150 µg/kg IV (adjuvant); 12.5–50 µg/kg/min (sedation/analgesia)
Contraindications:	↑ ICP, severe hypertension or coronary artery disease, ophthalmologic procedures (due to nystagmus), ↑ IOP
Drug Interactions:	Benzodiazepines, barbiturates, propofol, volatile anesthetics ↓ sympathetic response; volatile anesthetics prolong recovery; ↑ nondepolarizing neuromuscular blockers; aminophylline ↓ seizure threshold
Key Points:	Use to induce sedation and hypnosis in patients without IV access; ↑ CNS stimulants ↓ seizure threshold; small doses (75–200 µg/kg) ↓ opioid analgesic requirements during perioperative period

MEPROBAMATE

Trade Names:	**Equinil, Meprospan, Miltown, Neuramate**
Indications:	Preoperative sedation, anxiety
Pharmacokinetics:	Onset: <0.5 h; peak: 1–2 h; protein binding: 20%; duration: 6–8 h; $T_{1/2}$ β: 6–17 h; crosses placental barrier; metabolized in liver, excreted in urine
Pharmacodynamics:	Nonselective CNS depression of thalamus, limbic system, spinal cord
CNS:	Drowsiness, ataxia, dizziness, slurred speech
CV:	↓ BP, ↑ HR, palpitations
GI:	Nausea, vomiting, diarrhea
Other:	Pancytopenia, pruritus, urticaria
Dosage:	400 mg PO initially, then 0.3–0.4 g qid (max. 2.4 g/d); 200 mg PO, 100–200 mg PO tid (children)
Contraindications:	Porphyria, pregnancy, breast-feeding
Drug Interactions:	Antihistamines, barbiturates, opioids ↑ CNS depression
Key Points:	↑ CNS depression produced by general anesthetics and other sedative-hypnotic drugs, prolonging recovery and ↑ hypotensive and respiratory depression

METHOHEXITAL

Trade Name:	**Brevital**
Indications:	Induction and maintenance of general anesthesia
Pharmacokinetics:	Onset: <60 sec; peak: 1–2 h; duration: 5–15 min; Vd: 1.1–2.2 L/kg; Cl: 10.9–12.1 mL/kg/min; $T_{1/2}$ α: 6 min, γ: slow, 58 min, β: 1.6–3.9 h; metabolized in liver, excreted in urine
Pharmacodynamics:	Ultra short-acting barbiturate, produces generalized CNS depression
CNS:	Headache, emergence delirium, seizures, myoclonic activity
CV:	↑ HR, ↓ BP
GI:	Nausea, vomiting, abdominal pain
Pulmonary:	↓ Respiration rate, transient apnea
Other:	Pain on injection, ↑ salivation, hiccups
Dosages:	*Induction:* 1–2 mg/kg IV; 15–30 mg/kg pr (children) *Maintenance:* 50–100 µg/kg/min infusion
Contraindications:	Acute intermittent porphyria, seizure disorders
Drug Interactions:	Phenytoin ↓ effect

METHOHEXITAL *continued*

Key Points: ↑ CNS depression produced by anesthetics and other sedative-hypnotics; less prolongation of recovery from anesthesia than other barbituates; ↑ CNS stimulant effects of drugs that ↓ seizure threshold

PHOSPHONOMETHYL PROPOFOL

Trade Name: **Aquavan (investigational)**

Indications: Conscious sedation (for diagnostic and therapeutic procedures)

Pharmacokinetics: Onset: 3–5 min; protein binding: 97%; duration: 10–20 min; Vd: 60 L/kg; Cl: 40 mL/kg/min; $T_{1/2}$ β: 2.5–5 h; metabolized in liver (by alkaline phosphatases), excreted in urine

Pharmacodynamics: CNS depressant with GABAergic receptor activity
CV: ↓ BP, ↑ HR
Pulmonary: ↓ Respiratory ventilation, ↑ $Paco_2$
Other: Transient pain in anal and genital region

Dosage: 7.5–10 mg/kg IV (sedation); 10–15 mg/kg (hypnosis)

Contraindications: Coma

Drug Interactions: ↑ CNS depression with benzodiazepines, opioids and sedatives

Key Points: Water-soluble prodrug of propofol, which has slower onset and recovery; potent opioids minimize peritoneal discomfort

PROPOFOL

Trade Names: **Diprivan, Ampofol (investigational)**

Indications: Induction and maintenance of anesthesia, sedation during local and regional anesthesia, ICU sedation

Pharmacokinetics: Onset: <45 sec; peak: 1–2 min; protein binding: 95%; duration: 10–15 min; Vd: 60 L/kg; Cl: 23–50 mL/kg/min; $T_{1/2}$ β: 1–3 min, γ: 45 min, β: 30–90 min (bolus) and 1–2 d (after prolonged infusion); metabolized in liver, excreted in urine

Inactive Ingredients: *Diprivan:* soybean oil: 100 mg/mL; egg lecithin: 12 mg/mL, EDTA preservative; generic contains metabisulfate as preservative
Ampofol: soybean 50 mg/mL, egg lecithin 6 mg/mL, no preservative

PROPOFOL *continued*

Pharmacodynamics:	Dose-dependent CNS depression due to ↑ GABAergic activity
CNS:	Sedation-hypnosis, amnesia, ↓ CBF, ↓ ICP, ataxia
CV:	↓ BP, direct myocardial depression, ↓ CO, ↓ HR
GI:	↓ Nausea, ↓ vomiting
Pulmonary:	↓Ventilation (↑ end-tidal CO_2), transient apnea
Other:	Pain on injection, ↑ triglyceride levels (less with Ampofol)
Dosage:	*Induction:* 1.0–2.5 mg/kg IV *Maintenance:* 75–200 µg/kg/min infusion *Sedation:* 0.5–1 mg/kg, then 12.5–75 µg/kg/min
Contraindications:	Coma, allergic to intralipids, soybeans, and/or egg lecithin
Drug Interactions:	Opioids, benzodiazepines, barbiturates, inhalation anesthetics, other sedative-hypnotics ↑ CNS depression; do not coadminister in same IV catheter with blood products
Key Points:	IV anesthetics with most rapid recovery and fewest postoperative side effects after surgery; coadministration with lidocaine 1% to ↓ pain on injection

THIOPENTAL

Trade Name:	**Pentothal**
Indications:	Induction of general anesthesia, status epilepticus
Pharmacokinetics:	Onset: <30 sec; peak: 30–60 sec; duration: 15–30 min; protein binding: 80%; Vd: 1.5–2.5 L/kg; Cl: 3.4–3.6 mL/kg/min; $T_{1/2}$ α: 5.5 min, γ: 54 min, β: 5–11 h; metabolized in liver, excreted in urine
Pharmacodynamics:	Barbiturate which ↑ GABA activity in CNS
CNS:	Sedation, hypnosis, ↓ CBF, ↓ ICP, ↓ $CMRO_2$
CV:	↓ BP, ↑ HR, ↓ venous return
Pulmonary:	↓ Respiratory rate, transient apnea, coughing, sneezing
Other:	Muscle relaxation, gangrene (intra-arterial injection)
Dosage:	*Induction*: 3–5 mg/kg IV; 4–7 mg/kg (children)
Contraindications:	Acute intermittent porphyria
Drug Interactions:	Alcohol ↑ CNS depressive effect
Key Points:	Use with opioids, benzodiazepines, inhalational anesthetics, other sedative-hypnotics ↑ CNS depression; recovery is slower and ↑ nausea and vomiting compared with propofol

ZALEPLON

Trade Name:	**Sonata**
Indications:	Insomnia
Pharmacokinetics:	Onset: 1 h; peak: 1 h; protein binding: 60%; duration: 3–4 h; $T_{1/2}$ β: 1 h; extensively metabolized in liver, excreted in urine
Pharmacodynamics:	Interacts with GABA and benzodiazepine receptor complexes
CNS:	Dizziness, depression, hallucinations, headache, somnolence
CV:	Chest pain (angina), peripheral edema
GI:	Dry mouth, dyspepsia, anorexia, nausea
Other:	Dysmenorrhea, pruritus, rash, myalgia
Dosage:	5–20 mg PO hs
Contraindications:	Severe hepatic impairment
Drug Interactions:	Carbamazepine, phenobarbital, phenytoin, rifampin ↓ level; cimetidine ↑ level; imipramine and alcohol ↑ CNS effects
Key Points:	Preoperative use with general anesthetics and opioid analgesics ↑ CNS depression, delaying initial recovery

ZOLPIDEM

Trade Name:	**Ambien**
Indications:	Premedication, sedation, insomnia
Pharmacokinetics:	Onset: <30 min; peak: 0.5–2 h; protein binding: 92.5%; $T_{1/2}$ β: 2.6 h
Pharmacodynamics: *CNS:*	Interacts with a GABA-B_2 receptor, ↑ GABA activity Somnolence, amnesia, headache, drowsiness
Dosage:	5–10 mg PO hs
Contraindications:	NK
Drug Interactions:	NK
Key Points:	Use with general anesthetics will ↑ CNS depressant effects; ↓ anesthetic induction dose requirement

30

Local Anesthetics

BENZOCAINE

Trade Names:	**Hurricaine, Cetacaine**
Indications:	Topical analgesia
Pharmacokinetics:	Onset: <30 sec; duration: 12–15 min; elimination by plasma pseudocholinesterase (forms alcohol and PABA), excreted in urine
Pharmacodynamics:	Reversible blockade of nerve conduction via membrane stabilization
CNS:	Analgesia, seizures (overdose)
CV:	Myocardial depression, vasodilation, ↑ HR
Other:	Muscle weakness, methemoglobinemia, localized reactions
Dosage:	2% aerosol spray, 200–400 mg (1–2 sec)
Contraindications:	IV or intraocular use
Drug Interactions:	PABA inhibits sulfonamides
Key Points:	Most commonly used for topical analgesia involving mucosal membranes

BUPIVACAINE

Trade Names:	**Marcaine, Sensorcaine**
Indications:	Peripheral nerve blocks, epidural (and spinal) anesthesia
Pharmacokinetics:	Onset: <30 min; peak: 30–45 min; protein binding: 95%; duration: 240–480 min; Vd: 73 L; Cl: 0.58 L/min; $T_{1/2} \beta$: 2.7 h; metabolized in liver, excreted in urine
Pharmacodynamics:	Blocks nerve conduction by ↑ threshold for nerve excitation
CNS:	Analgesia, restlessness, confusion, tremors, seizures, tinnitus, dizziness, blurred vision, drowsiness, muscle weakness
CV:	↓ HR, arrhythmias, (–) inotrope, ↓ BP, cardiac arrest
GI:	Nausea, vomiting
Pulmonary:	Respiratory arrest, status asthmaticus
Dosage:	0.25–0.75% 15–30 mL solutions (max. 2 mg/kg)
Contraindications:	Sensitivity to para-aminobenzoic acid (PABA) or parabens, avoid 0.75% bupivacaine for epidural analgesia in parturients
Drug Interactions:	↑ Toxic effects with antiarrhythmic drugs; epinephrine in combination with MAOIs and TCAs ↑ BP; butyrophenones and phenothiazines ↓ pressor effect of epinephrine; chloroprocaine ↓ efficacy

BUPIVACAINE *continued*

Key Points: Most commonly used for local (incisional) anesthesia to prevent postoperative pain; use of high concentrations (0.75%) or large volumes of 0.5% bupivacaine with volatile anesthetics and ketamine may cause cardiac arrhythmias; 4× more potent than lidocaine

2-CHLOROPROCAINE

Trade Name: **Nesacaine**

Indications: Peripheral nerve blocks, spinal and epidural anesthesia

Pharmacokinetics: Onset: <10 min; peak: 30 min; duration: 45–60 min; rapidly hydrolyzed by plasma cholinesterase, excreted in urine

Pharmacodynamics: Reversible blockade of nerve conduction
CNS: Analgesia, restlessness, circumoral paresthesia, disorientation, tonic-clonic seizures, drowsiness, tinnitus, blurred vision
CV: ↓ BP, ↓ HR, (−) inotrope, arrhythmias, cardiac arrest
Pulmonary: Respiratory arrest
Other: Muscle weakness, myalgias, pain at injection site

Dosage: 1–3% solutions 15–30 mL (max. 1 g); spinal: 30–60 mg IT

Contraindications: Myasthenia gravis, concurrent use of bupivacaine

Drug Interactions: 4-amino-2-chloroprocaine metabolite impairs action; sodium bisulfate (antioxidant)-produced neurologic deficits after spinal-epidural administration

Key Points: Central neuroaxis blockade with antioxidant-free 2-chloroprocaine associated with most rapid recovery; ↓ transient neurologic symptoms (TNS) compared with lidocaine (e.g., back pain)

COCAINE

Other Name: **Cocaine (viscous)**

Indications: Topical anesthesia of nasal mucosal, local vasoconstriction

Pharmacokinetics: Onset: <2 min; peak: 3–5 min; duration: 1–2 h; $T_{1/2}$ β: 60–90 min; metabolized by liver and plasma pseudocholinesterase, excreted in urine

Pharmacodynamics: Blocks initiation and conduction of nerve impulses by inactivating sodium channels and reuptake of dopamine and norepinephrine

COCAINE *continued*

CNS:	Analgesia, excitement (euphoria), depression, tremors, seizures, mydriasis, fever, respiratory failure
CV:	↑ BP, ↑ HR, tachyarrhythmias, cardiac arrest
Other:	Pulmonary edema, ↓ uterine blood flow

Dosage: 4% topical solution 0.5–4 mL (max. 3 mg/kg)

Contraindications: Addictive personality, CAD, intraocular or IV use; traumatized mucosa

Drug Interactions: Sensitizes myocardium to circulating catecholamines; MAOI and epinephrine ↑ cardiotoxicity

Key Points: Rapid absorption can result in cardiovascular collapse; use with volatile anesthetics and sympathomimetics should be avoided

ETIDOCAINE

Trade Name: **Duranest**

Indications: Local infiltration, peripheral nerve blocks, caudal/lumbar epidural blocks

Pharmacokinetics: Onset: <15 min; peak: 30–60 min; protein binding: 95%; duration: l5–10 h after infiltration; Vd: 134 L; Cl: 1.1 L/min; $T_{1/2}$ β: 2.7 h

Pharmacodynamics: Inhibition of neuronal ion fluxes; ↓ nerve impulse conduction

CNS:	Analgesia, restlessness, confusion, tremors, shivering, drowsiness, tinnitus, lightheadedness, blurred vision, muscle weakness
CV:	↓ HR, myocardial depression, ↓ BP, cardiovascular collapse
GI:	Nausea, vomiting
Pulmonary:	Respiratory arrest, trimus

Dosage: 1–1.5% solution 5–40 mL (max. 300 mg; 400 mg with epinephrine)

Drug Interactions: NK

Key Points: Regional anesthesia with etidocaine may ↑ side effects compared with lidocaine and bupivacaine

LEVOBUPIVACAINE

Trade Name: **Chirocaine**

Indications: Local (infiltration) anesthesia, peripheral nerve blocks, central neuroaxis blockade

LEVOBUPIVACAINE *continued*

Pharmacokinetics:	Onset: 15 min; peak: 30–60 min; protein binding: 97%; duration: 8–10 h; Vd: 66 L; Cl: 39 L/h; $T_{1/2}$ β: 3.3 h; extensively metabolized in liver, excreted 1° in urine
Pharmacodynamics:	S-enantiomer of bupivacaine; blocks generation and conduction of nerve impulses
CNS:	Hypokinesia, tremor, confusion, dizziness
CV:	↓ BP, arrhythmia
GI:	Nausea, vomiting
Other:	Anemia, low back pain (myalgias)
Dosage:	0.25–0.75% solution 15–30 mL, 0.5–2 mg/kg (max. 570 mg)
Contraindications:	Sensitivity to amide-type local anesthetic drugs
Drug Interactions:	Cytochrome P_{450} inhibitors ↑ toxicity, inducers (e.g., phenytoin, phenobarbital, rifampin) ↓ levels
Key Points:	Levoisomer of bupivacaine may have ↓ risk of cardiotoxicity compared with racemic bupivacaine

LIDOCAINE

Trade Name:	**Xylocaine**
Indications:	Topical anesthesia, local infiltration anesthesia, peripheral nerve blocks, central neuroaxis block, IV regional anesthesia (Bier block)
Pharmacokinetics:	Onset: <10 min; peak: 30 min; protein binding: 70%; duration: 1–3 h (± epinephrine); Vd: 1.7 L/kg; Cl: 0.64 L/kg/min; $T_{1/2}$ β: 1.5–2 h; metabolized in liver by oxidative *N*-dealkylation, excreted in urine
Pharmacodynamics:	Inhibition of sodium flux, ↓ conduction of nerve impulses
CNS:	Analgesia, lightheadedness, euphoria, confusion, seizures, drowsiness, tinnitus, blurred vision, tremor, TNS
CV:	↓ HR, ↓ BP, cardiovascular collapse/arrest
GI:	Nausea, vomiting
Pulmonary:	Respiratory depression
Other:	Urticaria, pruritus, angioneurotic edema, anaphylactoid reactions
Dosage:	Topical 2–4% (10–20 mL); inhalational 4–10%; parenteral 1–2% 15–30 mL (max. dose: 4.5 mg/kg; 300 mg), 25–100 mg IT
Contraindications:	Sensitivity to amide-type local anesthetics, preservative (parabens), advanced heart block (without pacemaker), sepsis

LIDOCAINE *continued*

Drug Interactions: Additive effect with phenytoin, procainamide, propranolol quinidine; ↓ clearance with β-blockers and cimetidine, benzodiazepines ↑ seizure threshold

Key Points: Use of mini-dose (15–30 mg) in combination with potent opioid (fentanyl 25 μg, sufentanil 5 μg) for spinal anesthesia facilitates recovery process and ↓ peripheral neuropathic TNS symptoms; ↑ neuromuscular-blocking drugs; regional anesthetic blocks with lidocaine associated with ↓ side effects

LIDOCAINE-BUPIVACAINE

Trade Name: **Duocaine**

Indications: Local or regional anesthesia (ophthalmology)

Pharmacokinetics: Peak: 20 min; protein binding: 60%–80%; $T_{1/2}$ β: 1.5–2 h (lidocaine), 2.7 h (bupivacaine); hepatic metabolism, excreted in urine

Pharmacodynamics: Blocks generation and conduction of nerve impulses; ↑ threshold for electrical excitation

  CNS: ↓ Seizure threshold, dizziness, restlessness, tremors, blurred vision, papillary constriction

  CV: ↓ CO, ↓ BP (due to ↓ PVR), arrythmias (bupivacaine)

  Other: Metallic taste, nausea, vomiting

Dosage: 1% lidocaine 2–5 mL + 0.375% bupivacaine

Contraindications: Sensitivity to amide-type local anesthetics, Stokes-Adams syndrome, Wolff-Parkinson-White syndrome, advanced heart block

Drug Interactions: MAOIs, TCA ↑ sympathetic response to epinephrine (phenothiazine, butyrophenone ↓ response); ergot-type oxytocics ↑ CV stimulation; ↑ digitalis toxicity; β-blockers ↓ clearance

Key Points: Achieves faster onset than bupivacaine and longer duration of analgesic than lidocaine

LIDOCAINE-PRILOCAINE

Trade Name: **EMLA Cream**

Indications: Topical analgesia

Pharmacokinetics: Onset: 1–2 h (after application); peak: 3–4 h; duration: 1–2 h after removal; systemic local anesthetic levels extremely low

LIDOCAINE-PRILOCAINE *continued*

Pharmacodynamics:	Inhibition of neuronal ion fluxes, $\downarrow$ nerve conduction
CNS:	Analgesia, $\downarrow$ sensory perception
Skin:	Hyperpigmentation, blanching, erythema, edema, itching, warm sensation
Other:	Methemoglobinemia
Dosage:	Apply 2–3 g over 10–30 cm^2 under occlusive dressing (each gram contains lidocaine, 25 mg; prilocaine, 25 mg)
Contraindications:	Sensitivity to amide local anesthetics, methemoglobinemia, G-6-PD deficiency, breast-feeding
Drug Interactions:	Sulfonamides, acetaminophen, nitrates, nitrites, nitrofurantoin, nitroglycerin, nitroprusside, phenacetin, phenobarbital, phenytoin $\uparrow$ methemoglobinemia
Key Points:	Topical analgesia requires 90–120 min and fails to block "pressure" sensation; systemic absorption from topical application, supplemental regional blocks $\uparrow$ tendency to produce CNS and cardiac side effects

MEPIVACAINE

Trade Name:	**Carbocaine**
Indications:	Local (infiltration) anesthesia, peripheral nerve block, central neuroaxis blockade
Pharmacokinetics:	Onset: 3–10 min; protein binding: 75%; duration: 60–120 min (after infiltration), longer duration than plain lidocaine; Vd: 84 L; Cl: 0.78 L/min; $T_{1/2}$ β: 1.9 h; metabolized in liver, excreted in urine
Pharmacodynamics:	Inhibition of sodium flux, $\downarrow$ conduction of nerve impulses
CNS:	Analgesia, restlessness, confusion, tremors, seizures, drowsiness, tinnitus, dizziness, blurred vision, muscle weakness
CV:	$\downarrow$ HR, (–) inotrope, $\downarrow$ BP, cardiovascular collapse/arrest
GI:	Nausea, vomiting
Pulmonary:	Respiratory arrest, apnea (overdose)
Dosage:	1–2% solution 15–30 mL (max. 4–7 mg/kg)
Contraindications:	Allergic to sodium metabisulfite, amide-type local anesthetics
Drug Interactions:	Bupivacaine may $\downarrow$ binding of mepivacaine to α_1-acid glycoprotein and $\uparrow$ risk of systemic toxicity
Key Points:	Used as alternative to lidocaine for central neuroaxis blockade in outpatient surgery setting to facilitate earlier ambulation

PRILOCAINE

Trade Name:	**Citanest**
Indications:	Local (infiltration) anesthesia, peripheral nerve blockade, extradural anesthesia, IV regional anesthesia (Bier block)
Pharmacokinetics:	Onset: <10 min; protein binding: 55%; duration: 1–3 h (after infiltration); Vd: 191 L; Cl: 2.37 L/min; $T_{1/2}$ β: 1.6 h; crosses both blood-brain and placental barriers; rapid hepatic metabolism to *o*-toluidine, which can produce methemoglobin; excreted in urine
Pharmacodynamics:	Inhibition of sodium flux, ↓ conduction of nerve impulses
CNS:	Analgesia, restlessness, confusion, dizziness, tremors, seizures, drowsiness, paresthesias, tinnitus, blurred vision, muscle weakness
CV:	↓ HR, (−) inotrope, ↓ BP, cardiovascular collapse/arrest
GI:	Nausea, vomiting
Pulmonary:	Respiratory arrest
Other:	Methemoglobinemia (>600 mg)
Dosage:	0.25–4% solutions 15–30 mL (max. 8 mg/kg <600 mg)
Contraindications:	Anemia, methemoglobinemia sensitivity to amide-type local anesthesias
Drug Interactions:	NK
Key Points:	Persistent paresthesias may occur after central and peripheral blocks; methemoglobinemia is treated with methylene blue, 1–2 mg/kg IV

PROCAINE

Trade Name:	**Novocaine**
Indications:	Central neuroaxis block, differential spinal blocks, peripheral nerve block, local (infiltration) anesthesia
Pharmacokinetics:	Onset: <5 min; protein binding: 6%; duration: 45–90 min after infiltration; rapidly hydrolyzed by plasma cholinesterase to para-aminobenzoic acid (PABA); $T_{1/2}$ β: 40 sec; excreted in urine
Pharmacodynamics:	Inhibition of sodium flux in response to nerve impulses
CNS:	Analgesia, restlessness, disorientation, tonic-clonic convulsions, drowsiness, tinnitus, dizziness, blurred vision
CV:	↓ HR, ↓ BP, arrhythmias, cardiac collapse
GI:	Nausea, vomiting

PROCAINE *continued*

Other:	Skin discoloration, pain at injection site, muscle relaxation
Dosage:	1–10% solutions 15–30 mL (max. 14 mg/kg); 50–200 mg IT
Contraindications:	Sensitivity to ester-type local anesthetics, PABA, sodium bisulfite
Drug Interactions:	↓ Effects of sulfonamides and aminosalicylic acid, ↑ effects of succinylcholine, anticholinesterases digitalis
Key Points:	Short-acting local anesthetic for spinal anesthesia where rapid recovery and early ambulation is very important

ROPIVACAINE

Trade Name:	**Naropin**
Indications:	Local (infiltration) anesthesia, major regional anesthesia for surgical procedures, labor analgesia, acute postoperative pain management
Pharmacokinetics:	Onset: <15 min; peak: 15–30 min; protein binding: 94% (α_1-acid glycoprotein); duration: 2–14 h; Vd_{ss}: 47 L; Cl: 440 mL/min; $T_{1/2}$ β: 4.2 h (epidural), >24 h (infiltration); hepatic metabolism (cytochrome P_{450}) to inactive metabolites, excreted in urine
Pharmacodynamics:	S (−) enantiomer blocks generation and conduction of nerve impulses
CNS:	Analgesia, restlessness, tremors, paresthesias, seizures, headache
CV:	↓ HR, AV block, (−) inotrope (↓ cardiac output, ↓ BP), arrhythmias
GI:	Nausea, vomiting
Other:	Back pain, muscle weakness
Dosage:	0.2–1% solutions 10–30 mL; for major nerve block ↑ 250 mg; for cesarean delivery ↑ 150 mg (e.g., 30 mL 0.5%)
Contraindications:	Sensitivity to amide-type local anesthetics
Drug Interactions:	May ↑ effect of cytochrome P_{450} (1A) metabolized drugs and other amide-type local anesthetics
Key Points:	Theoretically, greater "safety" margin than racemic bupivacaine with respect to cardiotoxicity; may produce greater separation between sensory and motor blockade

TETRACAINE

Trade Name:	**Pontocaine**
Indications:	Spinal anesthesia, local anesthesia for ophthalmologic surgery, adjuvant to local anesthetic solutions
Pharmacokinetics:	Onset: <10 min; protein binding: 85%; duration: 2–3 h after infiltration; metabolized by plasma esterases to aminobenzoic acid and diethylaminoethanol, excreted in urine
Pharmacodynamics:	Inhibition of sodium flux in response to nerve impulses
CNS:	Analgesia, disorientation, seizures, drowsiness, tinnitus, lacrimation, photophobia, keratitis
CV:	Cardiac arrest, ↓ HR, (–) inotrope, ↓ BP, arrhythmias
GI:	Nausea, vomiting
Other:	Urticaria, contact dermatitis (topical), respiratory arrest
Dosage:	1–2% solution 1–2 mL (adjuvant); 0.5% (ophthalmic use; max. 1.5 mg/kg); 5–15 mg IT
Contraindications:	Ophthalmic infection; sensitivity to ester-type local anesthetic
Drug Interactions:	↓ Effects of aminosalicylic acid and sulfonamides
Key Points:	Potent local anesthetic (4× lidocaine) with long duration of action in subarachnoid space (75–150 min)

31

Metabolic Therapies

ACARBOSE

Trade Name:	**Precose**
Indications:	Diabetes mellitus; adjunct to insulin, melformin, sulfonylureas
Pharmacokinetics:	Onset: <10 min; peak: 1 h; duration: 2–4 h; $T_{1/2}$ β: 2 h; acts locally in the GI tract; metabolized in GI tract by intestinal bacteria, excreted in feces as unabsorbed drug and in urine as metabolites
Pharmacodynamics:	Oligosaccharide that inhibits pancreatic α-amylase and membrane-bound intestinal α-glucoside hydrolase
GI:	Pain, diarrhea, flatulence, ↑ LFTs
Other:	Hypocalcemia, vitamin B_6 deficiency
Dosage:	25–100 mg PO tid
Contraindications:	Diabetic ketoacidosis, cirrhosis, renal failure, colonic ulceration, intestinal obstruction, pregnancy, breast-feeding
Drug Interactions:	↓ Digoxin level; ↑ effect of insulin and sulfonylureas; charcoal, amylase, pancreatin ↓ effect; CCB, steroids, estrogens, isoniazid, nicotine, phenytoin, phenothiazines, sympathomimetics, thiazides, thyroid drugs ↓ effect
Key Points:	No known interactions with anesthetic drugs

ACETYLCYSTEINE

Trade Names:	**Mucomyst, Mucosil, Acetadote**
Indications:	Acute and chronic bronchopulmonary disease, acetaminophen toxicity
Pharmacokinetics:	Onset: <2 h; protein binding: 83%; Vd: 0.54 kg; Cl: 0.11 L/kg/h; $T_{1/2}$ β: 5–6 h; metabolized in liver to cysteine and disulfides, excreted in urine
Pharmacodynamics:	↓ Viscosity of mucus by splitting disulfide bonds in mucoprotein; inactivates acetaminophen metabolite; ↑ glutathione levels in liver
CV:	↑ HR, vasodilation
GI:	Nausea, vomiting, LFTs
Pulmonary:	Bronchospasm, watery secretions
Other:	Anaphylactoid reactions, rash, pruritus
Dosage:	10 or 20% solution 1–2 mL q 1–2 h (reduce viscosity); 140 mg/kg, followed by 70 mg/kg q 4 h (acetaminophen toxicity)

ACETYLCYSTEINE *continued*

Contraindications:	Severe respiratory insufficiency, sensitivity to cysteine/disulfides
Drug Interactions:	Activated charcoal $\downarrow$ effect; incompatible with oral antibiotics, rubber, metals
Key Points:	Need to initiate treatment <8 h after acetaminophen overdose

AGALSIDASE BETA

Trade Name:	**Fabrazyme**
Indications:	Fabry's disease
Pharmacokinetics:	Onset: rapid; duration: 2 wk; Vd: 0.35 L/kg; Cl: 2–4 mL/kg/min; $T_{1/2}$ β: 45–100 min
Pharmacodynamics:	Recombinant α-galactosidase A, enzyme replacement therapy, $\downarrow$ globotriaosylceramide (GL-3) deposits
CV:	$\uparrow$ BP, CHF
Other:	Fever, chills, myalgias, pharyngitis, anxiety
Dosage:	1 mg/kg IV q 2 wk
Contraindications:	Anaphylactic reaction
Drug Interactions:	Acetaminophen, antihistamines, NSAIDs $\downarrow$ side effects
Key Points:	No known interactions with anesthetic drugs

ALENDRONATE, ETIDRONATE, RISEDRONATE

Trade Names:	**Didronel (etidronate), Fosamax (alendronate), Actonel (risedronate)**
Indications:	Paget's disease, heterotopic ossifications, hypercalcemia of malignancy, severe osteoporosis
Pharmacokinetics:	Onset: 1 h; peak: 2–3 h; duration: 1–7 d; $T_{1/2}$ β: 1–6 h; not metabolized, excreted in urine and feces
Pharmacodynamics:	Suppresses osteoclast activity, reduces bone turnover
GI:	Metallic (or altered) taste, diarrhea, nausea, dyspepsia
Musculoskeletal:	Bone pain, poor healing of fractures, arthralgia
Other:	Electrolyte disturbances, $\downarrow$ renal function, bleeding tendency
Dosages:	*Etidronate:* 5–10 mg/kg/d
	Alendronate: 5–10 mg/d (or 35–70 mg/wk)
	Risedronate: 5 mg/d (or 35 mg/wk)

ALENDRONATE, ETIDRONATE, RISEDRONATE *continued*

Contraindications:	Renal and cardiac failure, severe osteomalacia, upper GI disorders
Drug Interactions:	↓ Efficacy with mineral supplements and antacids; ↑ warfarin effect
Key Points:	Use rapid induction sequence due to ↓ lower esophageal sphincter tone

ALLOPURINOL

Trade Names:	**Aloprim, Zyloprim**
Indications:	Gouty arthritis, hyperuricemia (due to neoplastic disease or chemotherapy), uric acid nephropathy, Ca^{2+} oxalate renal calculi
Pharmacokinetics:	Onset: <30 min; bioavailability: 85%; peak: 0.5–2 h; duration: 1–2 wk; $T_{1/2}$ β: 1–3 h (oxipurinol 12–30 h); hepatic metabolism to active metabolite (oxipurinol), excreted in urine
Pharmacodynamics:	Inhibits xanthine oxidase, hypouricemia
CNS:	Drowsiness, headache, paresthesia (peripheral neuritis)
GI:	Nausea, vomiting, diarrhea, anorexia, taste loss, ↑ LFTs
GU:	Renal failure, xanthine calculi (stones), uremia
Other:	Gout, bone marrow suppression, rash, fever, vasculitis, Stevens-Johnson syndrome, epistaxis, arthralgia, myopathy
Dosage:	100–400 mg PO (max. 600 mg/d); 50–100 mg tid (children)
Contraindications:	Idiopathic hemochromatosis
Drug Interactions:	↑ Levels of coumarin, azathioprine, mercaptopurine; ↓ clearance of theophylline and chlorpropamide; cyclophosphamide ↑ risk of bone marrow suppression; thiazides ↑ risk of anaphylaxis
Key Points:	Use with volatile anesthetics may ↑ risk of hepatic damage

BROMOCRIPTINE

Trade Name:	**Parlodel**
	See Chapter 20, "Central Stimulants"

CHENODIOL

Trade Name:	**Chenix**
Indications:	Cholesterol gallstones
Pharmacokinetics:	Onset: <30 min; peak: 50–120 min; duration: 12–24 h; metabolized to taurine and glycine conjugates, excreted in bile
Pharmacodynamics:	Naturally occurring bile acid
CV:	↑ Atherosclerosis
GI:	Constipation, anorexia, nausea, vomiting, cramps, ↑ LFTs
Other:	↑ Serum cholesterol (↑ LDL)
Dosage:	250 mg/d PO (max. 10 mg/kg bid)
Contraindications:	Pregnancy, hepatic impairment, bile duct disorders (1° biliary cirrhosis, cholangitis, cholestasis, fistulas, cholecystitis, pancreatitis)
Drug Interactions:	Antacids ↓ absorption
Key Points:	Use with volatile anesthetics may ↑ risk of liver damage

CHOLESTYRAMINE

Trade Name:	**Questran**
Indications:	Primary hyperlipidemia/hypercholesterolemia; pruritus (due to biliary obstruction); digitalis overdose, steatorrhea (due to ileal resection, hyperoxaluria)
Pharmacokinetics:	Onset: 1–2 d; peak: 1–2 wk; duration: 2–4 wk; not absorbed, eliminated in feces
Pharmacodynamics:	Binds to bile acid forming insoluble compound
GI:	Constipation, fecal impaction, nausea, vomiting, ↑ LFTs, GI bleeding, gallstones, malabsorption syndrome
Other:	Hypochloremic acidosis; electrolyte disturbances; ↓ lipid levels; osteoporosis; hypoprothrombinemia; vitamin K, A, D, and E deficiencies; bleeding tendency; anemia; hematuria
Dosage:	4 g PO qid (max. 32 g/d); 80 mg/kg tid (children)
Contraindications:	Complete biliary obstruction, children (< 2 yr), phenylketonuria (contains phenylalanine)
Drug Interactions:	↓ Absorption of fat-soluble vitamins, propranolol, chlorothiazide, acetaminophen, warfarin, digitalis, ursodiol, thyroid, steroids, tetracycline, penicillin G, vancomycin, phenobarbital, phenylbutazone, folic acid

CHOLESTYRAMINE *continued*

Key Points: Coagulation and electrolyte profile should be assessed before surgery

CILIARY NEUROTROPHIC FACTOR

Trade Name:	**Axokine (investigational)**
Indications:	Morbid obesity
Pharmacokinetics:	NK
Pharmacodynamics:	Stimulates satiety center in brain, ↓ food intake
GI:	Nausea
Pulmonary:	Coughing
Other:	Pain at injection site
Dosage:	1–2 mg/kg/d SC (×12 wk)
Contraindications:	NK
Drug Interactions:	Neutralizing antibodies occurred in 17% of subjects
Key Points:	No known adverse interactions with anesthetic drugs

CINACELCET

Trade Name:	**Sensipar**
Indications:	Hyperparathyroidism (due to chronic renal disease)
Pharmacokinetics:	Peak: 2–6 h; protein binding: 95%; $T_{1/2}$ β: 30–40 h; hepatic metabolism, excreted in urine
Pharmacodynamics:	↓ PTH levels by ↑ sensitivity of Ca^{2+}-sensing receptors
CNS:	↓ Seizure threshold, paresthesias
Other:	Myalgias, cramping, tetany, hypocalcemia
Dosage:	30 mg/d initially, then ↑ in 30-mg increments at 2- to 4-wk intervals (max. 180 mg/d)
Contraindications:	Hepatic failure (↓ dose)
Drug Interactions:	NK
Key Points:	Check preoperative Ca^{2+} levels and renal function

CLOFIBRATE

Trade Name:	**Atromid-S**
Indications:	Hyperlipidemia, hypertriglyceridemia, diabetes insipidus

CLOFIBRATE *continued*

Pharmacokinetics:	Onset: 1–2 h; peak: 4–6 h; $T_{1/2}$ β: 12–25 h (↑ to 113 h with hepatorenal disease); deesterification in GI tract, metabolized in liver to clofibric acid (active form), excreted in urine
Pharmacodynamics:	↓ Serum triglycerides level by ↑ catabolism of LDL
CNS:	Headache, dizziness, fatigue
CV:	Arrhythmias, thromboembolism, intermittent claudication
GU:	Renal toxicity (i.e., dysuria, hematuria, proteinuria, oliguria)
GI:	Stomatitis, gastritis, nausea, vomiting, diarrhea, ↑ LFTs, cholelithiasis
Other:	Impotence, ↓ libido, anemia, leukopenia, hypoglycemia, myalgias, myopathy, flulike syndrome, rhabdomyolysis
Dosage:	0.5–1 g PO bid
Contraindications:	Pregnancy, breast-feeding, hepatorenal impairment, 1° biliary cirrhosis
Drug Interactions:	↑ Effects of coumarin, furosemide, hypoglycemics, phenytoin; ↓ clearance with probenecid; cholestyramine ↓ absorption
Key Points:	Hepatorenal function, electrolytes, coagulation status should be carefully evaluated before surgery

COLCHICINE

Trade Name:	**None**
Indications:	Gouty arthritis, Mediterranean fever, amyloidosis, Paget's disease, dermatitis herpetiformis, primary biliary cirrhosis
Pharmacokinetics:	Onset: <1 h; peak: 6–12 h; duration: 24–48 h; $T_{1/2}$ β: 1 h; metabolized in liver, excreted in bile
Pharmacodynamics:	Inhibits leukocyte migration, ↓ lactic acid production, ↓ phagocytosis and inflammatory response
CNS:	↓ Central ventilatory drive, peripheral neuropathy
CV:	MI, (−) inotropic (↓ CO, ↓ BP), profound shock
GI:	Nausea, vomiting, diarrhea, hemorrhagic gastroenteritis, ↑ LFTs
GU:	Renal failure, hematuria, oliguria, azoospermia
Pulmonary:	Respiratory depression
Other:	Bone marrow suppression, coagulopathy, DIC, metabolic acidosis (↓ Na^+, ↓ K^+), alopecia, dermatitis, myopathy, muscle weakness

COLCHICINE *continued*

Dosages:	1–2 mg/d PO (max. 8 mg/d); 2 mg IV initially, then 0.5 mg IV q 6 h
Contraindications:	Severe cardiac, hepatic and renal disorders, blood dyscrasias
Drug Interactions:	↑ Toxicity with alcohol, erythromycin, anticoagulants, phenylbutazone, antineoplastics, radiation therapy; ↑ pressor effects with sympathomimetics; loop diuretics, alcohol, ↓ effect; vitamin B ↓ absorption
Key Points:	Use with anesthetic drugs ↑ CNS depressant effects, resulting in enhanced respiratory depression and delayed recovery

COLESTIPOL

Trade Name:	**Colestid**
Indications:	Primary hypercholesterolemia and xanthomas, pruritus (with biliary obstruction), digitalis overdose, steatorrhea (after ileal resection)
Pharmacokinetics:	Onset: 24–48 h; peak: 1 wk; duration: 1 mo; not absorbed, excreted in feces
Pharmacodynamics:	Binds to bile acid forming insoluble compound
CNS:	Headache, dizziness, anxiety, tinnitus
GI:	Constipation, fecal impaction, nausea, vomiting, ↑ LFTs, GI bleeding, gallstones, malabsorption syndrome
Other:	Hypochloremic acidosis; electrolyte disturbances; anemia; rash; ↓ PT; vitamin K, A, D, E deficiencies; bleeding tendency
Dosage:	1–5 g PO bid (max. 16 g/d)
Contraindications:	Biliary obstruction and bowel obstruction
Drug Interactions:	↓ Absorption of fat-soluble vitamins, propranolol, chlorothiazide, warfarin, digitalis, ursodiol, thyroid hormones, tetracycline, furosemide, penicillin G, gemfibrozil, vancomycin
Key Points:	Check electrolytes and coagulation profile prior to surgery

DARBEPOETIN ALFA

Trade Name:	**Aranesp**
	See Chapter 26, "Hormones"

DIMERCAPROL, DIMERCAPTOPROPANOL

Trade Name:	**BAL (British Anti-Lewisite)**
Indications:	Arsenic and gold poisoning, inorganic mercury and lead toxicity
Pharmacokinetics:	Onset: <30 min; peak: 30–60 min; duration: 4 h; eliminated as metal-dimercprol (BAL) complex in urine and bile
Pharmacodynamics:	Forms heterocyclic ring complexes with heavy metals
CNS:	Drowsiness, convulsions, blepharospasm, ↑ lacrimation, conjunctivitis, paresthesia, anxiety
CV:	↑ HR, ↑ BP
GI:	Nausea, vomiting, abdominal pain, ↑ LFTs
GU:	Nephrotoxicity
Other:	↓ ^{131}I thyroid uptake, oral burning, myalgias, neutropenia, rhinorrhea, diaphoresis, hemolysis (with G-6-PD deficiency)
Dosage:	2–3 mg/kg IM qid × 3 d, then bid × 7 d
Contraindications:	Arsine gas, iron, cadmium, selenium poisoning; hepatic or renal impairment; pregnancy
Drug Interactions:	Forms toxic complexes with cadmium, iron, selenium, uranium
Key Points:	No adverse interactions with anesthetic drugs

DORNASE ALFA

Trade Name:	**Pulmozyme**
Indications:	Cystic fibrosis
Pharmacokinetics:	Onset: 3–7 d; peak: 9 d (achieves therapeutic sputum levels <15 min)
Pharmacodynamics:	Enzyme that reduces sputum viscosity
CV:	Chest pain (angina)
Other:	Rash, urticaria, pharyngitis, laryngitis, conjunctivitis
Dosage:	2.5 mg/d with nebulizer
Contraindications:	NK
Drug Interactions:	NK
Key Points:	No known interaction with anesthetic drugs

EDETATE (EDTA) CALCIUM

Trade Name:	**Calcium Disodium Versenate**
Indications:	Lead poisoning, heavy metal poisoning

EDETATE (EDTA) CALCIUM *continued*

Pharmacokinetics:	Onset: 1 h; peak: 12–24 h; duration: 24–48 h; distributed primarily in extracellular fluid; excreted in urine as metal chelate
Pharmacodynamics:	Forms a water-soluble complex with heavy metals
CNS:	Tremor, headache, numbness, tingling, malaise
CV:	↓ BP, thrombophlebitis
GI:	Nausea, vomiting, anorexia
GU:	Proteinuria, hematuria, nephrotoxicity
Other:	Myalgia, arthralgia
Dosage:	1.5 g/m^2/d for 5 d; 1 g/m^2/d for 3–5 d (children)
Contraindications:	Anuria, hepatitis, acute renal disease
Drug Interactions:	Interferes with insulin by binding with zinc
Key Points:	Check glucose and electrolyte levels prior to surgery

EDETATE (EDTA) DISODIUM

Trade Names:	**Disotate, Endrate**
Indications:	Hypercalcemia, cardiac glycoside (digitalis) toxicity
Pharmacokinetics:	Excreted rapidly in urine
Pharmacodynamics:	Binds divalent and trivalent ions, forms stable water-soluble complexes
CNS:	Seizures, anxiety, confusion, numbness, circumoral paresthesia
CVS:	Arrhythmias, ↑ QT interval, postural hypotension, thrombophlebitis
GI:	Abdominal pain and cramps, diarrhea
GU:	Nephrotoxicity, dysuria, proteinuria
Pulmonary:	Dyspnea, laryngeal stridor
Other:	Hypoglycemia, hypokalemia, hypomagnesemia, exfoliative dermatitis, muscle spasms, tetany, muscle weakness
Dosage:	50 mg/kg/d IV over 24 h; 40 mg/kg IV over 24 h (children)
Contraindications:	Hypocalcemia, severe renal impairment, TB, seizure disorders
Drug Interactions:	Chelation of zinc in insulin; Ca^{2+} antagonizes inotropic and chronotropic effects of digitalis
Key Points:	Use with general anesthetics and muscle relaxants ↑ cardiac and neuromuscular depressant effects

EZETIMIBE

Trade Name:	**Zetia**
Indications:	Hypercholesterolemia
Pharmacokinetics:	Onset: 1–2 h; bioavailability: 35%–60%; peak: 4–12 h; duration: 24 h; $T_{1/2}$ β: 22 h; excreted 1° in feces
Pharmacodynamics:	Inhibits intestinal absorption of cholesterol and phytosterols
CNS:	Dizziness, headache
CV:	Chest pain
GI:	Abdominal pain, diarrhea
Pulmonary:	Coughing, pharyngitis, sinusitis
Other:	Fatigue, arthralgia, back pain
Dosage:	10 mg/d PO
Contraindications:	Hepatic dysfunction (due to HMG-CoA inhibitor); pregnancy
Drug Interactions:	Cholestyramine ↓ effect; fenofibrate and gemfibrozil ↑ effect
Key Points:	No known perioperative concerns

FAT EMULSIONS

Trade Names:	**Intralipid, Liposyn**
Indications:	Fatty acid deficiency (with anemia, dermatitis, hepatic dysfunction, impaired wound healing, hair loss, thrombocytopenia)
Pharmacokinetics:	Onset: <10 min; peak: <30 min; contains phosphatides (cholines) and glycerin; hepatic metabolism (analogous to chylomicrons)
Pharmacodynamics:	Neutral triglycerides are hydrolyzed to essential free fatty acids (linoleic, linolenic, arachidonic acid) and glycerol by lipoprotein lipase
CNS:	Dizziness, fever, flushing, focal seizures
GI:	Diarrhea, hepatomegaly, ↑ LFTs, pancreatitis
Other:	Sepsis, thrombophlebitis, hypercoagulability, ↓ renal function
Dosage:	0.5–1 mL/min infusion (max. 500 mL over 4–6 h); 0.1 mL/min, max. 100 mL over 4–6 h (children)
Contraindications:	Allergic to soybean, egg, or safflower oil; primary hyperlipidemias with nephrosis and/or pancreatitis
Drug Interactions:	Heparin facilitates clearance, minimizing risks of a hypercoagulable state

FAT EMULSIONS *continued*

Key Points: Check electrolyte and coagulation status prior to
                                surgical procedures

FENOFIBRATE

Trade Name: **TriCor**

Indications: Hyperlipidemia (↑ triglyceride, cholesterol, LDL levels)

Pharmacokinetics: Onset: 1–2 h; peak level: 6–8 h; $T_{1/2}$ β: 20 h; highly
                        protein bound; rapidly hydrolyzed to active metabolite,
                        excreted in urine and feces

Pharmacodynamics: Inhibits triglyceride synthesis, ↓ VLDL and LDL levels
  CNS: Dizziness, asthenia, fatigue, paresthesia, blurred vision
  CV: Arrhythmias
  GI: ↑ Appetite, nausea, vomiting, flatulence, pancreatitis,
                        ↑ LFTs
  GU: Polyuria vaginitis, ↓ libido
  Other: Anemia, cough, rash, pruritus, urticaria

Dosage: 50–200 mg/d PO

Contraindications: Gallbladder disease, primary biliary cirrhosis, renal
                        insufficiency

Drug Interactions: Bile acid resins ↓ absorption; cyclosporin ↓
                        elimination; ↑ effects of anticoagulants

Key Points: Esterase inhibitors ↓ biotransformation to active
                        compound

GEMFIBROZIL

Trade Name   **Lopid**

Indications: Primary hyperlipidemia, pancreatitis (with
                        hypertriglyceridemia)

Pharmacokinetics: Onset: 2–5 d; peak: 4 wk; protein binding: 95%;
                        duration: 12 h; $T_{1/2}$ β: 1.5 h; metabolized by liver,
                        excreted in urine

Pharmacodynamics: Inhibits lipolysis and ↓ hepatic triglycerides synthesis
                        (↓ VLDL, ↑ HDL levels)
  CNS: Headache, dizziness, somnolence
  CV: Atrial fibrillation
  GI: Abdominal pain, nausea, vomiting, diarrhea, ↑ LFTs,
                        cholelithiasis
  GU: Renal toxicity (i.e., dysuria, hematuria, proteinuria,
                        oliguria)

GEMFIBROZIL *continued*

Musculoskeletal:	Myalgia, myositis, myopathy, flulike syndrome, rhabdomyolysis
Other:	Impotence, ↓ libido, anemia, leukopenia, eosinophilia, rash, pruritus
Dosage:	600 mg PO bid
Contraindications:	Hepatorenal impairment, 1° biliary cirrhosis, gallbladder disease
Drug Interactions:	↑ Effects of coumarin, ↑ risk of rhabdomyolysis with lovastatin, pravastatin, simvastatin
Key Points:	Check electrolyte panel and LFTs prior to surgery

GOLD THIOMALATE

Trade Name:	**Aurolate**
Indications:	Rheumatoid arthritis, psoriatic arthritis, pemphigus
Pharmacokinetics:	Onset: <1 h; peak: 3–6 h; protein binding: 87%; duration: 3–6 mo; $T_{1/2}$ β: 14–40 d; excreted in urine
Pharmacodynamics:	↓ Joint inflammation by ↓ immunoglobulins
CNS:	Confusion, encephalitis, hallucinations, seizures, corneal ulcer
CVS:	Angioedema, ↓ BP, ↓ HR
GI:	Glossitis, gingivitis, stomatitis, nausea, diarrhea, cramps
GU:	Nephrotic syndrome, glomerulitis, hematuria, acute renal failure
Hepatic:	Toxic hepatitis with jaundice, cholestasis, ↑ LFTs
Pulmonary:	Interstitial pneumonitis, "gold" bronchitis
Other:	↓ Phagocytic mechanisms, ↓ collagen biosynthesis, dermatitis, urticaria, vesicular lesions, photosensitivity
Dosage:	10–50 mg/wk (max. 50 mg/dose); 1 mg/kg/wk (children)
Contraindications:	Hepatitis, exfoliative dermatitis, toxicity from previous heavy metals exposure, breast-feeding, colitis, blood dyscrasias, vascular disease, SLE, Sjögren's syndrome
Drug Interactions:	Cross-sensitivity to other gold-containing substances; ↑ toxicity of aminoglycosides; ↑ hepatorenal impairment; penicillamine ↑ dimercaprol (BAL) chelates gold; sun exposure ↑ risk of photosensitivity
Key Points:	Check LFT and electrolyte panels prior to elective surgery due to prolonged effect of therapy

IARONIDASE

Trade Name:	**Aldurazyme**
Indications:	Mucopolysaccharide storage (MPS) disorders
Pharmacokinetics:	Onset: rapid; Vd: 0.4 L/kg; Cl: 2.2 mL/kg/min; $T_{1/2}$ β: 2.5 h
Pharmacodynamics:	Synthetic enzyme that ↑ catabolism of glycosaminoglycans (GAG) in lysosomes
Pulmonary:	URI, airway obstruction
Other:	Rash, anaphylactic (and local) reactions
Dosage:	0.58 mg/kg IV over 3–4 h q wk
Contraindications:	NK
Drug Interactions:	Antipyretic/antihistaminic pretreatment ↓ side effects
Key Points:	No known interactions with anesthetic drugs

IBANDRONATE

Trade Name:	**Boniva**
Indications:	Treatment and prevention of osteoporosis
Pharmacokinetics:	Onset: 30 min; bioavailability: <10%; peak: 1–2 h; protein binding: 95%; Vd: 1.5 L/kg; Cl: 80–160 mL/min; $T_{1/2}$ β: 10–60 h; excreted unchanged in urine and feces
Pharmacodynamics:	Inhibits osteoclast-mediated bone resorption
GI:	Dysphagia, esophagitis, diarrhea, dyspepsia, ulcers
Other:	Back pain, myalgias, bronchitis
Dosage:	2.5 mg/d PO
Contraindications:	Hypocalcemia, renal insufficiency, inability to stand
Drug Interactions:	Food ↓ absorption; ASA and NSAIDs ↑ GI irritation
Key Points:	Check Ca^{2+} levels and consider premedication with H_2-blocker or PPI

LEVOSIMENDAN

Trade Name:	**Simdax (investigational)**
Indications:	Chronic CHF, acute decompensation
Pharmacokinetics:	$T_{1/2}$ β: 80 h (active metabolite)
Pharmacodynamics:	Inodilator, ↑ affinity of cardiac troponin C for Ca^{2+} ([+] inotropic effect), activation of ATP-dependent K^+ channel on vascular smooth muscle (cardioprotective effect)

LEVOSIMENDAN *continued*

CNS:	Headache
CV:	↑ HR, ↓ BP (2° ↓ PVR), ↑ CI, ↓ PCWP, ↑ CBF
Pulmonary:	Vasodilator

Dosage: 3–12 µg/kg, followed by 0.05–0.2 µg/kg/min

Contraindications: Severe hepatorenal impairment, ↑ QT interval (torsades de pointes), breast-feeding

Drug Interactions: NK

Key Points: Need to assess and correct hypovolemia; 6–24 h infusion produces (+) inotropic effect for 7–10 d

LOVASTATIN, ATORVASTATIN, PRAVASTATIN, SIMVASTATIN, FLUVASTATIN

Trade Names: **Altocor, Mevacor (lovastatin); Pravachol (pravastatin); Zocor (simvastatin); Lipitor (atorvastatin); Lescol (fluvastatin)**

Indications: Hyperlipidemia, prevention of coronary artery disease (CAD)

Pharmacokinetics: Onset: <1 h; peak: 1–3 h; protein binding: 97%; duration: 12–24 h; $T_{1/2}$ β: 14 h; extensive 1st-pass hepatic extraction; excreted in feces; crosses placental and blood-brain barriers

Pharmacodynamics: Metabolized to β-hydroxy acid, which inhibits HMG-CoA reductase

CNS:	Fatigue, insomnia, blurred vision, dizziness, peripheral neuropathy
CV:	Chest pain (angina)
GI:	Dyspepsia, cramping, nausea, ↑ LFTs
Musculoskeletal:	Myalgia, myositis, rhabdomyolysis
Other:	Impotence, rash, pruritus, alopecia, photosensitivity

Dosage: 10–40 mg PO hs (max. 80 mg/d)

Contraindications: Pregnancy, breast-feeding, hepatic impairment

Drug Interactions: ↑ Rhabdomyolysis with immunosuppressants, gemfibrozil, niacin, erythromycin, amiodarone, verapamil; pectin, cholestyramine, colestipol ↓ absorption; isradipine ↑ clearance; itraonazol ↑ HMG-CoA reductase; ↑ effect of warfarin; alcohol and grapefruit ↑ side effects; sun exposure ↑ photosensitivity

Key Points: Due to risk of MH, avoid halogenated anesthetics, succinylcholine, other "triggering" agents

MESNA

Trade Name:	**Mesnex**
Indications:	Prophylaxis for ifosfamide-induced hemorrhagic cystitis, cyclophosphamide toxicity in bone marrow recipients
Pharmacokinetics:	Vd: 0.65 L/kg; plasma $T_{1/2}$ β: 0.5 h (metabolite 1.5 h); hepatic metabolism to active metabolite, excreted in urine
Pharmacodynamics:	Detoxifies antineoplastic drugs in GU tract
CNS:	Headache, fatigue, dizziness
CV:	↓ BP, ↑ HR, flushing
GI:	Nausea, vomiting, diarrhea
Pulmonary:	Dyspnea, cough
Other:	Diaphoresis, alopecia, bone marrow suppression
Dosage:	240–480 mg/m^2 at 2 h and 6 h
Contraindications:	Sensitivity to thiol-containing compounds
Drug Interactions:	Not compatible with cisplastin
Key Points:	No adverse interactions with anesthetic drugs reported

METFORMIN

Trade Name:	**Glucophage**
Indications:	Diabetes mellitus
Pharmacokinetics:	Onset: 1 h; peak: 6 h; duration: 12 h; not metabolized, excreted in urine
Pharmacodynamics:	↓ Hepatic glucose production and GI absorption, ↑ peripheral glucose uptake and utilization
CNS:	Headache
GI:	Metallic taste, diarrhea, nausea, vomiting, bloating, flatulence
Other:	Rash, dermatitis, megaloblastic anemia, lactic acidosis
Dosage:	500–1000 mg PO bid (max. 2.5 g/d)
Contraindications:	Severe heart failure, renal disease, metabolic acidosis
Drug Interactions:	Ca-blocker, corticosteroids, estrogens, OCPs, isoniazid, nicotinic acid, phenothiazines, phenytoin, sympathomimetics, diuretics, thyroid drugs, amiloride, cimetidine, digoxin, morphine, procainamide, quinidine, quinine, zanitidine, triamterene, trimethoprim, vancomycin ↑ glucose levels; iodinated contrast dye ↓ renal function; alcohol ↓ glucose levels

METFORMIN *continued*

Key Points:
Ringer's lactate should be avoided because of ↓ lactate metabolism; use of β-blocker may suppress hypoglycemic symptoms; carefully monitor glucose levels during perioperative period

METHIMAZOLE

Trade Name:	**Tapazole**
Indications:	Hyperthyroidism, thyrotoxic crisis
Pharmacokinetics:	Onset: <30 min; bioavailability: 93%; peak: 0.5–1 h; duration: 24 h; $T_{1/2}$ β: 4–5 h; crosses placenta and distributed into breast milk; metabolized in liver, excreted in urine
Pharmacodynamics:	Synthesis of thyroid hormone (interferes with incorporation of iodide into tyrosyl); ↓ iodothyronine
CNS:	Headache, drowsiness, vertigo, encephalopathy
CVS:	Periarteritis (SLE-like syndrome)
GI:	Nausea, vomiting, loss of taste, ↑ salivary glands
Hepatic:	Jaundice, fulminant hepatitis, ↑ LFTs
Musculoskeletal:	Peripheral neuritis (paresthesias), arthralgias, myalgia
Other:	Rash, urticaria, pruritus, alopecia, ↑ pigmentation, pancytopenia, fetal hypothyroidism (during pregnancy), nephritis, lupus-like syndrome
Dosage:	5–20 mg PO tid; 0.1 mg/kg qid (children)
Contraindications:	Acute hyperthyroidism, exogenous thyrotoxicosis; breast-feeding
Drug Interactions:	Potassium iodide, amiodarone, iodine, lithium ↑ effect; ↑ effect of warfarin; ↑ agranulocytosis with bone marrow suppressants; ↑ digoxin level
Key Points:	Check thyroid function tests and LFTs before surgery

METYRAPONE

Trade Name:	**Metopirone**
Indications:	Cushing syndrome, assess adrenal gland function
Pharmacokinetics:	Onset: <1 h; duration: <4 h; $T_{1/2}$ β: 25 min; hepatic metabolism to active compound (metyrapol), excreted in urine
Pharmacodynamics:	Inhibits cortisol synthesis
CNS:	Nervousness, confusion, somnolence
CV:	↑ BP, ↑ HR, arrhythmias, cardiovascular collapse
GI:	Nausea, vomiting, diarrhea, cramps

METYRAPONE *continued*

Other:	Adrenal insufficiency (addisonian crisis), muscle weakness, hirsutism, bone marrow suppression, hypokalemic alkalosis, pedal edema, weight gain, alopecia, diaphoresis, acne
Dosage:	250–750 mg PO q 4–8 h; 15 mg/kg q 4 h (children)
Contraindications:	Addisonian crisis, hypopituitarism, preeclampsia, pheochromocytoma
Drug Interactions:	↓ Efficacy of phenytoin, estrogens, progestins, corticosteroids, phenothiazines, chlordiazepoxide, chlorpromazine, amitriptyline, phenobarbital, methysergide
Key Points:	Check electrolyte panel and hydration status prior to surgery

METYROSINE (α-METHYLTYROSINE)

Trade Name:	**Demser**
Indications:	Pheochromocytoma
Pharmacokinetics:	Onset: <2 h; peak: 2–3 d; $T_{1/2}$ β: 3–8 h; excretion in urine
Pharmacodynamics:	Inhibits tyrosine hydroxylase, ↓ catecholamine synthesis
CNS:	Drowsiness, extrapyramidal movements
CV:	↓ BP
GI:	Dry mouth, nausea, vomiting, diarrhea
Other:	Impotence, interstitial pulmonary fibrosis, crystalluria
Dosage:	1 g PO qid for 5–7 d prior to surgery
Contraindications:	Hypotension, CHF
Drug Interactions:	↑ CV effect of phenothiazines and vasodilators
Key Points:	↑ arrhythmias during volatile anesthetics; maintain adequate hydration to avoid ↓ BP during surgery

MIGLITOL

Trade Name:	**Glyset**
Indications:	Diabetes mellitus
Pharmacokinetics:	Onset: 1 h; bioavailability: 60%; peak: 2–3 h; protein binding: 4%; duration: 10 h; $T_{1/2}$ β: 2 h; no metabolism, excreted in urine

MIGLITOL *continued*

Pharmacodynamics:	Reversible inhibition of α-glucosidase in small intestine, delayed glucose absorption, $\downarrow$ postprandial glucose levels
GI:	Diarrhea, abdominal pain, flatulence
Other:	Rash, $\downarrow$ iron level
Dosage:	25–50 mg PO tid (max. 100 mg bid)
Contraindications:	Diabetic ketoacidosis, renal impairment, colitis, intestinal obstruction
Drug Interactions:	$\downarrow$ Effect of digoxin, propranolol, ranitidine, charcoal, amylase
Key Points:	No known adverse interactions with anesthetic drugs

MIGLUSTAT

Trade Name:	**Zavesca**
Indications:	Gaucher's disease (type 1)
Pharmacokinetics:	Onset: <1 h; bioavailability: 97%; peak: 2 h; Vd: 80–100 L; $T_{1/2}$ β: 6–7 h; renal excretion unchanged
Pharmacodynamics:	Synthetic analog of D-glucose that inhibits glucosylceramide synthase, $\downarrow$ glucosylceramide
CNS:	Headache, paresthesias, back pain, tremor, incoordination
GI:	Black (tarry) stools, diarrhea, flatulence, cramps, nausea
Other:	Gingival bleeding, hematuria, pruritus, anorexia
Dosage:	100 mg PO tid ($\times$12 mo)
Contraindications:	Pregnancy, breast-feeding
Drug Interactions:	NK
Key Points:	Assess hydration and neurologic status prior to induction of general or regional anesthesia

ORLISTAT

Trade Name:	**Xenical**
Indications:	Obesity
Pharmacokinetics:	Onset: <1 h (minimal GI absorption); peak: 8 h; protein binding: 99%; metabolized within GI wall, excreted in feces
Pharmacodynamics:	Reversible inhibitor of gastric and pancreatic lipases; $\downarrow$ hydrolysis of dietary fat
CNS:	Headache, dizziness, fatigue, anxiety, otitis media

ORLISTAT *continued*

GI:	Fatty (oily stool), ↑ defecation, diarrhea, rectal pain
GU:	Menstrual irregularity, UTI
Other:	Rash, myalgia, URI, pedal edema
Dosage:	120 mg PO tid
Contraindications:	Cholestasis, chronic malabsorption syndrome
Drug Interactions:	↓ Absorption of fat-soluble vitamins; ↑ pravastatin level
Key Points:	Patients may need multivitamin supplements that contain fat-soluble vitamins; check glucose level prior to elective surgery

PAMIDRONATE

Trade Name:	**Aredia**
Indications:	Hypercalcemia, Paget's disease, osteolytic bone lesions
Pharmacokinetics:	Onset: <1 h; peak: <72 h; duration: 6 mo; not metabolized, excreted in urine
Pharmacodynamics:	Inhibits bone reabsorption
CNS:	Seizures, headache, fatigue, generalized pain
CV:	↑ BP, arrhythmias
GI:	Anorexia, nausea, vomiting, constipation
Other:	Bone marrow suppression, renal impairment, electrolyte disturbances
Dosage:	60–90 mg IV over 2–24 h, or 30 mg/d over 4 h × 3 d
Contraindications:	Sensitivity to bisphosphonates (etidronate), renal impairment
Drug Interactions:	Precipitates with Ca^{2+}-containing solutions
Key Points:	Check electrolyte panel and renal function prior to surgery

PENICILLAMINE

Trade Names:	**Cuprimine, Depen**
Indications:	Wilson's disease, heavy metal toxicity, rheumatoid arthritis, Felty's syndrome, cystinuria, 1° biliary cirrhosis
Pharmacokinetics:	Onset: <30 min; peak: 1 h; duration: 24 h; metabolized in liver to inactive compounds, excreted in urine and feces
Pharmacodynamics:	↓ IgM rheumatoid factor and immune complexes, ↓ T-cell function, forms water-soluble complexes with metal ions and cysteine

PENICILLAMINE *continued*

CNS:	Optic neuritis, peripheral neuropathy, diplopia, tinnitus
GI:	Oral ulcers, stomatitis, nausea, vomiting, diarrhea, cheilosis, glossitis, metallic taste, peptic ulcer, pancreatitis
Hepatic:	Intrahepatic cholestasis, toxic hepatitis, jaundice ↑ LFTs
Musculoskeletal:	Muscle weakness (myasthenia gravis–like syndrome), arthralgias
Pulmonary:	Obliterative bronchiolitis, Goodpasture's syndrome, pneumonitis
Other:	Skin friability, delayed wound healing, bone marrow suppression, TTP, drug fever, thyroiditis, hematuria, proteinuria

Dosage: 125–250 mg PO q 6 h; 30 mg/kg/d (children)

Contraindications: Bone marrow suppression, rheumatoid arthritis (with renal insufficiency), pregnancy, breast-feeding, hepatic insufficiency

Drug Interactions: ↑ Toxicity with gold salts, antimalarials, cytotoxic drugs, oxyphenbutazone, phenylbutazone; ↑ digoxin level; iron salts and antacids ↓ absorption

Key Points: Preoperative chest radiograph (to detect alveolitis); regional blocks should be performed only after neurologic assessment due to drug-induced neuropathy

PIOGITAZONE, ROSIGLITAZONE (± METFORMIN)

Trade Names: **Actos (piogitazone), Avandia (rosiglitazone), Avandamet (rosiglitazone + metformin)**

Indications: Diabetes mellitus (in combination with sulfonylureas or metformin)

Pharmacokinetics: Onset: <30 min; peak: 1–2 h; protein binding: 98%; $T_{1/2}$ β: 3–7 h; extensively metabolized in liver, excreted in urine and feces

Pharmacodynamics: Peroxisome proliferator–activated receptor-gamma (PPARγ) agonists at insulin-sensitive receptors in adipose tissue, skeletal muscle, liver; ↓ insulin resistance, ↓ glucose from liver

CNS:	Headache, fatigue
CV:	CHF, pedal edema
GI:	Nausea, vomiting, diarrhea, ↑ LFTs, lactic acidosis (metformin)
Pulmonary:	URI, sinusitis, dyspnea
Other:	Myalgia, anemia, hypoglycemia, weight gain

PIOGITAZONE, ROSIGLITAZONE
(± METFORMIN) *continued*

Dosages: *Piogitazone:* 15–30 mg/d PO (max. 45 mg/d)
Rosiglitazone: 4 mg/d PO (max. 8 mg/d)
Rosiglitazone 1–4 mg/d + metformin 0.5–1 g/d
(max. 2.5 g/d)

Contraindications: Type 1 diabetes; diabetic ketoacidosis; severe
cardiac, renal, or liver disease; alcohol abuse;
advanced age

Drug Interactions: Metformin ↑ renal impairment; ↓ effect of OCPs;
furosamide, CCBs, thiazides, phenytoin, phenothiazines
↓ effect

Key Points: Unless postoperative dietary intake is restricted,
continue use throughout perioperative period

POTASSIUM IODIDE

Trade Names: **KI, Pima, SSKI, Thyro-Block**

Indications: Thyrotoxic crisis, iodine replenishment, nuclear
radiation protection, expectorant, preoperative
thyroidectomy, cutaneous sporotrichosis

Pharmacokinetics: Onset: <24 h; peak: 10–15 d; rapid GI absorption,
excreted in urine

Pharmacodynamics: ↓ Synthesis and release of thyroid hormone, ↓ mucus
viscosity
    CNS: Metallic taste, severe headache, periorbital edema
    GI: Diarrhea, dyspepsia, burning in mouth, ↑ salivary
secretions
    Pulmonary: Laryngeal inflammation, productive cough, pulmonary
edema
    Other: Angioedema, mucosal hemorrhage, fever, arthralgias,
adenopathy, eosinophilia, SLE, fatal TTP, arteritis,
hypocomplementemic vasculitis, autoimmune thyroid
disease, paradoxical thyrotoxicosis (low doses), goiter,
hypothyroidism (with prolonged therapy)

Dosage: Saturated solution (SSKI); 1 g/mL Lugol's solution:
50–500 mg/d

Contraindications: Acute bronchitis, tuberculosis, hyperkalemia, sulfite
allergy

Drug Interactions: Lithium ↑ effect; K⁺ supplements (and K⁺-sparing
diuretics) cause hyperkalemia

Key Points: Sudden withdrawal may precipitate thyroid toxicosis;
careful monitoring of electrolytes required during
perioperative period

PRAVASTATIN

Trade Name:	**Pravigard (with aspirin)**
Indications:	Hypercholesterolemia (Fredrickson Types IIa and IIb)
Pharmacokinetics:	Onset: 0.5 h; bioavailability: 34%; peak: 1–2 h; $T_{1/2}$ β: 77 h; extensive 1st-pass metabolism, 1° excreted in feces
Pharmacodynamics:	HMG-CoA reductase inhibitor, ↓ cholesterol biosynthesis
GU:	Myoglobinuria (brown urine)
Other:	Rash, myalgias (↑ CPK), flulike syndrome
Dosage:	20–40 mg/d PO (max. 80 mg/d)
Contraindications:	Active hepatic disorders (↑ LFTs), pregnancy, breast-feeding, alcohol abuse
Drug Interactions:	Food ↓ absorption; fibric acid derivatives (clofibrate, gemfibrozil) ↑ risk of myopathy; immunosuppressive drugs ↓ dosage
Key Points:	Check LFTs and renal function preoperatively

PROBENECID

Trade Name:	**Benemid**
Indications:	Gouty arthritis, hyperuricemia, adjunct to antibiotics
Pharmacokinetics:	Onset: <1 h; bioavailability: 90%; peak: 2.5 h; protein binding: 75%; $T_{1/2}$ β: 3–12 h; metabolized in liver, excreted in urine
Pharmacodynamics:	Competitively inhibits reabsorption of uric acid and organic acids
CNS:	Dizziness, headache
GI:	Nausea, vomiting, anorexia, gingivitis, ↑ LFTs
GU:	Urate nephropathy, renal colic, nephrotic syndrome
Other:	Blood dyscrasias, hemolytic anemia (with G-6-PD deficiency), fever, urticaria, pruritus
Dosage:	250 mg PO bid for 1 wk, then 500 mg bid or 1 g (with antibiotic)
Contraindications:	Blood dyscrasias, uric acid stones, acute gouty attack, PUD
Drug Interactions:	↑ Toxicity of heparin, dapsone, lorazepam, oxazepam, temazepam, NSAIDs, methotrexate, chlorpropamide, sulfonamides, furosemide, penicillins, cephalosporins, ciprofloxacin, acetaminophen, rifampin, nitrofurantoin, sulfinpyrazone; ↑ effect with allopurinol; ↓ urate nephropathy with antineoplastics; ↓ natriuretic effects of bumetanide, ethacrynic acid, furosemide; alcohol ↓ level

PROBENECID *continued*

Key Points: Delays elimination of drugs via renal tubular secretion; maintain adequate hydration and alkalization of urine

PROBUCOL

Trade Name: **Lorelco**

Indications: Hyperlipidemia

Pharmacokinetics: Onset: 2–4 wk; peak: 4 min; duration: 12 h; $T_{1/2}$ β: >6 wk (slow biliary elimination), accumulates in fat

Pharmacodynamics: Antilipemic activity
CNS: Paresthesias, dizziness
CV: ↑ QT interval
GI: Diarrhea, flatulence, abdominal pain, nausea
Other: Angioneurotic edema, eosinophilia

Dosage: 500 mg PO bid

Contraindications: Acute MI, ventricular arrhythmias, pregnancy, breast-feeding

Drug Interactions: Interaction with antiarrhythmics that ↑ QT interval (e.g., amiodarone, beryllium, disopyramide, encainide)

Key Points: Use with volatile anesthetics and sympathomimetics ↑ arrhythmias; neurological exam should precede regional block techniques

PROPYLTHIOURACIL (PTU)

Trade Name: **Propyl-Thyracil**

Indications: Hyperthyroidism

Pharmacokinetics: Onset: <1 h; peak: 1–2 h; bioavailability: 75%; duration: 8–12 h; Vd: 0.4 L/kg; $T_{1/2}$ β: 1–2 h; readily crosses placenta, distributed into breast milk; metabolized by liver, excreted in urine

Pharmacodynamics: ↓ Synthesis of thyroid hormone, ↓ incorporation of I^- into thyroglobulin
CNS: Headaches, drowsiness, vertigo, peripheral neuropathy (paresthesias)
CV: Periarteritis (SLE-like syndrome)
GI: Nausea, vomiting, loss of taste, jaundice, ↑ LFTs
Pulmonary: Interstitial pneumonitis
Other: Rash, urticaria, pruritus, alopecia, hyperpigmentation, bone marrow suppression, arthralgias, myalgias, nephritis

PROPYLTHIOURACIL (PTU) *continued*

Dosage:	300–450 mg/d in divided doses; 5–7 mg/kg/d (children)
Contraindications:	Acute hyperthyroidism, thyrotoxicosis, pregnancy, breast-feeding
Drug Interactions:	Potassium iodide, amiodarone, iodine, lithium ↑ effects, ↑ PT with anticoagulants; ↑ agranulocytosis with bone marrow suppressants
Key Points:	Assess peripheral nerve function prior to regional nerve block

RALOXIFENE

Trade Name:	**Evista**
Indications:	Osteoporosis
Pharmacokinetics:	Onset: <1 h; highly protein bound; duration: 24 h; Vd: 2.3 L/kg; extensive 1st-pass metabolism, excreted in feces
Pharmacodynamics:	↓ Bone resorption and ↑ bone mineral density
CNS:	Depression, insomnia, headache
CV:	Hot flashes, chest pain, peripheral edema
GI:	Nausea, vomiting, gastroenteritis, diarrhea
GU:	UTI, vaginitis, leukorrhea
Other:	Weight gain, cough, rash, sweating, fever
Dosage:	60 mg/d PO
Contraindications:	Pregnancy, vein thrombosis
Drug Interactions:	Cholestyramine ↓ absorption; clifibrate, diazepam, diazoxide, indomethacin, naproxen ↑ level; ↓ warfarin effect
Key Points:	↑ Clinical effects of highly protein-bound IV anesthetics

ROSUVASTATIN

Trade Name:	**Crestor**
Indications:	Hypercholesterolemia, mixed dyslipidemia (Fredrickson types II and IV)
Pharmacokinetics:	Onset: 1 h; bioavailability: 20%; peak: 3.5 h; protein binding: 88%; Vd: 2 L/kg; $T_{1/2}$ β: 19 h; minimal metabolism; 1° excreted in feces
Pharmacodynamics:	Inhibits HMG-CoA reductase, ↓ cholesterol biosynthesis
Other:	Myalgia, pharyngitis, myopathy/rhabdomyolysis, UTI

ROSUVASTATIN *continued*

Dosage:	10-40 mg/d PO
Contraindications:	Active hepatic disease, pregnancy, alcoholism
Drug Interactions:	Antacid ↓ absorption; gemfibrozil, cyclosporine, OCP ↑ levels
Key Points:	Check LFTs and glucose level before surgery

SIBUTRAMINE

Trade Name:	**Meridia**
Indications:	Obesity
Pharmacokinetics:	Onset: <1 h; bioavailability: 80%; peak: 34 h; protein binding: 90%; extensive 1st-pass hepatic cytochrome P_{450} metabolism, excreted in urine
Pharmacodynamics:	Inhibits reuptake of norepinephrine, serotonin, dopamine
CNS:	Asthenia, headache, anxiety, paresthesia, somnolence, ear pain
CV:	↑ HR, vasodilation, ↑ BP, chest pain, generalized edema
GI:	Anorexia, bad taste, nausea, vomiting, constipation
GU:	Dysmenorrhea, UTI, vaginal candidiasis
Other:	Myalgia, tenosynovitis, cough, rash, sweating
Dosage:	5–10 mg/d (max. 15 mg/d)
Contraindications:	Use of MAOIs, centrally active appetite suppressants, anorexia nervosa, CAD, seizures, hepatorenal syndrome
Drug Interactions:	Inhibitors (e.g., erythromycin, ketoconazole) ↓ metabolism; ephedrine and psuedoephedrine ↑ BP; dextromethorphan, fentanyl, SSRIs, lithium, MAOIs, meperidine, paroxeline, pentazocine, sumatriptan ↑ side effects
Key Points:	↓ CNS depression associated with general anesthetics; sympathomimetics can trigger hypertensive crisis

SODIUM POLYSTYRENE SULFONATE (SPS)

Trade Name:	**Kayexalate**
Indications:	Hyperkalemia
Pharmacokinetics:	Onset: 2–12 h; not absorbed, excreted unchanged in feces

SODIUM POLYSTYRENE
SULFONATE (SPS) *continued*

Pharmacodynamics:	Cation-exchange resin that releases Na^+ in exchange for other cations in GI tract
CNS:	Confusion, irritability
CV:	Arrhythmia, CHF
GI:	Fecal impaction, abdominal cramping, nausea, vomiting, diarrhea
Pulmonary:	Pulmonary edema
Other:	Muscle weakness hypokalemia, hypocalcemia
Dosage:	15 g/d in 10–20 mL 70% sorbitol syrup (to prevent constipation); 25–100 g prn; 1–4 g/kg/d (children)
Contraindications:	Hypokalemia/calcemia, CHF, uncontrolled hypertension
Drug Interactions:	Laxatives ↑ systemic alkalosis; K^+-sparing diuretics and K^+ supplementation ↓ effect; ↑ toxicity of digitalis (due to ↑ K^+ level)
Key Points:	Preoperative assessment of electrolytes and fluid balance

SR141716

Trade Name:	**Rimonabant (investigational)**
Indications:	Morbid obesity, smoking cessation
Pharmacokinetics:	NK
Pharmacodynamics:	Centrally active cannabinoid (CB1) receptor antagonist
Other:	Weight loss
Dosage:	NA
Key Points:	Potentially could ↑ anesthetic requirement

SULFINPYRAZONE

Trade Name:	**Anturane**
Indications:	Gouty arthritis, hyperuricemia
Pharmacokinetics:	Onset: <1 h; peak: 1–2 h; protein binding: 99%; duration: 4–6 h; $T_{1/2}$ β: 1–5 h; active metabolites with uricosuric and antiplatelet activity
Pharmacodynamics:	Competitively inhibits renal tubule reabsorption of uric acid, adenosine diphosphate, 5-HT, ↓ platelet adhesiveness
CNS:	Convulsions, coma, dizziness
GI:	Peptic ulcers, nausea, vomiting, diarrhea, jaundice, ↑ LFTs
GU:	Urate nephropathy, renal colic

SULFINPYRAZONE *continued*

Other:	Bone marrow suppression, hypoglycemia, bleeding tendency, rash, ASA-induced bronchoconstriction
Dosage:	100–200 mg PO bid, then 200–400 mg bid
Contraindications:	Blood dyscrasias, peptic ulcer disease, colitis
Drug Interactions:	↑ Effects of sulfonamides, sulfonylureas, penicillin, β-lactam antibiotics, nitrofurantoin, insulin; ↑ effects of coumarin, heparin, thrombolytics, NSAIDs, verapamil, phenytoin; ↑ urate nephropathy with antineoplastic agents; ↑ antihyperuricemic effects with allopurinol; cholestyramine ↓ absorption; alcohol ↓ effect; probenecid ↓ renal excretion
Key Points:	↑ Anticoagulant drug effects; ↑ bleeding tendency due to antiplatelet effect

SULFONYLUREAS (CHLORPROPAMIDE, GLIPIZIDE, [+ METFORMIN], GLIMEPIRIDE, GLYBURIDE [± METFORMIN], TOLAZAMIDE, TOLBUTAMIDE)

Trade Names:	**Diabinese (chlorpropamide); Glucotrol (glipizide); Metaglip (glipizide + metformin); Glynase, Micronase (glyburide); Glucovance (glyburide + metformin); Orinase (tolbutamide); Tolinase (tolazamide), Amaryl (glimepiride)**
Indications:	Diabetes mellitus, non–insulin dependent (type 2) diabetes
Pharmacokinetics:	*Chlorpropamide:* Onset: 1 h; peak: 2–4 h; duration: 24 h *Glipizide:* Onset: <0.5 h; peak: 1–6 h; duration: 4–24 h *Glipizide + metformin:* Onset: 1 h; peak: 2–3 h; duration: 24 h *Glyburide:* Onset: 1–4 h; peak: 4 h; duration: 24 h *Glyburide + metformin:* Onset: 1 h; peak 2–4 h; duration: 24 h *Glimepiride:* Onset: 1 h; peak: 2–3 h; duration: >24 h *Tolazamide:* Onset: 4–6 h; peak: 3–4 h; duration: 12–24 h *Tolbutamide:* Onset: 0.5–1 h; peak: 3–5 h; duration: 6–12 h
Pharmacodynamics:	Stimulate insulin release from pancreas, ↑ peripheral sensitivity to insulin, ↓ hepatic glucose production; ↑ effect of vasopressin
CNS:	Drowsiness, coma, seizures, malaise, headache
CV:	CHF, edema, ↑ BP

SULFONYLUREAS
(CHLORPROPAMIDE, GLIPIZIDE,
[+ METFORMIN], GLIMEPIRIDE,
GLYBURIDE [± METFORMIN],
TOLAZAMIDE, TOLBUTAMIDE) *continued*

GI:	Nausea, vomiting, diarrhea, dyspepsia, jaundice, ↑ LFTs
Other:	Bone marrow suppression, aplastic anemia, hypoglycemia, angioedema, rash, pruritus, SIADH, muscle weakness, myalgias
Dosages:	*Chlorpropamide:* 250 mg/d PO (max. 750 mg/d) *Glimepiride:* 1–2 mg/d PO (max. 8 mg/d) *Glipizide:* 5 mg/d PO (max. 15 mg/d) *Glipizide + metformin:* 2.5–7.5 mg + 250–750 mg/d PO *Glyburide:* 2.5–5 mg/d PO (max. 20 mg/d) *Glyburide + metformin:* 1.25–2.5 mg + 500 mg/d PO *Tolazamide:* 100–250 mg/d PO (max. 500 mg/bid) *Tolbutamide:* 1–2 mg/d PO (max. 3 g/d)
Contraindications:	Metabolic acidosis; ketoacidosis; diabetic coma; severe infection, burn, or trauma; acute MI; renal failure; pregnancy; breast-feeding; sensitivity to sulfonylureas
Drug Interactions:	Disulfiram-like reaction with alcohol; ↑ effect of anticoagulants; β-blocker, sulfonamides, salicylates, miconazole, furosemide, coumarin, probenecid, MAOIs, chloramphenicol, ginkgo biloba ↑ hypoglycemia; CCB, corticosteroids, estrogens, isoniazid, nicotine, phenytoin, thiazides, thyroid drugs, sympathomimetics, phenothiazines ↓ effect
Key Points:	Check perioperative glucose levels and electrolytes; NSAIDs, β-blockers, coumarins, other highly protein-bound drugs ↑ hypoglycemic action

TROMETHAMINE

Trade Name:	**Tham**
Indications:	Metabolic acidosis, prime for cardiac pump-oxygenator
Pharmacokinetics:	Onset: <10 min; peak: <1 h; no metabolism, excreted in urine
Pharmacodynamics:	↓ Hydrogen ion concentration, ↑ flow of alkaline urine
Metabolic:	Acidosis, hypoglycemia, hyperkalemia
Pulmonary:	Respiratory depression
Other:	Thrombosis, skin necrosis
Dosage:	324 mg/kg IV (max. 500 mg/kg)

TROMETHAMINE *continued*

Contraindications:	Anuria, uremia, chronic respiratory acidosis, pregnancy
Drug Interactions:	CNS depressants, ↑ risk of respiratory depression
Key Points:	Check electrolyte and acid-base status before cardiac surgery requiring CBP

URSODIOL

Trade Name:	**Actigall**
Indications:	Cholesterol gallstones
Pharmacokinetics:	Onset: <30 min; bioavailability: 90%; peak: 1–3 h; protein binding: 70%; duration: 6–8 h; extensive 1st-pass hepatic metabolism to taurine and glycine, excreted in feces
Pharmacodynamics:	Naturally occurring bile acid
Hepatic:	↑ LFTs
Dosage:	8–10 mg/kg/d PO with meals
Contraindications:	Bowel obstruction, pancreatitis, cholecystitis
Drug Interactions:	Sensitivity to bile acids; ↓ efficacy with progestins, estrogens, cholestyramine, colestipol, antacids, clofibrate, neomycin
Key Points:	No interactions with anesthetic drugs reported

ZOLEDRONIC ACID

Trade Name:	**Zometa**
Indications:	Hypercalcemia (due to bone metastases)
Pharmacokinetics:	Onset: <1 h; protein binding: 22%; duration: 7–28 d; $T_{1/2} \beta$: 2–167 h; no metabolism, excreted in urine
Pharmacodynamics:	Inhibits bond resorption by ↓ osteoclast activity and osteoclastic resorption of mineralized bone
CNS:	Headache, insomnia, fatigue, paresthesia
CV:	↑ BP, pedal edema
GI:	Nausea, vomiting, dysphagia
GU:	↓ Serum creatinine, UTI
Pulmonary:	Dyspnea, cough
Other:	Bone marrow suppression, dehydration, dermatitis
Dosage:	4 mg IV (+200 mg mannitol) over 15 min q 3–4 wk

ZOLEDRONIC ACID *continued*

Contraindications: Severe renal impairment, hypercalcemia (due to malignancy)

Drug Interactions: Aminoglycosides and loop diuretics ↑ effects; thalidomide ↑ renal dysfunction

Key Points: Check electrolytes and renal function before surgery; avoid prolonged administration of N_2O in presence of bone marrow suppression

32

Minerals

CALCIUM

Trade Names:	**Calphron (calcium acetate), Citrical (calcium citrate)**
Indications:	Hypocalcemia, $\uparrow$ K^+, hypermagnesemia, hyperphosphatemia, osteoporosis prevention, cardiotonic use
Pharmacokinetics:	Duration: 0.5–2 h; no metabolism, excreted in feces
Pharmacodynamics:	Maintains functional integrity of the nervous and musculoskeletal systems, necessary for cell membrane and capillary permeability
CNS:	Tingling sensations, headache, irritability, weakness
CV:	Vasodilation, arrhythmias, syncope
GI:	Constipation, anorexia, rebound hyperacidity, nausea, vomiting
GU:	Polyuria, renal calculi
Other:	Hypercalcemia, local reactions, pruritus
Dosage:	0.25–1 g IV at 100 mg/min; 20 mg/kg/min (children); 0.5–2 g/d PO
Contraindications:	Arrhythmias, hypercalcemia, hypophosphatemia, renal calculi
Drug Interactions:	$\downarrow$ Absorption of atenolol, fluoroquinolones, tetracyclines; $\uparrow$ digitalis toxicity; $\downarrow$ effect of CCB; thiazides $\uparrow$ risk of hypercalcemia; caffeine, dairy products, alcohol $\downarrow$ calcium absorption
Key Points:	Check electrolyte panel (and calcium/phosphate levels) before surgery

CHROMIUM

Trade Name:	**None**
Indications:	Chromium deficiency, glucose intolerance, neuropathic disorders
Pharmacokinetics:	Poorly absorbed (<1%) unless chelated; protein binding to transferrin (15%); no metabolism, excreted in urine
Pharmacodynamics:	$\uparrow$ Action of insulin by $\uparrow$ insulin receptor kinase
Dosage:	50–200 mg/d PO; 0.14–0.2 µg/kg/d; 10–200 µg/d (children)
Contraindications:	NK
Drug Interactions:	$\downarrow$ Insulin requirement
Key Points:	Monitor perioperative blood glucose in diabetic patients

COPPER

Trade Name:	**None**
Indications:	Copper deficiency, anemia, neutropenia, bone demineralization
Pharmacokinetics:	Absorption 50% (stomach, duodenum); highly bound to ceruloplasmin (>90%); hepatic metabolism, excreted in feces
Pharmacodynamics:	Leukocytosis, bone mineralization, catecholamine metabolism, elastin and collagen cross-linking, myelin formation, oxidative phosphorylation
CNS:	Coma
GI:	Diarrhea, dyspepsia, vomiting, ↑ LFTs
Dosage:	1.5–3 mg/d PO; 0.4–1.5 mg/d (children)
Contraindications:	NK
Drug Interactions:	Penicillin ↑ concentrations; zinc supplements ↓ absorption
Key Points:	No known adverse interactions with anesthetic drugs

FLUORIDE

Trade Names:	**Fluoritab, Fluorodex, Flura, Karidium, Luride, Pediaflor**
Indications:	Prevention of dental caries
Pharmacokinetics:	Onset: <30 min; peak: 60 min; no metabolism, excreted in urine
Pharmacodynamics:	Remineralization of decalcified tooth enamel
GI:	Dyspepsia
Other:	Hypocalcemia, osteosclerosis/malacia, atrophic dermatitis, urticaria
Dosage:	0.25–1 mg/d PO (children)
Contraindications:	NK
Drug Interactions:	Aluminum and magnesium ↓ absorption
Key Points:	No known adverse interactions with anesthetic drugs

IODIDE

Trade Name:	**Iodopen**
Indications:	Iodine deficiency (due to diet or intestinal malabsorption)
Pharmacokinetics:	Rapidly absorbed from GI tract, skin, lungs; protein binding: 100%; eliminated in sweat, urine, feces

IODIDE *continued*

Pharmacodynamics:	Inhibits release of thyroid hormone
GI:	Nausea, diarrhea, vomiting, abdominal pain
Other:	Iodism, angioedemia, arthralgia, eosinophilia, urticaria
Dosage:	0.25–1 mg/d PO
Contraindications:	NK
Drug Interactions:	Ca^{2+} interferes with iodide absorption; antithyroid agents block oxidation of iodide to I^-; lithium ↑ hypothyroid effects
Key Points:	No known adverse interactions with anesthetic drugs

IRON

Trade Names:	**Femiron, Feosol, Feostat, Fer-In-Sol, Ferospace, Ferralet, Ferralyn, Ferra-TD, Fer-Iron, Fero-Gradumet, Fumasorb, Fumerin, Hemocyte, Hytinic, Mal-Iron, Niferex, Nu-Iron**
Indications:	Iron-deficiency anemia due to inadequate diet, malabsorption, burns, gastrectomy, pregnancy, and blood loss
Pharmacokinetics:	Onset 4 d; peak: 7–10 d; protein binding to transferrin (>90%); duration: 2–6 mo; $T_{1/2}$ β: 6 h (ferrous sulfate); 5–20 h (iron dextran); absorption from duodenum and proximal jejunum ↑ when iron depleted (or ↑ RBC production); heme iron readily absorbed (ferrous > ferric), stored in hepatocytes and reticuloendothelial system
Pharmacodynamics:	Formation of hemoglobin and myoglobin
CNS:	Headache, dizziness, paresthesias, anorexia
CV:	↓ BP, angina
GI:	Nausea, dyspepsia, cramps, vomiting, constipation, black stools
Other:	Teeth staining, myalgias, fever
Dosage:	50–300 mg/d PO; 25–100 mg IM; 3–16 mg/kg/d (children)
Contraindications:	Hemochromatosis, hemosiderosis, hemolytic anemia, peptic ulcer disease, regional enteritis, ulcerative colitis; blood transfusion
Drug Interactions:	Chelation with acetohydroxamic acid ↓ absorption; toxic complex with dimercaprol; ↓ absorption of etidronate and tetracyclines; chloramphenicol ↑ effect; vitamin C (ascorbic acid) ↑ absorption; black cohosh and St. John's Wort ↓ absorption
Key Points:	No known adverse interactions with anesthetic drugs

LITHIUM

Trade Names: **Eskalith, Lithane, Lithonale**

See Chapter 36, "Psychotropics."

MAGNESIUM

Other Names: **Mag sulfate, Epson salt**

See Chapter 7, "Anticonvulsants."
See also Chapter 4, "Antiarrhythmics," Chapter 11, "Anti-inflammatory Analgesics," and Chapter 22, "Dermatologic Drugs."

MANGANESE

Trade Name: **None**

Indications: Manganese deficiency (due to intestinal malabsorption or pregnancy)

Pharmacokinetics: Absorption is variable, bound to transport protein transmanganin; elimination in bile, enterohepatic recirculation, excreted in feces

Pharmacodynamics: Enzyme activation

Dosage: 2–5 mg PO; 0.2 mg/d IV (TPN); 1–3 mg PO (children)

Contraindications: NK

Drug Interactions: NK

Key Points: No known adverse interactions with anesthetic drugs

MOLYBDENUM

Trade Name: **Molypen**

Indications: Deficiency (due to nutrition or intestinal malabsorption)

Pharmacokinetics: Well absorbed, stored in major organs, excreted in urine

Pharmacodynamics: Component of xanthine, sulfite, aldehyde oxidases
Other: Hyperuricemia (gout)

Dosage: 75–250 µg/d; 20–150 µg/d (children)

Contraindications: NK

MOLYBDENUM *continued*

Drug Interactions: Mobilization of copper from tissue

Key Points: No known adverse interactions with anesthetic drugs

ZINC

Trade Names: **Orazinc (zinc gluconate), Verazinc (zinc sulfate),
                          Zincate (zinc sulfate)**

Indications: Zinc deficiency, inhibition of copper absorption
                          (Wilson's disease)

Pharmacokinetics: Rapid absorption; protein binding to albumin (60%) and
                          to α_2-macroglobulin (40% transferrin); excreted in
                          feces, urine, sweat

Pharmacodynamics: Maintenance of nucleic acid, protein, and cell
                          membrane structure

   GI: Nausea, vomiting, mucosal ulceration, diarrhea,
                          dyspepsia

   Other: Dehydration, neutropenia, leukopenia

Dosage: *Zinc chloride:* 2.5–4 mg/d IV
                          Zinc gluconate: 1–6 mg/d PO
                          Zinc chloride: 100 µg/kg/d IV
                          Zinc gluconate: 1–20 mg/d PO (children)

Contraindications: Renal failure, biliary obstruction

Drug Interactions: ↓ Copper absorption from intestine; ↓ absorption of
                          tetracycline; thiazide diuretics ↑ urinary excretion

Key Points: No known adverse interactions with anesthetic drugs

33

Miscellaneous Compounds

ALPROSTADIL, PROSTAGLANDIN E$_1$ (PGE$_1$)

Trade Names:	**Prostin, Edex, Muse, Caverject**
Indications:	Patent ductus arteriosus, pulmonary vasodilator, erectile dysfunction
Pharmacokinetics:	Onset: <10 min; protein binding: 81%; T$_{1/2}$ β: 5–10 min; rapid metabolism in lung, excreted in urine
Pharmacodynamics:	Relaxes or dilates smooth muscle of ductus arteriosus and trabecular smooth muscle, dilates cavernosal arteries in penis
CNS:	Seizures, fever, cerebral hemorrhage
CV:	Vasodilation, cardiac arrest, flushing, ↓ BP, edema
GI:	Stimulation of intestinal smooth muscle, diarrhea
Pulmonary:	Apnea in neonates with congenital heart disease
Other:	↑ Uterine contractions, ↓ platelet aggregation, ↓ activation of coagulation factor X, ↑ fibrinolysis, DIC, hypokalemia
Dosage:	2.5–5 µg IV q 1 h; 0.05–0.40 µg/kg/min (children)
Contraindications:	Neonatal RDS, bleeding disorders, priapism
Drug Interactions:	Anticoagulants ↑ risk of bleeding
Key Points:	Preoperative use ↑ hypotension during general anesthetia

BERACTANT

Trade Name:	**Survanta**
Indications:	RDS in premature infants
Pharmacokinetics:	Distributed across alveolar surface; undergoes surfactant pathway metabolism, alveolar clearance
Pharmacodynamics:	Natural lung surfactant-related protein, ↓ surface tension
CV:	Vasoconstriction, ↓ HR, ↓ BP, pallor
Pulmonary:	↓ SaO$_2$, apnea
Dosage:	25 mg/mL; 100 mg/kg intratracheal instillation
Contraindications:	Sensitive to bovine products
Drug Interactions:	NK
Key Points:	Potentially alters uptake and elimination of inhaled anesthetics

CARBOPROST

Trade Name:	**Hemabate**
Indications:	Postpartum hemorrhage, 2nd-trimester abortion
Pharmacokinetics:	Onset: <30 min; peak: 15–60 min; duration: 24 h; metabolized in liver, excreted in urine
Pharmacodynamics:	Prostaglandin, stimulates myometrial contractions of gravid uterus
CNS:	Headache, anxiety
CV:	Chest pain, arrhythmias
GI:	Vomiting, diarrhea, nausea
GU:	Uterine rupture, endometritis
Pulmonary:	Bronchospasm, cough
Other:	Rash, diaphoresis, hot flashes, uterine cramps
Dosage:	250 µg IV, (repeat dose at 2-h intervals)
Contraindications:	PID; pre-existing cardiac, pulmonary, renal, or hepatic diseases
Drug Interactions:	↑ Effects of oxytocin
Key Points:	Avoid using volatile anesthetics that relax uterus due to ↑ blood loss

CONTRAST DRUGS/DYES

Trade Names:	**Diatrizoate Meglumine, Indigo Carmine, Iodamide, Iodipamide, Iothalamate, Iopanoic acid (Telepaque); Ipodate (Orografin); Metrizamide, Propyliodone (Dionosil); Tyropanoate (Bilopague)**
Indications:	Radiographic contrast materials
Pharmacodynamics:	Visualization of internal structures
CNS:	Seizures
CV:	↓ BP (reflex ↑ HR), ↑ BP (with ↓ HR), arrhythmias, angina
GU:	↑ Urine output, renal impairment
Pulmonary:	Bronchospasm, laryngospasm, coughing
Dosage:	Volume used depends on radiologic procedure
Contraindications:	Sensitivity to contrast dye
Drug Interactions:	None reported
Key Points:	↑ Hypotensive effects of anesthetic drugs

CYCLODEXTRIN

Trade Name:	**Trappsol (Org 25969)—Investigational**
Indications:	Reversal of nondepolarizing muscle blockade

CYCLODEXTRIN *continued*

Pharmacokinetics:	Onset: <2 min; peak: 3–5 min; duration: 60–90 min; excreted in urine
Pharmacodynamics:	Cyclic oligosaccharide that encapsulates rocuronium in a water-soluble complex
Key Points:	Prompt reversal of rocuronium even from "deep" neuromuscular block

DIGOXIN IMMUNE FAB

Trade Names:	**Digibind, DigiFab**
Indications:	Digoxin intoxication
Pharmacokinetics:	Onset: <10 min; peak: 30 min; duration: 15–20 hr; excreted in urine
Pharmacodynamics:	Specific digoxin-binding antibodies ↓ free digoxin levels
CV:	CHF, arrhythmias
Other:	Hypokalemia
Dosage:	228 mg IV over 30 min (max. 760 mg)
Contraindications:	Sensitivity to ovine products
Drug Interactions:	↓ Cardiac glycoside (digitalis) levels
Key Points:	Redigitalization should not be attempted until antibody has been completely cleared from body (up to 1 wk)

DINOPROST

Trade Name:	**Prostin F2 alpha**
Indications:	Vasodilator for angiographic procedures, induction of labor
Pharmacokinetics:	Onset: <5 min; peak: <10 min; duration: 1–2 h; $T_{1/2}$ β: <5 min; undergoes enzymatic breakdown in maternal lungs and liver, excreted in urine
Pharmacodynamics:	Direct effect on uterine and vascular smooth muscle
CNS:	Dizziness, anxiety, paresthesia, double vision
CV:	Vasoconstriction, ↑ BP, heart block
GI:	Nausea, vomiting, adynamic ileus
GU:	Dysuria, hematuria, urinary retention
Pulmonary:	Bronchoconstriction
Other:	Myalgias, endometritis, uterine bleeding
Dosage:	2.5 μg/min IV, repeat q 1 h (max. 20 μg/min)
Contraindications:	NK

DINOPROST *continued*

Drug Interactions: NK

Key Points: Potential interactions with CV drugs during surgery

DINOPROSTONE (PROSTAGLANDIN E$_2$) [PGE$_2$]

Trade Names: **Cervidil, Prepidil, Prostin E$_2$**

Indications: 2nd-trimester abortion, intrauterine fetal demise, hydatidiform mole

Pharmacokinetics: Onset: <10 min; peak: 17 h; duration: 2–6 d; metabolized in lungs, liver, kidney, spleen, excreted in urine

Pharmacodynamics: Stimulates myometrial contractions in gravid uterus
CNS: Headache, dizziness, anxiety, paresthesia, blurred vision
CV: Chest pain, arrhythmias, syncope
GI: Nausea, vomiting, diarrhea
Pulmonary: Cough, dyspnea
Other: Diaphoresis, rash, leg cramps, fetal distress, ↓ HR, hot flashes

Dosage: 20 mg PR q 3–5 h (max. 240 mg)

Contraindications: Prolonged uterine contractions, placenta previa, acute pelvic inflammatory diseases, cardiopulmonary and hepatorenal diseases

Drug Interactions: ↑ Effect of oxytocin; alcohol ↓ effect

Key Points: Potential interactions with adjunctive CV drugs

EPOPROSTENOL

Trade Name: **Flolan**

Indications: Pulmonary hypertension, CHF

Pharmacokinetics: Extensively metabolized and excreted in urine

Pharmacodynamics: Direct vasodilation of pulmonary and systemic arterial vasculature, ↓ platelet aggregation
CNS: Headache, anxiety, agitation, dizziness, paresthesia
CV: Chest pain, flushing, ↓ BP, ↓ HR
GI: Nausea, vomiting, dyspepsia, diarrhea, abdominal pain
Other: Dyspnea, sweating, chills, thrombocytopenia, myalgia

Dosage: 2 ng/kg/min, ↑ by 1–2 ng/kg/min q 15 min

EPOPROSTENOL *continued*

Contraindications:	Long-term use, CHF, pulmonary edema
Drug Interactions:	Anticoagulants and antiplatelet drugs ↑ risk of bleeding; ↑ hypotension with vasodilators, diuretics, antihypertensives
Key Points:	Enhances hypotensive effect of anesthetic drugs

HYALURONAN

Trade Name:	**Orthovisc**
Indications:	Severe osteoarthritis (knee joint)
Pharmacokinetics:	NK
Pharmacodynamics:	Natural complex glycosaminoglycan from rooster combs
Other:	Arthralgias
Dosage:	30 mg IA q wk (×3)
Contraindications:	Hypersensitivity to avian products (e.g., eggs, poultry, feathers); avoid disinfectants containing quaternary ammonium salts
Drug Interactions:	NK
Key Points:	No known interactions with anesthetic drugs

LOXILAN

Trade Name:	**Oxilan**
Indications:	Cerebral and coronary arteriography, visceral angiography, excretory urography, contrast-enhanced CT
Pharmacokinetics:	Vd: 8 L; Cl: 98 mL/min; $T_{1/2}$ β: 120 min; excreted unchanged in urine
Pharmacodynamics:	Nonionic, water-soluble, tri-iodinated contrast agent
CNS:	Headache
Other:	Chemotoxic and idiosyncratic (anaphylaxic) reactions
Dosage:	300–350 mg/mL IA; 300 mg/mL IV
Contraindications:	Intrathecal use
Drug Interactions:	Hypotensive drugs ↑ side effects
Key Points:	Administration under general anesthesia associated with ↑ risk of adverse reactions

METHYLERGONOVINE

Trade Name:	**Methergine**
Indications:	Postpartum uterine hemorrhage (uterine atony)
Pharmacokinetics:	Onset: <10 min; peak: 30 min; duration: 1–3 h; extensive hepatic 1st-pass metabolism, excreted in urine
Pharmacodynamics:	Stimulates contractions of uterine and vascular smooth muscle
CNS:	Hallucinations, dizziness, seizures, headache
CV:	↑ BP (due to ↑ PVR), ↓ HR, coronary vasospasm, angina, arrhythmias, peripheral vasospasm, thrombophlebitis
GI:	Nausea, vomiting, diarrhea
Other:	Hematuria, dyspnea, uterine contraction, leg cramps
Dosage:	0.2 mg IV after delivery, then q 2–4 h; 0.2 mg PO tid (max. 1 wk)
Contraindications:	Severe hypertension, toxemia (preeclampsia/eclampsia), CVA, occlusive peripheral vascular disease, Raynaud's phenomenon
Drug Interactions:	↑ Vasoconstriction with sympathomimetics
Key Points:	Local anesthetics with vasoconstrictors produce ↑ vasoconstriction with risk of ischemia and serious CV complications

SILDENAFIL

Trade Name:	**Viagra**
Indications:	Erectile dysfunction
Pharmacokinetics:	Onset: <60 min; bioavailability: 40%; peak: 1–2 h; protein binding: 96%; duration: 4 h; Vd: 105 L; metabolized by hepatic CYP3A4 and CYP2CG isoenzymes, excreted by urine
Pharmacodynamics:	↑ Effect of NO by inhibiting phosphodiesterase
CNS:	Headache, dizziness, color blindness, photophobia
CV:	Flushing, angina, ventricular arrhythmias
GI:	Dyspepsia, diarrhea
GU:	UTI, priapism
Other:	Rash
Dosage:	25–50 mg PO 1 h before sexual activity
Contraindications:	Organic nitrates, recent MI, CVA

SILDENAFIL *continued*

Drug Interactions: Delavirdine, protease inhibitors, cimetidine, erythromycin, ketoconazole ↑ levels and side effects; ↑ hypotensive effects of nitrates; rifampin ↓ level; high-fat meal ↓ absorption

Key Points: Use before general or spinal anesthesia ↑ intraoperative hypotension

TADALAFIL

Trade Name: **Cialis**

Indications: Erectile dysfunction

Pharmacokinetics: Onset: <1 h; peak: 2 h; protein binding: 94%; duration: 24–36 h; Vd: 1 L/kg; $T_{1/2}$ β: 17 h; hepatic metabolism via cytochrome P_{450}, 1° excreted in feces

Pharmacodynamics: Selective inhibitor of cGMP-specific phosphodiesterase (PDE) type 5, ↑ penile blood flow
CNS: Headache, dyspepsia
CV: Vasodilation, ↓ BP (orthostatic hypotension)
GU: Priapism (>6 h), Peyronie's disease
Other: Myalgias, facial flushing

Dosage: 5–10 mg PO (max. 20 mg)

Contraindications: Nitrates ("poppers"), α-adrenergic antagonists

Drug Interactions: Ritonavir, ketoconazole ↑ levels; CYP inhibitors, hepatorenal dysfunction ↓ dosage

Key Points: Adequate hydration prior to induction of general anesthesia

TECHNETIUM Tc99m TETROFOSMIN

Trade Name: **Myoview**

Indications: Detection of myocardial ischemia, evaluate cardiac function

Pharmacokinetics: Onset: <5 min; peak: 30 min; physical $T_{1/2}$ β: 6 h; excreted in urine (40%) and feces (26%)

Pharmacodynamics: Myocardial perfusion imaging
CNS: Blurred vision, headache
Other: Rash, urticaria, flushing

Dosage: 5–33 mCi IV

TECHNETIUM Tc99m
TETROFOSMIN *continued*

Contraindications:	Breast-feeding
Drug Interactions:	NK
Key Points:	No interactions with anesthetic drugs

VARDENAFIL

Trade Name:	**Levitra**
Indications:	Erectile dysfunction
Pharmacokinetics:	Onset: 0.5 h; bioavailability: 15%; peak: 1–2 h; protein binding: 95%; Vd: 3 L/kg; Cl: 0.7 L/kg/h; $T_{1/2}\beta$: 4–5 h; hepatic metabolism; excreted 1° in feces
Pharmacodynamics:	↓ Cyclic guanosine monophosphate (cGMP) and phosphodiesterase; relaxes smooth muscle in corpus cavernosum
CNS:	Headache, dizziness
GI:	Dyspepsia, nausea
Other:	Flushing, rhinitis, priapism (>6 h)
Dosage:	5–10 mg/d PO (max. 20 mg)
Contraindications:	Aortic stenosis, IHSS, unstable angina
Drug Interactions:	Hepatic impairment, CYP, and protease inhibitors ↑ level (and ↑ duration of action); α-blockers, vasodilators, nitrates ↑ hypotension
Key Points:	Adequate hydration prior to induction of anesthesia to minimize any residual CV effects

34

Muscle Relaxants

ATRACURIUM

Trade Name:	**Tracrium**
Indications:	Tracheal intubation, muscle relaxation during surgery, facilitates mechanical ventilation
Pharmacokinetics:	Onset: 2–3 min; peak: 3–5 min; protein binding: 82%; duration: 35–50 min; Vd: 0.2 L; Cl: 5.5 mL/kg/min; $T_{1/2}$ β: 20 min; metabolism via ester hydrolysis and Hofmann elimination, active metabolite (laudanosine) with convulsant properties, excreted in urine
Pharmacodynamics:	↓ Response to ACh at neuromuscular junction, competitively blocks access of ACh to motor end-plate
CV:	↑ HR, ↓ BP, vasodilation (due to histamine release)
Pulmonary:	Bronchospasm (due to histamine release), dyspnea
Other:	Erythema, pruritus, flushing
Dosage:	0.3–0.5 mg/kg IV (intubation); 0.08–0.1 mg/kg q 25–50 min (maintenance)
Contraindications:	Sensitivity to benzylisoquinolines
Drug Interactions:	Prolonged action with inhalation agents; variable duration when combined with other nondepolarizing agents; ↓ clearance with antibiotics and anticonvulsants; opioids ↑ respiratory depression
Key Points:	Repeated bolus doses do not produce cumulative effects; ↑ laudanosine levels ↑ volatile anesthetic requirement

CISATRACURIUM

Trade Name:	**Nimbex**
Indications:	Tracheal intubation, muscle relaxation during surgery, facilitation of mechanical ventilation
Pharmacokinetics:	Onset: 1–2 min; peak effect: 3–4 min; protein binding: 82%; duration: 25–44 min; Vd at steady-state: 145 mL/kg; Cl: 5 mL/kg/min; $T_{1/2}$ β: 22–29 min; metabolized by nonspecific ester hydrolysis and Hofmann degradation, excreted in urine and feces
Pharmacodynamics:	Binds competitively to cholinergic receptors on the motor end-plate to antagonize the action of ACh, blocking membrane depolarization
CV:	↓ BP
Other:	Muscle weakness, dyspnea
Dosage:	0.15–0.25 mg/kg IV (intubation); 0.03 mg/kg boluses or 1–3 µg/kg/min (maintenance)
Contraindications:	Sensitivity to benzylisoquinolines

CISATRACURIUM *continued*

Drug Interactions: Blockade with inhalation (volatile) anesthetics, antibiotics, anticonvulsants, lithium, local anesthetics, magnesium; carbamazepine and phenytoin ↓ blockade

Key Points: If different nondepolarizing muscle relaxants are administered, 1st drug usually dictates recovery

DOXACURIUM

Trade Name: **Neuromax**

Indications: Tracheal intubation, muscle relaxation during prolonged surgery or mechanical ventilation in ICU

Pharmacokinetics: Onset: 2–4 min; peak: 36 min; protein binding: 30%; duration: 90–120 min; Vd: 0.2 L/kg; Cl: 2.5 mL/kg/min; $T_{1/2}$ β: 120 min; not metabolized, excreted unchanged in urine and bile

Pharmacodynamics: Binds to cholinergic receptors on motor end-plate to antagonize action of ACh, blocking neuromuscular transmission
Pulmonary: Dyspnea, respiratory depression
Other: Prolonged muscle weakness

Dosage: 0.05 mg/kg IV; 0.03–0.05 mg/kg (children)

Contraindications: Hepatorenal impairment, sensitivity to benzylisoquinolines, benzylalcohol

Drug Interactions: ↑ Blockade with inhalation (volatile) agents, aminoglycosides, anticonvulsants, CCB, magnesium salts, lithium, local anesthetics; carbamazepine and phenytoin ↓ duration

Key Points: Use with volatile anesthetics further prolongs duration of block; incompatible with alkaline solutions (precipitates)

METAXALONE

Trade Name: **Skelaxin**

Indications: Musculoskeletal pain

Pharmacokinetics: Onset: <1 h; peak: 3 h; duration: 6–12 h; Cl: 67 L/h; $T_{1/2}$ β: 3–9 h; hepatic metabolism, excreted in urine

Pharmacodynamics: CNS depression of spinal reflexes
CNS: Sedation, dizziness, headache, nervousness
GI: Nausea/vomiting, ↑ LFTs, jaundice
Other: Rash, bone marrow depression, hemolytic anemia

METAXALONE *continued*

Dosage: 400–800 mg PO q 6–8 h

Contraindications: Severe hepatorenal impairment, drug-induced hemolytic
                         anemia

Drug Interactions: ↑ Effects of alcohol and other CNS depressants

Key Points: Acute use ↓ anesthetic requirement; chronic use
                         ↑ anesthetic requirement

METHOCARBAMOL

Trade Names: **Robaxin, Skelex, Carbacot**

Indications: Musculoskeletal pain

Pharmacokinetics: Onset: <30 min; peak: 1–2 h; duration: 6–8 h; $T_{1/2}$ β:
                         1–2 h; metabolized in liver, excreted in urine

Pharmacodynamics: CNS depression of spinally mediated reflexes
CNS: Dizziness, headache, agitation, ataxia, confusion
CV: ↓ BP, ↓ HR
GI: Nausea, abdominal cramps

Dosage: 0.5–1.5 g PO qid; 0.5–1 g IV/IM; 1 g tid (max. 3 g/d)

Contraindications: Impaired renal function, seizure disorders, pregnancy

Drug Interactions: Alcohol and CNS depressants ↑ effect; ↑ weakness in
                         myasthenia gravis (with anticholinesterase drugs)

Key Points: ↑ CNS depressant effect of anesthetics, opioid
                         analgesics, benzodiazepines

METOCURINE

Trade Name: **Metubine**

Indications: Tracheal intubation, muscle relaxation during
                         surgery

Pharmacokinetics: Onset: 3–5 min; duration: 1–2 h; protein binding: 60%;
                         Vd: 0.4 L/kg; Cl: 1.3 mL/kg/min; $T_{1/2}$ β: 220 min;
                         hepatic metabolism, excreted in urine

Pharmacodynamics: Binds competitively to cholinergic receptors on
                         motor end-plate to antagonize action of ACh,
                         ↓ neuromuscular transmission
CV: ↑ HR, ↓ BP (due to histamine release)
Pulmonary: Bronchospasm (due to histamine release)

Dosage: 0.2–0.3 mg/kg IV (intubation)

Contraindications: Sensitivity to iodine

METOCURINE *continued*

Drug Interactions:　　↑ Blockade with inhalation (volatile) agents, antibiotics, anticonvulsants, local anesthetics, lithium

Key Points:　　↓ Dose or avoid in patients with renal disease and in those prone to histamine release (e.g., asthmatics, atopic seasonal allergies)

MIVACURIUM

Trade Name:　　**Mivacron**

Indications:　　Tracheal intubation, muscle relaxation during short surgical procedures

Pharmacokinetics:　　Onset: 2 min; peak: 3–5 min; protein binding: <10%; duration: 20–30 min; Vd: 0.2 L/kg; Cl: 4.2 mL/kg/min; $T_{1/2}$ β: 55 min; metabolism by plasma pseudocholinesterase hydrolysis, excreted in urine

Pharmacodynamics:　　Competes with ACh for receptor sites at motor end-plate, antagonizes action of ACh, reversed by cholinesterase inhibitors

CNS:　　Dizziness
CV:　　↑ HR, ↓ BP, vasodilation (due to histamine release)
Pulmonary:　　Bronchospasm due to histamine release
Other:　　Muscle weakness, rash, urticaria, phlebitis

Dosage:　　0.15–0.25 mg/kg (intubation); 0.075–0.15 mg/kg q 10–15 min, or 5–30 µg/kg/min (maintenance)

Contraindications:　　Severe hepatorenal impairment, ↓ plasma cholinesterase

Drug Interactions:　　↓ Dosage and prolonged action with inhalation (volatile) agents; carbamazepine and phenytoin ↓ blockade; glucocorticoids, hormonal contraceptives, MAOIs ↑ blockade due to ↓ plasma cholinesterase activity; ranitidine ↑ dosage requirement

Key Points:　　↓ Dosage requirements in patients with hepatorenal impairment; avoid in patients at risk to histamine release; two-step (split) intubating dose minimizes histamine release; most rapid spontaneous recovery of available nondepolarizing muscle relaxants

PANCURONIUM

Trade Name:　　**Pavulon**

Indications:　　Tracheal intubation, muscle relaxation during long surgical procedures or mechanical ventilation

PANCURONIUM *continued*

Pharmacokinetics:	Onset: 30–60 sec; peak: 2–4 min; protein binding: 87%; duration: 40–80 min; Vd: 0.3 L/kg; Cl: 1–2 mL/kg/min; $T_{1/2}$ β: 100–130 min; hepatic metabolism, excreted unchanged in urine
Pharmacodynamics:	Prevents ACh from binding to receptors on motor end-plate, blocking depolarization
CV:	↑ HR, ↑ BP, ↑ CO (due to vagolytic effects)
Other:	Excessive salivation, residual muscle weakness, rash, itching
Dosage:	0.06–0.12 mg/kg (intubation); 0.01 mg/kg q 30–60 min (maintenance)
Contraindications:	Hepatorenal impairment, CHF with coronary artery disease, sensitivity to bromides and steroid relaxants
Drug Interactions:	Prolonged action with inhalation (volatile) agents, antibiotics, β-blockers, lithium, magnesium, diuretics, anticonvulsants, TCAs; ↓ effect after steroid pretreatment
Key Points:	↓ Dosage requirement in patients with renal or hepatic insufficiency; useful for patients with slow HR (without cardiac disease)

PIPECURONIUM

Trade Name:	**Arduan**
Indications:	Tracheal intubation, muscle relaxation during long surgical procedures, mechanical ventilation in ICU setting
Pharmacokinetics:	Onset: 3–5 min; duration: 2–4 h; Vd: 0.3 L/kg; Cl: 2.4 mL/kg/min; $T_{1/2}$ β: 140 min; metabolized in liver, excreted in urine
Pharmacodynamics:	Prevents ACh from binding to receptors on motor end-plate, blocking depolarization at neuromuscular junction
Pulmonary:	Residual ventilatory depression
Other:	Prolonged muscle weakness
Dosage:	0.04–0.08 mg/kg IV (intubation)
Contraindications:	Severe hepatorenal impairment, sensitivity to steroid relaxants
Drug Interactions:	Prolonged action with inhalation (volatile) agents, ↑ relaxant effect with antibiotics, lithium, anticonvulsants, magnesium
Key Points:	↓ Dosage requirement in patients with renal or hepatic insufficiency, residual blockade may necessitate mechanical ventilatory support

ROCURONIUM

Trade Name:	**Zemuron**
Indications:	Tracheal intubation, muscle relaxation during surgical procedures, mechanical ventilation in ICU
Pharmacokinetics:	Onset: <1 min; peak: 2–3 min; duration: 45–90 min; Vd: 0.3 L/kg; Cl: 4.0 mL/kg/min; $T_{1/2}$ β: 130 min; hepatic metabolism, excreted in feces
Pharmacodynamics:	Binds competitively to cholinergic receptors on motor end-plate, antagonizes action of ACh at myoneural junction
CV:	↑ HR (children)
Other:	Anaphylactic-type reaction with histamine release (rare)
Dosage:	0.5–1.0 mg/kg (intubation); 0.1–0.3 mg/kg q 15–30 min, or 0.008–0.016 µg/kg/min (maintenance)
Contraindications:	Severe hepatic impairment, allergic reaction to steroid-type relaxants
Drug Interactions:	Prolonged action with inhalation (volatile) agents
Key Points:	Genetically susceptible individuals may experience severe allergic reactions; most rapid onset of action of available nondepolarizing muscle relaxants

SUCCINYLCHOLINE

Trade Names:	**Anectine, Quelicin**
Indications:	Rapid-sequence induction, tracheal intubation and muscle relaxation during short surgical procedures
Pharmacokinetics:	Onset: 1–2 min (IV), 3–5 min (IM); duration: 6–12 min; $T_{1/2}$ β: 2–4 min; rapidly hydrolyzed by plasma cholinesterase, excreted in urine
Pharmacodynamics:	Binds to ACh nicotinic receptors to produce prolonged depolarization at myoneural junction (i.e., depolarizing muscle relaxants)
CNS:	↑ ICP, ↑ intraocular pressure (transient)
CV:	↓ BP, arrhythmias (due to vagal stimulation), cardiac arrest (due to denervation hypersensitivity)
GI:	↑ Intragastric pressure, ↑ esophageal sphincter tone
Other:	↑ K+ after denervation (e.g., burns, tetanus, paraplegia, spinal cord or crush injury, neuromuscular disease, stroke, prolonged immobility), fasciculations, myalgias, masseter spasm, ↑ salivation
Dosage:	0.5–1.5 mg/kg IV (intubation); 2–4 mg/kg IM; 2–3 mg/kg (children)

SUCCINYLCHOLINE *continued*

Contraindications:	Malignant hyperthermia, plasma cholinesterase disorders, myopathies (especially Duchenne's), sensitivity to parabens
Drug Interactions:	↑ Effects by cholinesterase inhibitors, oxytocin, magnesium, local anesthetics, inhalational anesthetics, lithium; digitalis ↑ arrhythmias; contraceptives, glucorticoids, MAOIs ↓ cholinesterase activity
Key Points:	Given potential for vagal arrhythmias, anticholinergic drug is recommended prior to administration; produces myoglobinuria in children

TAAC3

Trade Name:	**None (investigational)**
Indications:	Tracheal intubation, muscle relaxation for brief surgical procedures
Pharmacokinetics:	Onset: 45–60 sec; duration: 3–30 min; lack of cumulative effect; metabolized by nonspecific plasma esterases, excreted in urine
Pharmacodynamics:	Ultra-short-acting nondepolarizing diester-type muscle relaxant
CV:	↑ HR
Dosage:	0.3–0.5 mg/kg IV
Contraindications:	NK
Drug Interactions:	NK
Key Points:	Possible nondepolarizing alternative to succinylcholine and mivacurium for short surgical procedures

TUBOCURARINE

Trade Name:	**Curare**
Indications:	Tracheal intubation, muscle relaxation during surgery, used as defasciculating agent prior to succinylcholine
Pharmacokinetics:	Onset: 1–2 min; peak: 3–5 min; protein binding: 42%; duration: 30–90 min; Vd: 0.3 L/kg; Cl: 1–3 mL/kg/min; $T_{1/2}\,\beta$: 102 min; hepatic metabolism, excreted unchanged in urine
Pharmacodynamics:	Prevents ACh from binding to muscarinic receptors on motor end-plate, blocks neuromuscular depolarization (fasiculations)
CNS:	↓ Autonomic ganglia activity

TUBOCURARINE *continued*

CV:	↑ HR, ↓ BP (due to histamine release), arrhythmias
Pulmonary:	Bronchospasm (due to histamine release)
Other:	↑ Salivation, residual muscle weakness
Dosage:	0.3–0.5 mg/kg IV; 2–4 mg (defasciculating)
Contraindications:	Asthma, severe hepatorenal disease
Drug Interactions:	Use with opioids ↑ respiratory depression; prolonged effects with volatile agents, antibiotics, β-blockers, local anesthetics, lithium, anticonvulsants, magnesium, thiazides
Key Points:	Small doses prevent succinylcholine-induced fasciculations but may not prevent postoperative myalgias.

VECURONIUM

Trade Name:	**Norcuron**
Indications:	Tracheal intubation, muscle relaxation during surgical procedures, mechanical ventilation in the ICU setting
Pharmacokinetics:	Onset: 1–3 min; peak: 3–5 min; protein binding: 75%; duration: 20–40 min; Vd: 0.3–0.4 L/kg; Cl: 3–4.5 mL/kg/min; $T_{1/2}$ β: 65–75 min; metabolized in liver, excreted 1° in feces
Pharmacodynamics:	Prevents ACh from binding to receptors on motor end-plate, blocking depolarization at neuromuscular junction
Other:	Residual muscle weakness
Dosage:	0.08–0.1 mg/kg IV (intubation); 0.02 mg/kg (maintenance)
Contraindications:	Sensitivity to bromide
Drug Interactions:	Prolonged action with inhalation (volatile) anesthetics, ↑ effect with some antibiotics, anticonvulsants, thiazides, magnesium
Key Points:	Requires reconstitution prior to use; slower onset than rocuronium

35

Opioid Agonists and Antagonists

ALFENTANIL

Trade Name:	**Alfenta**
Indications:	Adjunct during induction and maintenance periods
Pharmacokinetics:	Onset: 60–90 sec; peak: 2–3 min; protein binding: 92%; duration: 15–30 min; Vd: 0.86 L/kg; Cl: 6.4 mL/kg/min; $T_{1/2}$ β: 68 min; metabolized in liver, excreted in urine
Pharmacodynamics:	Synthetic agonist, interacts with ENS opioid μ-receptors
CNS:	Analgesia, drowsiness, dizziness, mood changes, ↓ CBF, ↓ ICP, miosis, tolerance/physical dependence
CV:	↓ HR, ↓ BP, arrhythmias
GI:	Nausea, vomiting, ↓ gastric emptying, ↑ intrabiliary pressure, constipation
Pulmonary:	↓ Ventilation, ↑ airway resistance, apnea, bronchospasm
Other:	Skeletal (truncal) muscle rigidity, ↑ ADH secretion, urinary retention
Dosage:	20–40 μg/kg IV (induction); 0.5–1.5 μg/kg/min (maintenance)
Contraindications:	Opioid intolerance, head injury (↑ ICP)
Drug Interactions:	Concurrent use of a benzodiazepine, N_2O, and volatile agents ↑ risk of cardiovascular and respiratory depression
Key Points:	Rapid, short-acting opioid that can facilitate early recovery process after ambulatory surgery due to its anesthetic-sparing effects

ALVIMOPAN

Other Name:	**Entereg**
Indications:	Postoperative ileus, acute and chronic opioid-related constipation
Pharmacokinetics:	Poorly absorbed (bioavailability 6%); duration 2–3 h; protein binding 75%; Vd 1L/kg; $T_{1/2}$ β: 3–8 h; does not cross blood-brain barrier
Pharmacodynamics:	Peripherally active μ-opioid receptor antagonist
GI:	Abdominal cramps, nausea, diarrhea, flatus
Dosage:	6–12 mg PO bid
Contraindications:	Mechanical bowel obstruction

ALVIMOPAN *continued*

Drug Interactions:	NK
Key Points:	Peripheral opioid antagonist that prevents bowel complications in patients receiving large doses of PCA opioids

BUPRENORPHINE

Trade Name:	**Buprenex**
Indications:	Acute and chronic pain, reverse opioid-induced side effects
Pharmacokinetics:	Onset: <2 min (IV), 15 min (IM); peak: 5 min (IV), 1 h (IM); duration: 6–12 h; protein binding: 96%; $T_{1/2}$ β: 7–8 h; metabolized in liver, excreted in feces
Pharmacodynamics:	Long-acting partial agonist-antagonist at μ-opioid receptors
CNS:	Analgesia, dizziness, sedation, confusion, euphoria, ↑ ICP, miosis
GI:	Nausea, vomiting, dry mouth
GU:	Urinary retention
Pulmonary:	Respiratory depression, dyspnea
Other:	Pruritus, diaphoresis, parasthesias
Dosage:	0.3 mg IM/IV initially, then repeat in 2–3 min (max. 1.2 mg/d), 0.2 mg intranasal
Contraindications:	None known
Drug Interactions:	MAOIs ↑ side effects; general anesthetics, barbiturates, benzodiazepines ↑ respiratory and CNS depression
Key Points:	If physically dependent on opioids, buprenorphine may cause "acute withdrawal syndrome" and reverse postoperative analgesia

BUTORPHANOL, LEVORPHANOL

Trade Name:	**Stadol (butorphanol), Levo-Dromoran (levorphanol)**
Indications:	Acute and chronic pain, opioid side effects during labor and delivery
Pharmacokinetics:	Onset: 2–3 min (IV), 10–15 min (IM); peak: 30–60 min; protein binding: 80%; Vd: 7 L/kg; Cl: 23.5 mL/kg/min; $T_{1/2}$ β: 150 min; hepatic metabolism, excreted in urine

BUTORPHANOL, LEVORPHANOL
continued

Pharmacodynamics:	Mixed opioid agonist-antagonist at μ-receptors and agonist at κ-receptors
CNS:	Acute withdrawal syndrome, dysphoria, drowsiness, ↑ ICP, paresthesia, dizziness, blurred vision, tinnitus, confusion, headache
CV:	↑ Pulmonary artery pressure, orthostatic hypotension (↓ PVR)
GI:	Nausea, vomiting, anorexia, constipation, dry mouth
Pulmonary:	↓ Ventilation (can partially reverse effect of agonist opioids)
Other:	Rash, diaphoresis, flushing
Dosage:	1–3 mg IV/IM, repeat 3–5 h
Contraindications:	Opioid-dependent chronic pain, allergic to benzethonium (preservative); acute MI, severe CHF, coronary artery disease
Drug Interactions:	Cimetidine, digoxin, phenytoin, rifampin ↑ effects; general anesthetics and other CNS depressants cause ↑ respiratory depression
Key Points:	In opioid-dependent or postoperative patients receiving large doses of opioid analgesics can precipitate acute withdrawal syndrome

CODEINE, DIHYDROCODEINE

Trade Names:	**See Appendix I, "Oral Analgesic Drug Combinations"**
Indications:	Acute pain, nonproductive (dry) cough
Pharmacokinetics:	Onset: <5 min (IV), 10–15 min (IM/SC), 30–45 min (oral); peak: 0.5–1 h (IM/SC), 1–2 h (PO); duration: 4–6 h; crosses blood-brain and placental barriers; metabolized in liver, excreted in urine
Pharmacodynamics:	μ-opioid receptor agonist, direct suppressant action on cough reflex
CNS:	Analgesia, drowsiness, dizziness, mood changes, abuse potential
CV:	↓ BP, ↓ HR, flushing
GI:	Nausea, vomiting, constipation, dry mouth
GU:	Urinary retention
Pulmonary:	Respiratory depression
Other:	Pruritus, physical/psychological dependence
Dosage:	10–20 mg q 4–6 h (antitussive), 0.25 mg/kg (children); 15–60 mg PO/SC/IM q 4–6 h (pain control); 0.5 mg/kg q 4–6 h (children)

CODEINE, DIHYDROCODEINE *continued*

Contraindications: Severe hepatorenal impairment, ↑ ICP, head injury

Drug Interactions: Anticholinergics cause paralytic ileus; antihistamines, MAOIs, phenothiazines, TCAs, CNS depressants ↑ sedation, respiratory depression, hypotensive effects

Key Points: Use with general anesthetics ↑ CNS and respiratory depression and PONV

DEZOCINE

Trade Name: **Dalgan**

Indications: Acute pain, postoperative analgesia

Pharmacokinetics: Onset: <15 min (IV), <30 min (IM); peak: 30–60 min; Vd: 8.8–10.7 L/kg; Cl: 3.3 L/h/kg; $T_{1/2}$ β: 1.7–2.4 hr; hepatic metabolism, excreted unchanged in urine

Pharmacodynamics: Mixed agonist-antagonist at CNS opioid receptors
  CNS: Analgesia, ↑ ICP, dysphoria, withdrawal reactions, drowsiness
  CV: Arrhythmias, pedal edema
  GI: Nausea, vomiting, ↑ sphincter of Oddi tone (biliary colic)
  Pulmonary: ↓ Ventilation (partially reverses effects of opioid agonists)
  Other: Dermatitis, thrombophlebitis

Dosage: 5–10 mg IM initially, then 10 mg q 3–6 h; 3–5 mg IV, then 5 mg q 2–4 h

Contraindications: Allergic to sodium metabisulfate (preservative), opioid-dependent chronic pain, severe CHF or CAD

Drug Interactions: General anesthetics, barbiturates, benzodiazepines ↑ respiratory and CNS depression

Key Points: Produces higher incidence of side effects than pure opioid agonist (e.g., PONV); if dependent on opioids, precipitates acute withdrawal syndrome

FENTANYL

Trade Names: **Sublimaze, Duragesic (TTS)**

Indications: Adjunct during induction and maintenance of anesthesia, postoperative analgesia, cancer pain (transdermal)

FENTANYL *continued*

Pharmacokinetics:	Onset: 1–2 min (IV), 7–15 min (IM), 12–24 h (TTS); peak: 3–5 min (IV), 20–30 min (IM), 12–24 h (TTS); duration: 0.5–1 h (IV), 1–2 h (IM), 1–3 d (TTS); Vd: 4.0 L/kg; Cl: 13.0 mL/kg/min. $T_{1/2}$ β: 3–4 hr; metabolized in liver, excreted in urine
Pharmacodynamics:	Opioid agonist, interacts with CNS μ-receptors
CNS:	Analgesia, somnolence, ↓ CBF, miosis, sedation, mood changes, dizziness, myclonis, tolerance/physical dependence
CV:	↓ HR (due to vagal effect), ↓ BP, brady-arrhythmias
GI:	Nausea, vomiting, ileus/constipation, ↓ gastric emptying, dry mouth, ↑ intrabiliary pressure
GU:	Urinary retention
Pulmonary:	↓ Ventilatory rate, ↑ airway resistance, apnea, bronchospasm
Other:	Muscle rigidity, physical dependence, ↑ ADH secretion, pruritus
Dosage:	2–75 μg/kg IV (anesthetic adjuvant); 25–100 μg TTS (for 72 h)
Contraindications:	Head injury, ↑ ICP, COPD, hepatorenal impairment
Drug Interactions:	Antihistamines, barbiturates, muscle relaxants, general anesthetics, benzodiazepines, phenothiazines, TCAs, cimetidine, protease inhibitors, sedative hypnotics ↑ CNS, cardiovascular, respiratory depression; droperidol ↓ BP
Key Points:	Potent IV and volatile anesthetic-sparing effects, facilitating faster emergence from general anesthesia; use in combination with volatile anesthetics and/or N_2O will ↑ PONV

HYDROCODONE

Trade Names:	**See Appendix I, "Oral Analgesic Drug Combinations"**
Indications:	Acute pain, antitussive
Pharmacokinetics:	Onset: <30 min; peak: 1.3 h; $T_{1/2}$ β: 4 h; hepatic metabolism, excreted in urine
Pharmacodynamics:	Semisynthetic μ-opioid receptor agonist
CNS:	Drowsiness, confusion, mood changes, dizziness, abuse potential
GI:	Nausea, vomiting, constipation/ileus, dry mouth
GU:	Urinary retention, ureteral spasm
Pulmonary:	Respiratory depression, ↓ SpO_2 and ↑ CO_2 levels

HYDROCODONE *continued*

Dosage:	2.5–10 mg PO q 4–6 h
Contraindications:	Head injury (↑ ICP), obstructive sleep apnea syndrome
Key Points:	Chronic use leads to tolerance to CNS effects of anesthetic and analgesic drugs

HYDROMORPHONE, OXYMORPHONE

Trade Names:	**Hydrostat, Dilaudid (hydromorphone), Numorphan (oxymorphone)**
Indications:	Acute postoperative pain, cancer pain, chronic cough
Pharmacokinetics:	Onset: <15 min (IM/IV), 30 min (oral); peak: 15–30 min (IV); 0.5–1 h (IM), 1–2 h (oral); duration: 2–3 h (IV), 3–4 h (IM), 4–6 h (oral); $T_{1/2} \beta$: 150 min; metabolized in liver, excreted in urine
Pharmacodynamics:	Stimulates μ-opioid receptors in CNS
CNS:	Analgesia, mood changes, drowsiness, ↓ CBF, miosis, dizziness, tolerance/physical dependence
CV:	↓ HR, ↓ BP
GI:	Nausea, vomiting, ↓ gastric emptying, ↑ intrabiliary pressure, constipation/ileus
GU:	Urinary retention
Pulmonary:	↓ Ventilatory rate, ↑ airway resistance, bronchospasm, apnea
Other:	Truncal rigidity, diaphoresis, ↑ ADH secretion, pruritus
Dosages:	*Hydromorphone:* 2–7.5 mg IM/IV (max. 40 mg/d); 1 mg PO q 3–4 h (antitussive) *Oxymorphone:* 1.5–5 mg IM/IV (max. 30 mg/d)
Contraindications:	Intracranial lesion (↑ ICP), COPD, cor pulmonale, status asthmaticus
Drug Interactions:	Anticholinergics ↑ paralytic ileus; cimetidine, barbiturates, antihistamines, benzodiazepines, general anesthetics, muscle relaxants, opioid analgesics, phenothiazines, sedative-hypnotics, TCAs ↑ CNS and respiratory depression
Key Points:	Bolus doses are highly effective for IV and epidural PCA, with fewer side effects than morphine

MEPERIDINE (PETHIDINE)

Trade Name:	**Demerol**
Indications:	Acute pain, postoperative pain
Pharmacokinetics:	Onset: 2–3 min (IV), 10–15 min (IM), 15–20 min (oral); peak: 5–7 min (IV), 30–50 min (IM), 1–2 h (oral); protein binding: 70%; duration: 2–4 h; Vd: 3.8 L/kg; Cl: 15 mL/kg/min; $T_{1/2}$ β: 180–264 min; metabolized to active metabolite (normeperidine), excreted in urine
Pharmacodynamics:	Synthetic μ-receptor agonist
CNS:	Analgesia, drowsiness, dizziness, euphoria, hyperactive reflexes, seizures, tremor, tolerance/physical dependence, high abuse potential
CV:	↓ BP (↓ PVR), myocardial depression, ↑ HR
GI:	Nausea, vomiting, ↓ gastric emptying, constipation/ileus, ↓ biliary tract spasms (↑ intrabiliary pressure)
GU:	Urinary retention
Pulmonary:	Respiratory depression, chest wall rigidity
Other:	Diaphoresis, pruritus, urticaria
Dosage:	50–150 mg PO q 3–4 h; 50–100 mg IM 1–3 h; 1–2 mg/kg q 4 h (children)
Contraindications:	Use of MAOIs (<14 d), head injury (↑ IOP), seizure disorders
Drug Interactions:	MAOIs can precipitate hypertension, tachycardia, fever, convulsions ("neuroleptic malignant syndrome" [NMS]); anticholinergics ↑ paralytic ileus; ↑ adverse effects of isoniazid; cimetidine, alcohol, antihistamines, barbiturates, benzodiazepines, anesthetics, phenothiazines, relaxants, sedative-hypnotics, TCAs ↑ CNS depression
Key Points:	Less efficacious analgesic than morphine or hydromorphone in postoperative period, associated with high incidence of PONV

METHADONE

Trade Names:	**Dolophine, Methadose**
Indications:	Acute and chronic pain, narcotic abstinence syndrome
Pharmacokinetics:	Onset: 10–20 min (IM), 0.5–1 h (oral); peak 0.5–1 h (IM), 1–2 h (oral); duration: 4–6 h; $T_{1/2}$ β: 7–14 h; metabolized in liver by *N*-demethylation, excreted in urine and feces

METHADONE *continued*

Pharmacodynamics:	Opioid μ-agonist, interacts with κ-opioid receptors
CNS:	Analgesia, ↓ CBF, miosis, drowsiness, seizures, mood changes, visual disturbances, dizziness
CV:	↓ HR, ↓ BP, edema
GI:	Nausea, vomiting, constipation, ↓ gastric emptying, dry mouth, anorexia, ↑ intrabiliary pressure
GU:	Urinary retention, ↓ libido
Pulmonary:	↓ Ventilatory rate, ↑ airway resistance
Other:	Truncal muscle rigidity, diaphoresis, pruritus, urticaria, flushing, ↑ ADH secretion

Dosage: 2.5–20 mg PO q 6–8 h; 15–40 mg/d (abstinence); 0.7 mg/kg PO q 4–6 h (children)

Contraindications: Hepatorenal impairment, BPH, ↑ ICP, asthma, COPD

Drug Interactions: Urinary acidifiers, phenytoin, rifampin ↑ elimination; nelfinavir, nevirapine, ritonavir ↓ effect; cimetidine, alcohol, CNS depressants ↑ respiratory and CNS depression

Key Points: Used in opioid detoxification programs and as adjunct for postoperative pain management; lower abuse potential than shorter-acting opioids

MORPHINE

Trade Names: **Duramorph, MS Contin**

Indications: Acute and postoperative pain, cancer pain, acute pulmonary edema

Pharmacokinetics: Onset: 5 min (IV), 20 min (IM), 45 min (epidural), 1 h (oral); peak: 20 min (IV), 30–60 min (IM), 60 min (epidural), 1–2 h (oral); duration: 4–5 h (IV/IM), 24 h (epidural), 6–12 h (oral); Vd: 3.2 L/kg; Cl: 15 mL/kg/min; $T_{1/2}$ β: 180 min; metabolized in liver, excreted in urine and bile

Pharmacodynamics:	Opioid agonist, interacts with μ-, Δ-, κ-, ς-opioid receptors
CNS:	Analgesia, mood changes, nightmares, ↓ CBF, miosis, drowsiness
CV:	↓ HR, ↓ BP
GI:	Nausea, vomiting, ↓ gastric emptying, ↑ intrabiliary pressure, ileus
GU:	Urinary retention, ↓ libido
Pulmonary:	Depressed ventilation, ↑ airway resistance, apnea

MORPHINE *continued*

Other:	Truncal muscle rigidity, pruritus, flushing, diaphoresis
Dosage:	1–3 mg IV, 2.5–10 mg IM, or 0.01–0.04 mg/kg h infusion (pain control); 10–15 mg IV (pulmonary edema)
Contraindications:	Acute bronchial asthma, severe hepatorenal impairment
Drug Interactions:	Benzodiazepines, general anesthetics, zidovudine, cimetidine, alcohol, barbiturates, antihistamines, phenothiazines, alcohol ↑ cardiovascular, respiratory, CNS depression; anticholinergics ↑ ileus
Key Points:	Commonly used opioid for patient-controlled analgesia (PCA); ↑ PONV with early ambulation; extended delivery systems (MS Contin) for cancer-related pain

NALBUPHINE

Trade Name:	**Nubain**
Indications:	Acute and chronic pain, analgesia in obstetrical patients
Pharmacokinetics:	Onset: 2–3 min (IV), 15 min (IM); peak: 30 min (IV), 1 h (IM); duration: 3–6 h; Vd: 2.9 L/kg; Cl: 19 mL/kg/min; $T_{1/2}$ β: 2–3 h; extensive 1st-pass metabolism in liver, excreted in urine
Pharmacodynamics:	Agonist at κ-opioid receptors, partial agonist at μ-receptors
CNS:	Analgesia, ↑ ICP, withdrawal reactions, sedation, dizziness, confusion, delusion, blurred vision, headache
GI:	Nausea, vomiting, ↑ sphincter of Oddi tone (biliary colic)
Pulmonary:	Respiratory depression, asthma, edema, dyspnea
Other:	Pruritus, urticaria, diaphoresis, dry mouth
Dosage:	5–20 mg IM/IV, repeat q 3–6 h
Contraindications:	Allergic to sodium metabisulfate (preservative)
Drug Interactions:	General anesthetics, barbiturates, benzodiazepines ↑ respiratory and CNS depression
Key Points:	Useful adjuvant for reversing pruritus and nausea related to epidural or intrathecal opioids; if opioid-dependent, precipitates withdrawal syndrome

NALMEFENE

Trade Name:	**Revex**
Indications:	Reversal of opioid overdose, UROD, respiratory depression due to spinal opioids
Pharmacokinetics:	Onset: <5 min; peak effect: <10 min (IV), 1 h (IM), 1.5 h (SC); high bioavailability; protein binding: 45%; Vd: 3.9 L/kg; Cl: 0.8 L/kg/h; $T_{1/2}$ β: 9–11 h; hepatic metabolism, excreted in urine
Pharmacodynamics:	Opioid receptor antagonist
CNS:	Dizziness, headache, agitation, opioid withdrawal syndrome
CV:	↑ BP, ↑ HR, vasodilation, arrhythmias
GI:	Nausea, vomiting, dry mouth, pharyngitis, diarrhea
Other:	Fever, chills, pruritus, urinary retention, tremors
Dosage:	0.1 mg IV (at 3-min intervals); 0.5–1.5 mg IV (opioid "overdose")
Contraindications:	CHF, acute and chronic pain conditions
Drug Interactions:	Reversal of adverse opioid effects on CNS, respiratory, cardiovascular, gastrointestinal, genitourinary systems
Key Points:	Side effects due to overdose with ultra–short-acting opioid (e.g., remifentanil) should be managed with succinylcholine

NALOXONE

Trade Name:	**Narcan**
Indications:	Reversal of opioid overdosage, UROD
Pharmacokinetics:	Onset: 1–2 min (IV), 2–5 (IM); peak: 5–15 min; duration: 60–90 min; Vd: 1.8 L/kg; Cl: 30.1 mL/kg/min; $T_{1/2}$ β: 64 min; hepatic metabolism (extensive 1st-pass effect), excreted in urine
Pharmacodynamics:	Pure opiate receptor antagonist
CNS:	Acute opioid withdrawal syndrome, dysphoria, tremors, seizures
CV:	↑ BP, ↑ HR, arrhythmias
GI:	Nausea, vomiting, abdominal cramps
Pulmonary:	↑ Respiratory rate, ↑ pulmonary edema
Other:	Diaphoresis, chills
Dosage:	0.1–0.2 mg IV q 2–3 min; 0.4–1.0 mg IV, repeat at 2- to 3-min intervals (max. dose 10 mg); 0.005–0.01 mg/kg IV/IM (children)

NALOXONE *continued*

Contraindications:	Severe CHF, acute and chronic pain conditions
Drug Interactions:	Morphine and methadone outlast the antagonist action of naloxone (requiring repeated dosing or continuous infusion)
Key Points:	For treatment of remifentanil-induced chest wall rigidity (and apnea), succinylcholine is preferable; ↑ doses of opioid agonists are required to produce analgesia after administration

NALTREXONE

Trade Names:	**Depade, Trexan, ReVia**
Indications:	Ultrarapid detoxification of opioid dependency (UROD), short-term therapy for alcoholism
Pharmacokinetics:	Onset: <30 min; peak: 1 h; duration: 24 h; protein binding: 24%; $T_{1/2}$ β: 4 h (13 h for active metabolite); extensive 1st-pass hepatic metabolism, excreted in urine
Pharmacodynamics:	Pure opiate receptor antagonist
CNS:	Acute withdrawal syndrome, insomnia, anxiety, dizziness, suicidal ideation, seizures, tremulousness, blurred vision, confusion, malaise
CV:	↑ BP, ↑ HR
GI:	Nausea, vomiting, anorexia, abdominal cramps, ↑ LFTs
Pulmonary:	↑ Respiratory rate
Other:	Rash, chills, lymphocytosis, delayed ejaculation
Dosage:	25–50 mg IV/IM initially, then 50 mg q 24 h
Contraindications:	Acute pain management, acute hepatitis or liver failure
Drug Interactions:	↓ Hepatic metabolism ↑ level; thioridazine ↑ lethargy and somnolence
Key Points:	↑ Doses of opioid agonists required to produce acute analgesia after reversal; not recommended for reversal of opioid overdose with short-acting opioid analgesics

OXYCODONE, PROPOXYPHENE

Trade Names:	**Percodan, OxyContin (oxycodone), Darvocet, Darvon (propoxyphene; also see Appendix I)**
Indications:	Acute and chronic pain
Pharmacokinetics:	Onset: 10–60 min; peak: 1–2 h; duration: 4–12 h; metabolized in liver, excreted in urine

OXYCODONE, PROPOXYPHENE *continued*

Pharmacodynamics:	Opioid agonist activity at CNS μ-receptor
CNS:	Analgesia, somnolence, euphoria, dizziness, headache, high abuse potential
CV:	↓ BP, ↓ HR
GI:	Nausea, vomiting, constipation, dry mouth
GU:	Urine retention
Pulmonary:	Respiratory depression
Other:	Diaphoresis, pruritus, rash
Dosages:	*Oxycodone:* 2.5–15 mg PO q 6 h
	Propoxyphene: 60–120 mg PO q 4 h
Contraindications:	Head injury (↑ ICP), COPD, asthma, BPH
Drug Interactions:	Anticholinergics ↑ paralytic ileus; cimetidine, barbiturates, antihistamines, phenothiazines, TCAs ↑ respiratory and CNS depression
Key Points:	General anesthetics, muscle relaxants, opioids, benzodiazepines ↑ postoperative respiratory and cardiovascular depression; chronic use ↑ perioperative opioid analgesic requirements

PENTAZOCINE

Trade Name:	**Talwin**
Indications:	Acute and chronic pain
Pharmacokinetics:	Onset: 2–3 min (IV), 15–20 min (IM),15–30 min (oral); peak: 15–30 min (IV), 30–60 min (IM), 1–4 h (oral); duration: 2–3 h; extensive 1st-pass metabolism in liver, excreted in urine and feces
Pharmacodynamics:	Partial agonist-antagonist at opioid μ-receptors and antagonist at κ-opioid receptors
CNS:	Analgesia, visual disturbances, drowsiness, dizziness, dysphoria, nystagmus, headache, confusion, tinnitus
CV:	↓ BP
GI:	Dry mouth, nausea, vomiting
GU:	Urine retention
Pulmonary:	↓ Ventilation, dyspnea
Other:	Diaphoresis, pruritus
Dosage:	30–50 mg PO q 4 h (max. 600 mg); 30 mg IM/IV q 3–4 h (max. 360 mg)
Contraindications:	Opioid dependence, pregnancy
Drug Interactions:	Cimetidine ↑ toxicity; general anesthetics, barbiturates, benzodiazepines ↑ respiratory and CNS depression

PENTAZOCINE *continued*

Key Points:	With opioid dependence, may cause acute withdrawal symptoms; physical dependence may develop with chronic usage

REMIFENTANIL

Trade Name:	**Ultiva**
Indications:	Adjunct for induction and maintenance of anesthesia, analgesia during local anesthesia and diagnostic procedures
Pharmacokinetics:	Onset: 30–60 sec; protein binding: 70%; Vd: 0.35 L/kg; Cl: 40 mL/kg/min; $T_{1/2}\beta$: 10–15 min; metabolized by nonspecific esterases
Pharmacodynamics:	Synthetic opioid agonist, interacts with μ-receptors
CNS:	Analgesia, sedation, tremors, acute tolerance
CV:	↓ HR, ↓ BP
GI:	Nausea, vomiting
Pulmonary:	↓ Respiratory rate, ↓ central ventilatory drive
Other:	Urinary retention, muscle rigidity, twitching, pruritus
Dosage:	0.5–2 μg/kg (induction); 0.05–0.2 μg/kg/min (maintenance)
Contraindications:	Adjunct with central neuroaxis blockade (formulation in glycine)
Drug Interactions:	↑ CNS depressant effects with sedative-hypnotics and inhaled anesthetics; no metabolic interactions with other esterase-hydrolyzed drugs (e.g., succinylcholine, mivacurium, esmolol)
Key Points:	Ultra-rapid and short-acting opioid associated with rapid development of tolerance, useful for short painful surgical procedures

SUFENTANIL

Trade Name:	**Sufenta**
Indications:	Adjunct for induction and maintenance of anesthesia
Pharmacokinetics:	Onset: 1–2 min; peak: 3–5 min; protein bound: 90%; Vd: 2.9 L/kg; Cl: 12.7 mL/kg/min; $T_{1/2}\beta$: 164 min; metabolized in liver and small intestine, excreted in urine
Pharmacodynamics:	Synthetic opioid agonist, interacts with μ-receptors in CNS

SUFENTANIL *continued*

CNS:	Analgesia, drowsiness, dizziness, depression, mood changes
CV:	↓ BP, ↓ HR
GI:	Nausea, vomiting, ↓ gastric emptying, ↑ intrabiliary pressure, ileus
GU:	Urinary retention
Pulmonary:	↓ Ventilatory rate, ↑ airway resistance, chest wall rigidity
Other:	Truncal rigidity, pruritus, ↑ ADH secretion, tolerance/physical dependence
Dosage:	0.5–5 µg/kg (induction) and 0.5–1 µg/kg/h (maintenance)
Contraindications:	NK
Drug Interactions:	Anesthetics and benzodiazepines ↑ cardiovascular and respiratory depression; anticholinergics ↑ paralytic ileus
Key Points:	Potent opioid analgesic that produces minimal cardiovascular depression; useful in hemodynamically unstable patients

TRAMADOL

Trade Names:	**Ultram, Ultracet**
Indications:	Acute and chronic pain
Pharmacokinetics:	Onset: 1 h; peak: 2 h; protein binding: 20%; duration: 4–8 h; $T_{1/2}$ β: 6–7 h; extensively metabolized, excreted in urine
Pharmacodynamics:	Synthetic analgesic; low affinity for opioid receptors, inhibits CNS reuptake of norepinephrine and serotonin
CNS:	Analgesia, dizziness, malaise, headache, mood changes, insomnia, seizures
CV:	Vasodilation, flushing
GI:	Nausea, vomiting, dyspepsia, dry mouth, constipation, anorexia
GU:	Urine retention
Pulmonary:	Respiratory depression
Other:	Diaphoresis, rash, hypertonia
Dosage:	50–100 mg PO q 4–6 prn (max. 400 mg/d)
Contraindications:	Acute alcohol intoxication; sedative-hypnotics, opioids, psychotropic drugs ↑ CNS and respiratory depression

TRAMADOL *continued*

Drug Interactions: Carbamazepine ↑ metabolism; MAOIs and neuroleptics
                          ↑ seizures

Key Points: Can prolong recovery of anesthesia and may partially
                          antagonize effects of opioid analgesics; discontinue at
                          least 24 h before surgery

36

Psychotropics

AMITRIPTYLINE, AMOXAPINE, CLOMIPRAMINE, DESIPRAMINE, DOXEPIN, IMIPRAMINE, NORTRIPTYLINE, TRIMIPRAMINE

Trade Names:	**Elavil (amitriptyline), Asedin (amoxapine), Anafranil (clomipramine), Tofranil (imipramine), Norpramin (desipramine), Aventyl, Pamelor (nortriptyline), Sinequan (doxepin), Surmontil (trimipramine)**
Indications:	Depression, enuresis, psychoneurotic anxiety, OCD, panic attack, anorexia (or bulimia), neurogenic pain
Pharmacokinetics:	Peak: 2–12 h; (amitriptyline), 0.5–2 h (imipramine), 2–4 h (desipramine, clomipramine), 7–8 h (nortryptyline), 1–2 h (amoxapine), 2 h (doxepin, trimipramine); protein binding: 92%–98%; duration: 2–4 wk; $T_{1/2}$ β: 10–50 hr; metabolized by liver (1st-pass effect) to active metabolites, excreted in urine
Pharmacodynamics:	TCAs that inhibit reuptake of neurotransmitters NE and 5-HT
CNS:	Drowsiness, confusion, disorientation, mood change; extrapyramidal symptoms, mydriasis, cycloplegia, seizures, tinnitus, ↑ IOP, peripheral neuropathy, headache, fatigue
CV:	Postural hypotension, ↑ HR, palpitations, pedal edema, angina, MI
GI:	Diarrhea, nausea, dry mouth, anorexia, constipation/ileus, ↑ LFTs
GU:	Urinary frequency (at high doses), urinary retention (at low doses)
Other:	Bone marrow suppression, hyperglycemia, diaphoresis, rash, urticaria, photosensitivity, SIADH
Dosages:	*Amitriptyline:* 75 mg/d PO (max. 300 mg), ↑ 500 mg/d, 20–30 mg IM qid; 30 mg/d (children) *Amoxapine:* 50 mg q 12 (max. 300 mg/d) *Clomipramine:* 25 mg/d, ↑ 100 mg/d (max. 250 mg/d); 25 mg/d, max. 3 mg/kg/d (children) *Desipramine:* 100–200 mg/d (max. 300 mg); 25–100 mg/d (children) *Doxepine:* 25–100 mg/d (max. 300 mg) *Imipramine:* 75–100 mg/d (max. 300 mg); 25–75 mg/d (children) *Nortriptyline:* 25 mg q 6–8 h; 30–50 mg/d (children) *Trimipramine:* 50–100 mg/d (max. 200 mg)
Contraindications:	BPH, angle-closure glaucoma, hyperthyroidism, MI, advanced heart block, use of MAOI (<14 d)

AMITRIPTYLINE, AMOXAPINE, CLOMIPRAMINE, DESIPRAMINE, DOXEPIN, IMIPRAMINE, NORTRIPTYLINE, TRIMIPRAMINE *continued*

Drug Interactions: MAOIs and TCAs can trigger hyperpyrexic crisis; ↓ effect of clonidine; ↑ effects of alcohol, hypnotics, sympathomimetic drugs; SSRI can cause serotonin syndrome; ↑ coumadin levels; ↑ cardiotoxicity of pimozide, procainamide, quinidine, disopyramide, levothyroxine; ↑ delirium with central anticholinergics

Key Points: ↑ CNS depressant effects of anesthetic and analgesic drugs; quinidine-like cardiotoxic effects ↑ arrhythmias during perioperative period; sympathomimetics can precipitate hypertensive crisis

ARIPIPRAZOLE

Trade Name: **Abilify**

Indications: Schizophrenia

Pharmacokinetics: Onset: 3–5 h; bioavailability: 87%; peak: 3–5 h; duration: 24 h; Vd: 4.9 L/kg; $T_{1/2}$ β: 75 h; metabolized by CYP to active metabolite ($T_{1/2}$ β: 94 h), excreted in urine and feces

Pharmacodynamics: Psychotropic activity at D_2 and 5-HT$_{1A}$ receptors; antagonist at 5-HT$_{2A}$ receptors

CNS: Headache, weakness, anxiety, dizziness, drowsiness, insomnia, akathisia (tardive dyskinesia), restlessness, fever, confusion, blurred vision, seizure activity

CV: Orthostatic hypotension, cardiac dysrrythmias

GI: Dysphagia, nausea, vomiting, constipation

GU: Urinary incontinence, renal failure, myoglobinuria

Pulmonary: Rhinitis, coughing

Other: Rash, asthenia, diaphoresis, thabdomyolysis (↑ CPK)

Dosage: 10–15 mg/d (max. 30 mg/d)

Contraindications: Risk of neuroleptic malignant syndrome (NMS)

Drug Interactions: Carbamazepine ↓ effect; ketoconazole, quinidine, fluoxetine, paroxetine ↑ effect

Key Points: Avoid drugs that can trigger NMS (e.g., meperidine); maintain adequate hydration and avoid "over-warming"

ATOMOXETINE

Trade Name: **Strattera**

Indications: Attention-deficit hyperactivity disorder

ATOMOXETINE *continued*

Pharmacokinetics:	Onset: <1 h; peak: 1–2 h; protein binding: 98%; duration: 5 h; Vd: 0.85 L/kg; Cl: 0.35 L/hr/kg; $T_{1/2}$ β: 5 h; extensive hepatic metabolism, excreted in urine
Pharmacodynamics:	Inhibition of presynaptic norepinephrine transporter
CNS:	Headache, somnolence, crying, irritability, aggression, mood swings, insomnia, mydriasis, fatigue
CV:	↑ HR, palpitations, ↑↓ BP, "hot flashes," chest pain
GI:	Upper abdominal pain, constipation, dyspepsia, nausea, vomiting, dry mouth, flatulence, ↓ appetite
GU:	Dysmenorrhea, impotence, prostatitis, urinary retention
Pulmonary:	Coughing, rhinorrhea
Other:	Ear infection, dermatitis, urticaria/edema, fever, rigors
Dosage:	0.5–1.2 mg/kg/d PO (max. 100 mg/d)
Contraindications:	Avoid MAOIs; narrow-angle glaucoma; breast-feeding; caution with cardiovascular diseases
Drug Interactions:	Albuterol ↑ HR, BP; fluoxetine, paroxetine, quinidine ↑ effect; ↑ effect of pressor drugs
Key Points:	Enhances cardiovascular responses to anesthetic drugs

BUPROPION

Trade Names:	**Wellbutrin, Zyban**
Indications:	Depression, smoking cessation
Pharmacokinetics:	Onset: 1 h; peak: 2 h; protein binding: 80%; duration: 8–12 h; $T_{1/2}$ β: 8–24 h; metabolized in liver, excreted in urine
Pharmacodynamics:	Mood stabilizer that inhibits NE, dopamine, and serotonin re-uptake in CNS
CNS:	Headache, seizures, anxiety, euphoria, insomnia, tremor, blurred vision
CV:	Arrhythmias
GI:	Dry mouth, ↑ appetite, constipation
GU:	Impotence, urine retention/frequency, ↓ libido
Other:	Hyperglycemia, rash, diaphoresis, photosensitivity
Dosage:	100 mg PO bid, max. 450 mg (depression); 150 mg/d for 3 d, max. 300 mg/d (smoking cessation)
Contraindications:	Seizure disorder; use of MAOIs (<14 d); anorexia nervosa
Drug Interactions:	Levodopa, MAOIs, phenothiazines, benzodiazepines, TCAs ↑ side effects
Key Points:	Avoid anesthetic drugs with stimulant properties (e.g., ketamine, etomidate, enflurane)

BUSPIRONE

Trade Name:	**BuSpar**
Indications:	Anxiety disorders, emotional lability
Pharmacokinetics:	Onset: <30 min; peak: 70 min; protein binding: 95%; duration: 8–12 h; extensive 1st-pass hepatic metabolism, excreted in urine
Pharmacodynamics:	Anxiolytic that ↓ serotonin activity; ↑ NE metabolism; presynaptic dopamine antagonist; indirect effects on GABA-chloride receptors
CNS:	Dizziness, drowsiness, insomnia, headache, blurred vision
CV:	↑ HR
GI:	Dry mouth, vomiting, anorexia
Other:	Diaphoresis
Dosage:	7.5 mg PO bid (max. 60 mg/d)
Contraindications:	Use of MAOIs (≤14 d); breast-feeding
Drug Interactions:	↑ Sedation with CNS depressants and alcohol; ↑ digoxin and haloperidol levels; grapefruit ↑ levels
Key Points:	↑ CNS depressant effects of anesthetics and ↑ residual sedation

CITALOPRAM

Trade Names:	**Celexa, Lexapro**
Indications:	Depression
Pharmacokinetics:	Onset: 1 h; bioavailability: 80%; peak: 2 h; protein binding: 80%; duration: 12–24 h;. $T_{1/2}$ β: 35 hr; metabolized by CYP enzymes to inactive metabolites, excreted in urine
Pharmacodynamics:	SSRI that ↑ CNS serotonergic activity by inhibiting neuronal reuptake of serotonin
CNS:	Somnolence, agitation, amnesia, tremor, dizziness, headache, insomnia
CV:	↑ HR, orthostatic hypotension (↓ PVR)
GI:	Dry mouth, nausea, vomiting, anorexia, ↑ appetite, constipation
GU:	Dysmenorrhea, impotence, ejaculation disorder, polyuria, ↓ libido
Pulmonary:	Cough, URI
Other:	↑ Salivation, diaphoresis, rash, pruritus, blurred vision
Dosage:	20 mg/d PO (max. 40 mg/d)
Contraindications:	Use of MAOIs (≤14 d), breast-feeding

CITALOPRAM *continued*

Drug Interactions: CNS depressants and alcohol ↑ effect; warfarin ↑ PT;
                      carbamazepine ↑ clearance; CYP inhibitors ↓ clearance;
                      lithium ↑ serotonergic effect

Key Points: ↑ Sedative effect of centrally acting anesthetic drugs

FLUOXETINE

Trade Names: **Prozac, Sarafem**

Indications: Depression, bipolar disorder (depressive phase),
                      affective mood disorder; bulimia; cataplexy,
                      obsessive-compulsive disorder

Pharmacokinetics: Onset: 1–2 h; bioavailability: 70%; peak: 6 h; protein
                      binding: 95%; duration: 24 h; Vd: 35–40 L/kg;
                      Cl: 400–600 mL/min; $T_{1/2}$ β: 48–72 h; metabolized
                      in liver, excreted in urine

Pharmacodynamics: SSRI that inhibits neuronal reuptake of serotonin in CNS
  CNS: Anxiety, headache, insomnia, nervousness, tremor,
                      somnolence
  GI: Nausea, ↑ appetite, dry mouth, ↓ libido
  Other: Rash, urticaria, hyperthyroidism, hypoglycemia,
                      hyponatremia, ↑ ACTH, ↑ corticosterone, ↑ vasopressin,
                      diaphoresis

Dosage: 5–20 mg/d PO (max. 80 mg/d) insufficiency

Contraindications: Hepatorenal impairment, use of MAOIs (≤14 d),
                      seizure disorder

Drug Interactions: MAOIs cause hyperthermia, delirium, coma, autonomic
                      instability; TCAs ↑ anticholinergic response; tryptophan
                      causes agitation, nausea, diarrhea, paresthesias; TCAs,
                      benzodiazepines, lithium ↑ ataxia and dysarthrias;
                      carbamazepine, quinidine, CYP inhibitors, warfarin,
                      St. John's Wort ↑ level

Key Points: Droperidol ↑ extrapyramidal side effects during peri-
                      operative period

LITHIUM

Trade Names: **Eskalith, Lithane, Lithonate**

Indications: Bipolar disorder, major depression, acute mania,
                      schizoaffective disorders, chronic cluster headaches

Pharmacokinetics: Onset: 5–10 d; peak: <3 wk; duration: 8–12 h; $T_{1/2}$ β:
                      20–25 h; no metabolism, excreted as unchanged drug
                      in urine

LITHIUM *continued*

Pharmacodynamics:	Mood stabilizer, competitively inhibits cations at Na$^+$-K$^+$ pump
CNS:	Lethargy, pseudotumor cerebri, ↓ neurotransmitters, epileptiform seizures, ataxia, coma, tinnitus, blurred vision, tremors
CV:	Arrhythmias, ↓ BP, ↓ HR, edema
GI:	Diarrhea, dry mouth, dyspepsia, vomiting
GU:	Nephrogenic DI, polyuria, renal tubular acidosis, ↓ renal concentrating ability
Other:	Hypothyroidism, 1° hyperparathyroidism, leukocytosis, muscular weakness, hyponatremia, pruritus, rash
Dosage:	20–30 mg/kg PO bid, then 900–1200 bid; 0.5–1.5 g/m^2 (children)
Contraindications:	Hemodialysis, pregnancy, breast-feeding
Drug Interactions:	Thiazide diuretics, antacids, aminophylline, caffeine, calcium, tetracycline, methyldopa, phenytoin, metronidazole ↑ level; ↓ effects of opiates and chlorpromazine; ↓ absorption with antacids; haloperidol ↑ side effects
Key Points:	↑ Effects of anesthetics, analgesics, muscle relaxants; avoid ketamine and enflurane due to ↑ risk of seizures; neurologic exam should precede regional nerve blocks; insure adequate fluid replacement before surgery

MIRTAZAPINE

Trade Name:	**Remeron**
Indications:	Depression
Pharmacokinetics:	Onset: <1 h; bioavailability: 50%; peak: 2 h; protein binding: 85%; duration: 24 h; T$_{1/2}$ β: 20–40 h; extensively metabolized in liver, excreted in urine
Pharmacodynamics:	TCA with antagonistic actions at 5-HT$_2$ and 5-HT$_3$ receptors
CNS:	Somnolence, dizziness, confusion
CV:	↓ BP, pedal edema
GI:	Nausea, dry mouth, ↑ appetite, constipation
GU:	Urinary frequency
Other:	Weight gain, rash, myalgia
Dosage:	15 mg/d PO hs (max. 45 mg/d)
Contraindications:	Concomitant use of MAOIs (<14 d)
Drug Interactions:	Benzodiazepines cause additive CNS depressant effects
Key Points:	↑ CNS depressant effects of anesthetics and sedatives, prolonging recovery

NEFAZODONE, TRAZODONE

Trade Names:	**Desyrel (trazodone), Serzone (nefazodone)**
Indications:	Depression, panic disorder, aggressive behavior
Pharmacokinetics:	Onset: <1 h; bioavailability: 20%; peak: 1–2 h; protein binding: 95%; duration: 12–24 h; $T_{1/2}$ β: 2–4 h; metabolized in liver (1st-pass effect), excreted in urine
Pharmacodynamics:	TCAs that inhibit neuronal uptake of serotonin and norepinephrine; antagonizes 5-HT$_2$ and α$_1$-adrenergic receptors
CNS:	Headache, somnolence, dizziness, confusion, amnesia, paresthesia, ataxia, blurred vision, tonic-clonic seizures, asthenia, insomnia
CV:	Orthostatic hypotension, vasodilation, ↑ HR, pedal edema
GI:	Dry mouth, nausea, vomiting, dyspepsia, thirst, constipation
GU:	UTI, vaginitis, urinary frequency/retention, ↓ libido
Other:	Hyponatremia, hypoatremia, arthralgia, rash, pruritus, chills
Dosages:	*Nefazodone:* 100 mg PO bid (max. 600 mg/d) *Trazodone:* 150 mg/d PO (max. 400 mg/d)
Contraindications:	Use of MAOI (<14 d), angina, acute MI
Drug Interactions:	↑ Effect of alprazolam, triazolam; MAOIs ↑ excitation and fever; ↑ digoxin and phenytoin levels; SSRIs ↑ risk of serotonin syndrome; antihypertensives, sedatives, opiates, St. John's Wort ↑ side effects
Key Points:	Chronic use prior to surgery may increase intraoperative hypotension and prolong recovery from general anesthesia

PAROXETINE, SERTRALINE

Trade Names:	**Asimia, Paxil (paroxetine); Zoloft (sertraline)**
Indications:	Major depressive disorder, panic disorder, OCD, anxiety disorders, PTSD, premature ejaculation
Pharmacokinetics:	Onset: 1 h; peak: 4–10 h (paroxetine), 5–9 h (sertraline); protein binding: 95%; duration: 24 h; $T_{1/2}$ β: 26 h (sertraline); metabolized in liver, excreted in urine and feces
Pharmacodynamics:	SSRI inhibits neuronal reuptake of serotonin, ↑ 5-HT$_2$ activity
CNS:	Somnolence, dizziness, insomnia, anxiety, headache, visual disturbances, asthenia, "restless legs"
CV:	Orthostatic hypotension (↓ PVR), ↑ HR
GI:	Dry mouth, nausea, vomiting, constipation, dyspepsia, ↑ LFTs

PAROXETINE, SERTRALINE *continued*

GU:	↓ Libido, ↓ ejaculation, urinary frequency
Other:	Diaphoresis, myalgia, pruritus, rash, NMS
Dosages:	*Paroxetine:* 10–20 mg/d PO (max. 60 mg/d) *Sertraline:* 25 mg/d PO (max. 200 mg/d)
Contraindications:	Use of MAOIs <14 d, tryptophan (↑ toxicity), sumatriptan, thioridazine
Drug Interactions:	Cimetidine, type 1C anti-arrhythmics ↑ side effects; MAOIs potentially ↑ fatal reactions; ↑ theophylline level; ↓ digoxin level; phenobarbital ↓ level; warfarin ↑ risk of bleeding; St. John's Wort ↑ risk of serotonin syndrome
Key Points:	Prolongs effects of benzodiazepines due to ↓ clearance

PHENELZINE, TRANYLCYPROMINE

Trade Names:	**Parnate (tranylcypromine), Nardil (phenelzine)**
Indications:	Depression, morbid preoccupation, psychomotor retardation
Pharmacokinetics:	Onset: <1 h; peak: 2–4 h; duration: 8–12 d; Vd: 1–6 L/kg; $T_{1/2}$ β: 2.5 h; metabolized in liver, excreted in urine
Pharmacodynamics:	MAOIs block CNS reuptake of norepinephrine and serotonin
CNS:	Headache, parkinsonian-like symptoms, vertigo, anxiety, agitation, manic symptoms, weakness, blurred vision
CV:	↑ HR, palpatations, orthostatic hypotension, pedal edema
Other:	Diaphoresis, weight gain, blood dyscrasias, ↑ LFTs
Dosages:	*Phenelzine:* 15 mg tid PO (max. 60 mg/d) *Tranylcypromine:* 10 mg tid PO (max. 60 mg/d)
Contraindications:	CHF, hepatorenal insufficiency, uncontrolled hypertension, cerebrovascular insufficiency, diabetes mellitus (DM), pheochromocytoma, Parkinson's disease, schizophrenia
Drug Interactions:	Tyramine, tryptophan, sympathomimetic, buspirone, catecholamine-releasing agents (e.g., cocaine, ephedrine, amphetamine, guanethidine) can cause hypertensive crisis, stroke, MI; ↑ effect of insulin and oral hypoglycemics; fatal reactions with concurrent TCAs (due to hypertension, fever, seizures); SSRIs cause serotonin syndrome (i.e., coma, seizures, fever); meperidine causes fever crisis, confusion, seizures; ↑ effects of anticholinergics

PHENELZINE,
TRANYLCYPROMINE *continued*

Key Points: Discontinue MAOIs at least 2 wk before elective
                            surgery requiring general anesthesia; avoid local
                            anesthetics containing epinephrine (or vasoconstrictors)
                            and hypovolemia due to diuretic therapy

VENLAFAXINE

Trade Name: **Effexor**

Indications: Depression, generalized anxiety disorder

Pharmacokinetics: Onset: 1 h; bioavailability: 92%; peak: 4–6 h; protein
                            binding: 27%; duration: 12–24 h; $T_{1/2}$ β: 5 h (11 h for
                            active metabolite); extensively metabolized in liver,
                            excreted in urine

Pharmacodynamics: Mood stabilizer that inhibits neuronal reuptake of
                            serotonin and norepinephrine, weak inhibitor of CNS
                            dopamine receptors

CNS: Headache, somnolence, dizziness, anxiety, paresthesia,
                            insomnia
CV: ↑ BP, vasodilation (↓ PVR), ↑ QT interval
GI: Dry mouth, nausea, vomiting, dyspepsia, diarrhea
GU: Impotence, abnormal ejaculation, urinary frequency
Other: Diaphoresis, weight loss, yawning

Dosage: 75 mg/d PO (max. 225 mg/d)

Contraindications: Use of MAOIs (<14 d)

Drug Interactions: Cimetidine ↑ level; St. John's Wort ↑ sedative-hypnotic
                            effects

Key Points: ↑ CNS depressant effects of anesthetic drugs, prolonging
                            recovery

37

Steroids

ANDROSTENEDIONE

Trade Name:	**Primobolan**
Other Names:	**4-Hydroxy-4-Androstenedione, androstenediol, norandrostenedione**
Indications:	↑ Muscle size and strength, ↑ libido
Pharmacokinetics:	Onset/peak/duration: NK; protein binding 90%; excreted in urine
Pharmacodynamics:	Testosterone precursor, ↑ protein anabolism, ↓ protein catabolism, stimulates production of RBCs
CNS:	Depression, anxiety, behavioral changes, headaches
GI:	Cholestatic jaundice, nausea, vomiting, ↑ LFTs
Other:	↑Cholesterol, ↓ HDL, ↓ thyroxin-binding globulin, hyperglycemia, electrolyte imbalance, water retention, polycythemia, ↓ clotting factors II, V, VII, X
Dosage:	50–200 mg/d PO
Contraindications:	Breast or prostate carcinoma, pregnancy, CHF, hepatorenal disease, use of hypoglycemic agents
Drug Interactions:	↑ Insulin dosage; ↑ bleeding with anticoagulants; ↓ thyroxine levels
Key Points:	Preoperative assessment of electrolytes, hemoglobin, PT/PTT, LFTs to minimize CV complications; avoid volatile anesthetics if ↑ LFTs

BUDESONIDE

Trade Names:	**Pulmicort, Rhinocort, Entocort**
Indications:	Allergic rhinitis, chronic asthma, active Crohn's disease
Pharmacokinetics:	Onset: <1 h; peak: 0.5–10 h; protein binding: 88%; Vd: 200 L; metabolized in liver, excreted in urine
Pharmacodynamics:	Inhibits cell types producing inflammatory mediators
CNS:	Headache
GI:	Dry mouth, dyspepsia, oral candidiasis, nausea, ↑ BP
Pulmonary:	Cough, dyspnea, nasal irritation, URI
Other:	Alopecia, acne
Dosage:	6–9 mg/d PO (Crohn's); 1–2 puffs, (200–400 μg) bid (32 μg/metered dose)
Contraindications:	Septal ulcer, nasal surgery, tuberculosis, diabetes, breast-feeding
Drug Interactions:	Prednisone ↑ hypothalamic-pituitary-adrenal suppression; CYP3A4 inhibitors ↑ toxicity; grapefruit ↑ level
Key Points:	Steroid coverage recommended during perioperative period

CLOBETASOL

Trade Names: **Clobevate, Cormex, Embeline E, Olux, Temovate**

See Chapter 22, "Dermatologic Drugs"

CORTISONE, HYDROCORTISONE, METHYLPREDNISOLONE, PREDNISOLONE, DEXAMETHASONE, BETAMETHASONE, TRIAMCINOLONE

Trade Names: **Cortone (cortisone); Diprolene, Celestone (betamethasone); Cortone, Solu-Cortef (hydrocortisone); Prelone, Delta-Cortef Cotolone (prednisolone); Decadron (dexamethasone); Azmacort, Kenacort, Kenalog (triamcinolone); Medrol, Solu-Medrol (methylprednisolone)**

Indications: Adrenal insufficiency, inflammatory/allergic reactions, immunosuppressant effects, shock, cerebral edema, tuberculous meningitis, prevention of PONV

Pharmacokinetics: Readily absorbed from GI tract; reversibly bound to corticosteroid-binding globulin and albumin; only unbound drug is pharmacologically active; crosses placenta and is distributed into breast milk, metabolized by liver, and excreted by kidneys
Cortisone: Onset: 1–2 h; peak: 24 h; duration: 48 h
Hydrocortisone: Onset: <0.5 h; peak: 1–2 h; duration: 6–12 h
Methylprednisolone: Onset: 1 h; peak: 2–3 h; duration: 30–36 h
Prednisolone: Onset: <0.5 h; peak: 1–2 h; duration: 12–36 h
Dexamethasone: Onset: <1 h; peak: 1–2 h; duration: 2–6 d
Betamethasone: Onset: <1 h; peak: 2–3 h; duration: 4–12 d
Triamcinolone: Onset: 0.5 h; peak: 1–2 h; duration: 18–36 h

Pharmacodynamics: Steroids with glucocorticoid and mineralocorticoid activity except methylprednisolone (lacks mineralocorticoid activity)

CNS: Euphoria, insomnia, psychic disturbances, vertigo, paresthesia, seizures, glaucoma, ↑ ICP, headache, ↓ hypothalamic-pituitary-adrenal axis

CV: CHF, ecchymoses, ↑ BP, arrhythmias, thromboembolism

CORTISONE, HYDROCORTISONE, METHYLPREDNISOLONE, PREDNISOLONE, DEXAMETHASONE, BETAMETHASONE, TRIAMCINOLONE *continued*

GI:	Mucosal irritation, ↑ appetite, pancreatitis, fatty liver, ↑ LFTs
Musculoskeletal:	Muscle weakness, cramps, atrophy, ↑ bone resorption/fractures
Other:	Menstrual irregularities, hypercholesterolemia, ↓ (ACTH), ↓ adrenal androgen, hyperglycemia, ↑ lipolysis, ↓ inflammation, ↓ immune responses, electrolyte disturbances, fluid retention, ↑ surfactant production
Dosages:	*Cortisone:* 25–300 mg/d or qod; 0.5–10 mg/kg/d (children) *Hydrocortisone:* 5–30 mg PO q 6–12 h; 100–500 mg IM/IV; 0.2–1 mg/kg/d (children) *Prednisolone:* 5–20 mg/d; 0.1–2 mg/kg/d (children) *Triamcinolone:* 4–12 mg/d; 1–2 puffs (50 µg/metered spray); 0.12–2 mg/kg/d (children) *Methylprednisolone:* 2–60 mg/d or 80 mg PO qod; 10–80 mg/d IM; 100–250 mg IV q 2–6 h; 0.2–2 mg/kg/d PO, 0.25–1.25 mg/m^2/d IM (children) *Betamethasone:* 0.6–1.2 mg PO q 6–8 h; 0.5–9 mg/d IM/IV 0.017–0.25 mg/kg/d (children) *Dexamethasone:* 0.25–6 mg PO q 6–12 h, 10 mg IM, then 2–4 mg IM q 6–8 h; 4–8 mg IV (antiemetic); 0.235–1.25 mg/m^2/d (children)
Contraindications:	Coagulopathy, osteoporosis, CHF, hypertension, systemic fungal infections, Cushing's syndrome
Drug Interactions:	NSAIDs and alcohol ↑ GI bleeding; amphotericin B and diuretics ↑ hypokalemia; digitalis ↑ arrhythmias; ritodine ↑ maternal pulmonary edema; antacids, cholestyramine, colestipol, barbiturates, phenytoin, rifampin ↓ levels; ↑ insulin requirement; ↓ effect of warfarin
Key Points:	Adequate steroid coverage should be performed for anticipated perioperative stress; ↓ efficacy of cholinesterase inhibitors

DANAZOL

Trade Name:	**Danocrine**
Indications:	Endometriosis, fibrocystic breast disease, hereditary angioedema

DANAZOL *continued*

Pharmacokinetics:	Onset: <1 d; peak 6–8 wk; $T_{1/2}$ β: >15 h; highly concentrated in liver, kidneys, adrenals; excreted in urine and feces
Pharmacodynamics:	Antiestrogenic and androgenic actions
CNS:	↑ ICP, dizziness, insomnia, tremor, blurred vision
CV:	↑ BP (due to volume expansion), flushing, peripheral edema
GI:	Gastric irritation, nausea, vomiting, jaundice, ↑ LFTs
GU:	↑ Creatine kinase (due to rhabdomyolysis), hematuria, vaginitis
Other:	↓ Platelets, ↑ PT, muscle cramps, hirsutism, acne, amenorrhea
Dosage:	100–400 mg PO bid for 2–6 mo
Contraindications:	Severe cardiac, hepatic and renal dysfunction, genital bleeding, pregnancy, breast-feeding, porphyria
Drug Interactions:	↑ Effects of anticoagulants; ↑ blood glucose level (due to resistance to insulin); ↑ carbamazepine and cyclosporine levels
Key Points:	Unstable perioperative glucose levels in insulin-dependent diabetics

DEHYDROEPIANDROSTERONE

Other Name:	**DHEA**
Indications:	Depression, erectile dysfunction, SLE, immune activator, menopause, memory aid, ↑ athletic performance
Pharmacokinetics:	Duration: 6–12 h; $T_{1/2}$ β: 8–11 h
Pharmacodynamics:	Anabolic steroid (↑ protein synthesis); inhibits glucose-6-phosphate
CNS:	Irritability, restlessness, headache, insomnia
CV:	Atherosclerosis, arrhythmias
GI:	Jaundice, ↑ LFTs, ↑ IGF
GU:	Hypogonadism, menstrual irregularities, gynecomastia
Other:	Hirsutism, acne, ↑ insulin requirement, ↓ platelet aggregation, ↑ Ca absorption, ↑ testosterone/estrone/estradiol/androstene
Dosage:	25–90 mg/d PO in divided doses
Contraindications:	Hormone-responsive breast, ovarian, endometrial cancers; lactation; pregnancy; BPH; endometriosis

DEHYDROEPIANDROSTERONE
continued

Drug Interactions: Synergism with corticosteroids, clonidine,
fluoxetine

Key Points: Careful monitoring of glucose levels is required in
insulin-dependent diabetics under general anesthesia
to avoid hyperglycemia

ESTRADIOL

Trade Names: **Alora, Climara, Esclim, Estrace, Vagifem, FemPatch,
Femring, Gynodiol, Valergen, Estrogel**

Indications: Estrogen deficiency, atrophic vaginitis, hypogonadism
(in females), vulvar hyperplasia, 1° ovarian failure,
vasomotor menopausal symptoms, uterine bleeding,
breast cancer, osteoporosis prophylaxis

Pharmacokinetics: Onset: 1–2 h; peak: 1–5 h; protein binding: 65%;
$T_{1/2}$ β: 13–27 h (72 h TTS); metabolized in liver,
excreted in urine

Pharmacodynamics: Mimics endogenous estrogen; inhibits hormone-sensitive
tumors
CNS: Dizziness, headache, depression, seizures
CV: Edema, angina, ↑ BP, pulmonary embolism,
thrombophlebitis
GI: Dyspepsia, cramps, bloating, nausea, vomiting,
pancreatitis, jaundice
GU: Dysmenorrhea, endometrial cancer, impotence,
testicular atrophy
Other: Hyperglycemia, hypercalcemia, gynecomastia
(breast pain), inhibited bone resorption, rash,
hirsutism (or alopecia), ↓ libido

Dosage: 1–10 mg/d PO; 30 mg IM q 2 wk; 0.05 mg/24 h TTS;
0.75 mg/d gel

Contraindications: Estrogen-dependent cancer, vaginal bleeding,
thromboembolism, pregnancy, breast-feeding

Drug Interactions: ↑ Side effects of glycocorticoids; ↓ effects of
bromocriptine and tamoxifen; ↓ metabolism of
cyclosporine (↑ toxicity); ↑ CV side effects with
smoking, ↓ effect of anticoagulants; carbamazepine,
barbiturates, phenytoin, rifampin ↓ effects; grapefruit
↑ level

Key Points: Avoid hepatotoxic anesthetic drugs with potential for
hepatotoxicity and monitor glucose levels

ETONOGESTREL-ESTRADIOL

Trade Name:	Nuva Ring
Indications:	Prevention of pregnancy (contraception)
Pharmacokinetics:	Peak: 59 h (estradiol), 200 h (etonogestrel); protein binding: 98%; $T_{1/2}$ β: 45 h (estradiol), 29 h (etonogestrel); hepatic metabolism, excreted in urine and feces
Pharmacodynamics:	Suppression of gonadotropins, inhibition of ovulation
CNS:	Depression, cerebral hemorrhage/thrombosis, migraine
CV:	Pulmonary embolism, hypertension, MI, thromboembolism
GI:	Hepatic adenomas, jaundice, nausea, vomiting, cramps
Other:	Menstrual disturbance, edema, vaginal candidiasis, weight gain, breast tenderness, dry eyes
Dosage:	0.12 mg/d estronogestrel + 0.015 mg/d estradiol for 3 wk
Contraindications:	Thrombophlebitis/thromboembolic disorders, cerebral artery disease or CAD, severe hypertension or diabetes, cholestatic jaundice, heavy smoker (>35 yr of age), hepatic tumor, hepatitis
Drug Interactions:	Same as for estradiol (e.g., antibiotics, antifungals, anticonvulsants ↑ clearance)
Key Points:	Check glucose levels and LFTs prior to surgery

FINASTERIDE

Trade Names:	Propecia, Proscar
Indications:	BPH, male pattern baldness
Pharmacokinetics:	Onset: <30 min; bioavailability: 63%; peak: 1–2 h; protein binding: 90%; metabolized by liver, excreted in urine and feces
Pharmacodynamics:	Competitively inhibits steroid 5α-reductase, ↓ androgen dihydrotestosterone
GU:	Impotence, ↓ ejaculate volume, ↓ libido
Dosage:	1–5 mg/d PO
Contraindications:	Pregnancy, children, severe hepatic impairment
Drug Interactions:	↑ Theophylline clearance (↓ effect)
Key Points:	Adjust dosage of bronchodilator prior to surgery

FLUDROCORTISONE

Trade Name:	**Florinef**
Indications:	Adrenocortical insufficiency (Addison's disease), adrenogenital syndrome, orthostatic hypotension
Pharmacokinetics:	Onset: <30 min; peak: 1.7 h; duration: 1–2 d; $T_{1/2}$ β: 3.5 h; hepatic metabolism, excreted in urine
Pharmacodynamics:	Synthetic glucocorticoid with potent mineralocorticoid activity
CV:	Arrhythmias, ↑ BP (due to ↑ intravascular volume)
GI:	Nausea, vomiting, anorexia, peptic ulcer, abdominal distention
Other:	↓ K$^+$, ↑ Na$^+$, hyperglycemia, glycosuria, water retention, muscle weakness/cramping, bruising, diaphoresis, urticaria, menstrual irregularities, cataracts
Dosage:	0.05–0.2 mg/d PO
Contraindications:	Coronary artery disease, CHF, hypertension, fungal infections
Drug Interactions:	Cardiac glycosides, amphotericin B, thiazide diuretics ↑ risk of hypokalemia and arrhythmias; barbiturates, phenytoin, rifampin ↓ effect; lithium antagonizes mineralocorticoid effect
Key Points:	Loop diuretics ↑ risk of hypokalemia; perioperative steroid coverage indicated if received drug <6 mo prior to surgery

NANDROLONE, OXANDROLONE, OXYMETHOLONE, STANOZOLOL

Trade Names:	**Anadrol (oxymetholone); Deca-Durabolin (nandrolone); Oxandrin (oxandrolone); Winstrol (stanozolol)**
Indications:	Severe trauma, anemia, breast cancer, hereditary angioedema
Pharmacokinetics:	Onset: <1 h; peak: 0.5–1.5 h (oxandrolone), 6–14 h (nandrolone); $T_{1/2}$ β: 9 h (oxandrolone), β: 6–8 d (nandrolone); duration: 24 h–2 wk; metabolized in liver, excreted in urine
Pharmacodynamics:	Inhibits hormone-responsive breast tumor and metastases; ↑ erythropoietin (kidney), ↑ RBC mass/volume; ↓ corticosteroid-induced catabolism
CV:	Pedal edema
GI:	Gastric irritation, nausea, vomiting, jaundice, ↑ LFTs
GU:	Bladder irritability, prostatic hypertrophy, hypoestrogenic and virilism (women), renal impairment, priapism

NANDROLONE, OXANDROLONE, OXYMETHOLONE, STANOZOLOL *continued*

Other:	↑ Protein anabolism, (+) nitrogen balance, ↓ glucose level, electrolyte imbalance, ↑ cholesterol, ↑ erythropoietin, ↑ hemoglobin, iron-deficiency anemia, suppression of clotting factors, muscle cramps, gynecomastia
Dosages:	*Nandrolone:* 25–200 mg/wk IM/IV *Oxandrolone:* 2.5–20 mg/d *Oxymetholone:* 1–5 mg/kg/d *Stanozolol:* 4–6 mg/d; 1–2 mg/d (children)
Contraindications:	Breast cancer, hepatic dysfunction, hypercalcemia, nephrosis, prostate cancer, breast-feeding, pregnancy
Drug Interactions:	↑ Effects of warfarin; ↑ hypoglycemia with insulin and sulfonylureas
Key Points:	Glucose level and electrolyte status should be carefully evaluated preoperatively in insulin-dependent diabetics receiving steroids

PROGESTERONE, MEDROXYPROGESTERONE, MEGESTROL, NORETHINDRONE, NORGESTREL

Trade Names:	**Aygestin, Amen, Crinone (progesterone), Provera, Depo-Provera (medroxy progesterone), Megace (megestrol), Micronor, Aygestin (norethindrone), Ovrette (norgestrel)**
Indications:	Amenorrhea, dysfunctional uterine bleeding, corpus luteum insufficiency, endometriosis, contraception, cachexia
Pharmacokinetics:	Onset/peak/duration: highly variable; $T_{1/2}$ β: 5–14 h; metabolized in liver, excreted in feces and urine
Pharmacodynamics:	Suppress ovulation, thicken cervical mucus, endometrial sloughing
CNS:	Headache, somnolence, CVA, depression
CV:	Thrombophlebitis/embolism, pulmonary embolism, edema
GI:	Nausea, vomiting, jaundice
GU:	Menstrual irregularity, nocturia, ↓ sodium reabsorption
Pulmonary:	↑ Ventilation, respiratory alkalosis

PROGESTERONE, MEDROXYPROGESTERONE, MEGESTROL, NORETHINDRONE, NORGESTREL *continued*

Other:	↑ Lipoprotein lipase, ↑ fat deposition, ↑ basal insulin, ↑ insulin response to glucose, breast tenderness, ↑ amino acids, hyperglycemia, galactorrhea, ↑ breast cancer, rash, pruritis, muscle weakness, ↑ glycogen storage, ↑ ketogenesis
Dosages:	*Medroxyprogesterone:* 5–10 mg/d; 500–1000 mg/wk IM *Megestrol:* 100–600 mg (cachexia); 40–80 mg PO qid *Norethindrone:* 0.35 mg/d (OCP); 2.5–10 mg/d (endometriosis) *Norgestrel:* 0.075 mg/d PO *Progesterone:* 5–10 mg/d IM
Contraindications:	Breast or reproductive organ cancer, severe hepatic dysfunction, thromboembolic disorders, pregnancy, vaginal bleeding
Drug Interactions:	↓ Effects of bromocriptine (amenorrhea/galactorrhea)
Key Points:	CNS depressant effects (analogous to pregnancy) can ↓ IV and volatile anesthetic requirements

TESTOSTERONE, METHYLTESTOSTERONE, FLUOXYMESTERONE

Trade Names:	**Andro, Testred (methyltestosterone); Halotestin (fluoxymesterone); Delatestryl, Testopel, Testoderm TTS, Virilon (testosterone)**
Indications:	Androgen deficiency, delayed male puberty, breast cancer, male hypogonadism, menopause-related vasomotor symptoms, postpartum breast engorgement
Pharmacokinetics:	Onset: <1 h; peak: 1–2 h; protein binding: 99%; duration: 9–24 h; $T_{1/2}$ β: longer with synthetics (fluoxymesterone, methyltestosterone); metabolized in liver (1st-pass effect), excreted in urine
Pharmacodynamics:	Endogenous androgen, promotes growth and development of male sexual organs and secondary characteristics, inhibits antiestrogenic effects on hormone-responsive breast tumors
CNS:	Headache, dizziness, anxiety, depression, paresthesia, fatigue
CV:	Peripheral edema
GI:	Nausea, vomiting, jaundice, ↑ LFTs

TESTOSTERONE,
METHYLTESTOSTERONE,
FLUOXYMESTERONE *continued*

GU:	Bladder irritability, prostatic hypertrophy, hypoestrogenic effects (in women), priapism, gynecomastia
Other:	Hypoglycemia, electrolyte imbalances, ↑ erythropoietin (↑ RBC mass), leukopenia, ↓ clotting factors, muscle cramps, hirsuitism, male pattern baldness, acne
Dosages:	*Fluoxymesterone:* 2–20 mg PO q 6–24 h (male); 10–40 mg/d (cancer); 2–5 mg/d (females) *Methyltestosterone:* 10–50 mg/d IM *Testosterone:* 10–25 mg IM qod; 25–400 mg IM q 3 wk; 5 mg TTS/24 h
Contraindications:	Breast and prostate cancer, hypercalcemia, severe cardiac, hepatic or renal impairment, pregnancy, breast-feeding
Drug Interactions:	Anticoagulants, ↑ PT (and INR); insulin, ↑ hypoglycemia
Key Points:	Carefully monitor glucose and electrolyte levels

38

Substance Abuse

ALCOHOL

Other Names:	**Booze, "small carbon fragments"**
Pharmacokinetics:	Onset: 30 min; peak: 1–2 h; duration: 2–4 h; $T_{1/2}$ β: 2–3 h; metabolized by alcohol dehydrogenase in liver ($\downarrow$ in women)
Pharmacodynamics:	Prolongation of $GABA_A$ activity, activation of dopamine neurons in mesolimbic system, inhibits NMDA receptor
CNS:	Somnolence, disinhibition, Wernicke-Korsakoff encephalopathy, DTs
CV:	$\uparrow$ BP, cardiomyopathy
GI:	Cirrhosis, alcoholic hepatitis, pancreatitis, gastric or duodenal ulcer, esophageal varices
Pulmonary:	Respiratory depression
Other:	Diabetes, erectile dysfunction, pernicious anemia, vitamin deficiencies, gynecomastia
Dosage:	1.5–4.5 fl oz
Contraindications:	Hepatic dysfunction, use of disulirm, concurrent use of CNS depressant drugs
Drug Interactions:	Didanosine $\uparrow$ risk of fatal pancreatitis; ecstasy $\uparrow$ risk of death; chronic alcohol consumption $\uparrow$ risk of liver damage with acetaminophen and halogenated (volatile) anesthetics; $\uparrow$ side effects with furazolidone, griseofulvin, metronidazole; $\downarrow$ levels warfarin, isoniazid, tolbutamide, rifampin; $\uparrow$ level of TCAs, warfarin, phenytoin; $\uparrow$ sedation effect with antihistamines, benzodiazepines, opioids
Key Points:	Therapeutic aids include disulfiram and naltrexone; β-blockers, α_2-agonists, benzodiazepines are used to treat withdrawal symptoms; acute intoxication considered as "full stomach" with reflux prophylaxis and rapid-sequence induction technique; polyneuropathy is relative contraindication to regional anesthesia; premedication with clonidine patch may prevent DTs; $\uparrow$ volatile anesthetic requirement in chronic alcoholics

CANNABIS, HASHISH, MARIJUANA, TETRAHYDROCANNABINOL (THC)

Trade Name:	**Ceramet, Nabilone**
Other Names:	**Grass, hash, herb, dope, ganja, kif, kind bud, Mary Jane, pot, reefer, skunk, weed**
Indications:	Chemotherapy-induced nausea and vomiting, HIV-induced cachecia

CANNABIS, HASHISH, MARIJUANA, TETRAHYDROCANNABINOL (THC) *continued*

Pharmacokinetics: Onset: <1 h; peak: 1–2 h; duration: 3–6 h; $T_{1/2}$ β: 30 h

Pharmacodynamics: Stimulates CB_1 and CB_2 cannabinoid receptors ($\downarrow$GABA, $\uparrow$ serotonin)

CNS: Sedation, mood changes, hallucinations, impaired motor coordination, conjunctival injection

CV: $\uparrow$ HR, $\uparrow$ BP, $\uparrow$ myocardial O_2 demand

GI: Dry mouth, $\uparrow$ appetite

Pulmonary: Bronchospasm (if inhaled)

Dosage: 1–2 mg/d PO

Contraindications: Severe hepatic impairment, pregnancy, breast-feeding

Drug Interactions: $\uparrow$ Sedative effect of barbiturates; protease inhibitors $\downarrow$ efficacy; cocaine $\uparrow$ CV side effects ($\uparrow$ HR)

Key Points: Acute intoxication $\downarrow$ anesthetic requirement; impairs learning and memory

COCAINE

Other Names: **Crack, nose candy, snow, rock, blow, devil's dandruff, Colombian marching powder, flake**

Pharmacokinetics: Onset: <1 min; bioavailability: 40%; peak: 2–5 min; duration: 0.5–1 h; Vd: 1.5–2 L/kg; Cl: 20–30 mL/min/kg; $T_{1/2}$ β: 6–8 h; metabolized by plasma and hepatic cholinesterase, excreted in urine

Pharmacodynamics: Blocks catecholamine (dopamine) reuptake, local anesthetic action due to Na^+ channel blockade, $\downarrow$ nerve conduction velocity

CNS: Excitation, hyperactivity, psychosis, hallucinations (nightmares), dyskinesia, mydriasis, convulsions, cerebral hemorrhage, psychological dependence, local analgesia

CV: $\uparrow$ HR, $\uparrow$ contractility, $\uparrow$ BP, arrhythmias, coronary vasoconstriction, angina, MI

GI: $\downarrow$ Appetite, abdominal pain, nausea, vomiting

GU: Placenta previa, abruptio placentae, premature labor

Pulmonary: Wheezing pulmonary edema, pneumomediastinum

Other: Fever, chills, diaphoresis, mucosal ulcerations

Dosage: 1–4 mL of solution (max. 3 mg/kg)

Contraindications: Sensitivity to ester-type local anesthetics

COCAINE *continued*

Drug Interactions:	β-blockers ↑ coronary vasoconstriction; ketamine and MAOIs ↑ CV toxicity; prolonged paralysis with succinylcholine; SSRIs ↑ risk of serotonin syndrome; caffeine and theophylline ↑ risk of seizures
Key Points:	Acute intoxication ↑ anesthetic requirement; sensitizes myocardium to catecholamine; sympathomimetics and volatile anesthetics ↑ arrhythmias and CV instability

GAMMA HYDROHYBUTYRATE (GHB)

Other Names:	**Fantasy, soap, liquid ecstasy, "date rape" drug, nature's quaalude, blue nitro, gamma G, vita-G, wolfies**
	See Chapter 29, "Intravenous Anesthetics and Sedatives"

HEROIN

Other Names:	**Smack, black tar, brown sugar, horse, junk, skag**
Pharmacokinetics:	Onset: <2 min; peak: <5 min; $T_{1/2}$ β: 5–10 min; metabolized in liver to active metabolites (morphine), excreted in urine and feces
Pharmacodynamics:	Activates μ-opioid receptor, ↑ dopaminergic transmission in limbic system, rapidly converted into morphine
CNS:	Euphoria, analgesia, drowsiness, tolerance/physical and psychological dependence, miosis, profound analgesia
CV:	↓ HR, ↓ BP
GI:	Nausea, vomiting, constipation
GU:	Premature ejaculation
Pulmonary:	Cough suppression, respiratory depression
Drug Interactions:	Protease inhibitors ↓ potency; cocaine ↑ risk of death; benzodiazepines, sedative-hypnotics, alcohol ↑ risk of CNS, respiratory and CV depression
Key Points:	A high-soluble prodrug of morphine with extremely high addition (abuse) potential; clonidine ↓ side effects associated with withdrawal

KETAMINE

Other Names:	**Special K, angel dust, bump, psychedelic heroin**
	See Chapter 29, "Intravenous Anesthetics and Sedatives"

LSD, MESCALINE, MUSHROOMS

Other Names:	**Acid, sugar cubes (LSD), buttons, beans (mescaline); blotter, microdot, tabs, trips, pallocylin, los niños (mushrooms)**
Pharmacokinetics:	Onset: <30 min; duration: 8–12 h (LSD, mescaline); 6–8 h (mushrooms); $T_{1/2}$ β: 110 min (LSD); metabolized in liver, excreted into bile (LSD) and urine (mescaline)
Pharmacodynamics:	Partial agonist activity at postsynaptic 5-HT receptors
CNS:	Anxiety, paranoia, tremor, depersonalization, visual illusion/hallucinations, mydriasis, flashbacks, seizures
CV:	↑ BP, ↑ HR, angina
Other:	Hyperthermia, rhabdomyalysis, myalgias, diaphoresis, uterine contractions, nausea
Drug Interactions:	SSRIs ↑ risk of serotonin syndrome, marijuana and ecstasy (MDMA) ↑ risk of seizures
Key Points:	Accentuates ketamine's psychomimetic activity and ↑ risk of seizures; ↑ confusion and disorientation after anesthesia

METHAMPHETAMINE

Other Names:	**Speed, crank, chalk, croak, grypto, crystal, glass, ice, meth, speedup, fast, whiz, white cross**
Pharmacokinetics:	Onset: 1–2 min (IV), 3 min (inhaled), 15–20 min (oral); $T_{1/2}$ β: 10–30 h; excreted unchanged in urine
Pharmacodynamics:	Blocks reuptake of NE and DA, weak MAO inhibitor
CNS:	Excitation, hyperactivity, mydriasis, psychosis, hallucinations (nightmares), dyskinesias, aggressive behavior
CV:	↑ HR, ↑ BP, arrhythmias, angina, MI, cardiomyopathy
Metabolic:	Fever, dehydration, ↓ appetite
Drug Interactions:	↓ Effect of antihypertensive drugs; protease inhibitors ↑ CNS effects; cocaine, MDMA, MAOIs ↑ cardiac arrhythmias; sympathomimetics ↑ BP
Key Points:	Use with volatile anesthetics ↑ risk of arrhythmias and hemodynamic instability

METHYLENEDIOXY-*N*-METHYLAMPHETAMINE (MDMA)

Other Names:	**Ecstasy, Adam, bean, roll, X**
Pharmacokinetics:	Onset: <1 h; peak: 2–3 h; duration: 4–6 h; metabolized in liver by CYP isoenzyme, excreted in urine
Pharmacodynamics:	Amphetamine-like hallucinogen, destroys serotonin neurons in CNS
CNS:	Impulsiveness, memory gaps, hallucinations, confusion, paranoia, nystagmus, blurred vision
CV:	↑ BP, ↑ HR
Other:	Sexual enhancement, muscle tension, nausea, sweating, hyperthermia
Drug Interactions:	Protease inhibitors ↑ CNS effects; SSRIs ↑ risk of serotonin syndrome; MAOIs and PCP ↑ arrhythmias and seizures
Key Points:	Ketamine can produce serious arrhythmias and seizure activity

PHENCYCLIDINE (PCP)

Other Names:	**Angel dust, ozone, wack**
Pharmacokinetics:	Onset: <10 min; peak: 30–60 min; $T_{1/2}$ β: 2–3 d; highly lipid soluble; metabolized in liver, excreted in urine
Pharmacodynamics:	NMDA antagonist, ↓ influx of Ca ions, ↑ dopaminergic activity
CNS:	Confusion, excitement, nystagmus, paranoia, hallucinations, seizures, ataxia, hyperacusis, unpredictable violence, ↓ response to painful stimuli (analgesic-like)
CV:	↑ HR, ↑ BP, angina, MI
GI:	↑ Salivation
Pulmonary:	Respiratory depression
Other:	Rabdomyalysis, muscle rigidity, fever, renal failure
Drug Interactions:	Alcohol, sedative-hypnotics, MDMA and cocaine ↑ side effects
Key Points:	A structural analog of ketamine with less sedative-hypnotic but greater psychomimetic properties

39

Vasodilators

AMRINONE, INAMRINONE

Trade Name:	Inocor
Indications:	CHF
Pharmacokinetics:	Onset: <5 min (IV); peak: 10 min; protein binding: 35%; Vd: 1.2 L/kg; $T_{1/2}$ β: 3.6 h; metabolized in liver, excreted in urine
Pharmacodynamics:	Inhibits phosphodiesterase, ↑ myocardial cAMP, arrhythmogenic properties
CV:	Vasodilator, (+) inotrope, ↓ LVEDP, ↓ BP, ↓ PCWP, angina, arrhythmias
GI:	Nausea, vomiting, diarrhea, anorexia, abdominal pain, ↑ LFTs, thrombocytopenia, fever
Dosage:	0.75 mg/kg IV; 5–10 µg/kg/min maintenance infusion (max. 10 mg/kg/d)
Contraindications:	Liver disease, severe thrombocytopenia, obstructive cardiomyopathy (e.g., IHSS), bisulfite allergic
Drug Interactions:	↑ Inotropic activity of cardiac glycosides; ↑ hypotension with disopyramide; incompatible with dextrose and furosemide
Key Points:	Volatile anesthetics, sympathomimetics, cardiac glycosides ↑ arrhythmias; mix with saline and protect from light

AMYL NITRATE, ISOSORBIDE

Trade Names:	Coronex, Novosorbide, Sorbitrate
Indications:	Angina, adjunct in cyanide poisoning (amyl nitrate)
Pharmacokinetics:	*Amyl nitrate:* Onset: <30 sec; peak: 1–2 min; duration: 3–5 min *Isosorbide:* Onset: <60 sec; peak: 2–3 min; duration: 0.5–6 min; $T_{1/2}$ β: 5 h; metabolized in liver, excreted in urine
Pharmacodynamics:	Vascular smooth muscle relaxation, peripheral vasodilation
CNS:	Headache (throbbing), dizziness, weakness, syncope
CV:	Orthostatic hypotension, tachycardia, flushing, ↑ BP
GI:	Nausea, vomiting
Other:	Cutaneous vasodilation, methemoglobinemia (amyl nitrate)
Dosages:	*Amyl nitrate:* 0.3 mL per inhalation, repeat 5–10 min *Isosorbide:* 20 mg bid; 30–60 mg/d ER (max. 120 mg/d)
Contraindications:	Pregnancy, severe anemia, angle-closure glaucoma, ↑ ICP, shock

AMYL NITRATE, ISOSORBIDE *continued*

Drug Interactions:	Antihypertensives, phenothiazines, alcohol ↑ hypotension
Key Points:	Use with general anesthetics and major central neuroaxis blockade may result in profound intraoperative hypotension

DIAZOXIDE

Trade Names:	**Hyperstat, Proglycem**
Indications:	Hypertensive crisis, hypoglycemia (due to hyperinsulinism)
Pharmacokinetics:	Onset: 1 min (IV), 1 h (oral); protein binding: >90%; duration: 2–12 h (IV); $T_{1/2}$ β: 30 h; metabolized by liver, excreted in urine
Pharmacodynamics:	Directly relaxes arteriolar smooth muscle, ↓ pancreatic insulin secretion
CNS:	Tinnitus, headache, extrapyramidal symptoms, confusion
CV:	Arteriolar vasodilation (↓ PVR), ↓ BP, ↑ HR
GU:	Nephrotic syndrome, Na^+ and H_2O retention, hematuria
Other:	Thrombocytopenia, thrombosis, hyperglycemia, ketoacidosis, hirsuitism, paresthesias, ↑ CO, pedal edema, angina, acute MI
Dosage:	1–3 mg/kg PO tid; 1–5 mg/kg IV q 5–15 min, 3–15 mg/kg IV bid
Contraindications:	Hypertension (coarctation or AV shunt), sensitive to sulfonamides
Drug Interactions:	↑ Effects of warfarin; droperidol and physostigmine can ↑ parkinsonian-like syndrome; α- and β-blockers and diuretics ↑ hypotensive effects; corticosteroids ↑ hyperglycemic effects
Key Points:	Vasoactive drugs, general anesthetics, acute intraoperative blood loss ↑ hypotensive effects; carefully monitor perioperative glucose levels

DIPYRIDAMOLE

Trade Names:	**Aggrenox, Persantine**
Indications:	Prevention of thromboembolic complications, inhibition of platelet adhesion with prostatic heart valves, coronary perfusion imaging
Pharmacokinetics:	Onset: <30 min; bioavailability: 43%; peak: 75 min; protein binding: 94%; duration: 6–24 h; Cl: 2.3–3.5 mL/min; $T_{1/2}$ β: 1–2 h; metabolized in liver, excreted in feces

DIPYRIDAMOLE *continued*

Pharmacodynamics:	Coronary vasodilator and platelet adhesion inhibitor, inhibits serum adenosine deaminase, phosphodiesterase, thromboxane A_2
CNS:	Headache, dizziness
CV:	Flushing, orthostatic hypotension, $\uparrow$ HR, chest pain
GI:	Nausea, vomiting, diarrhea
Other:	$\uparrow$ Bleeding time, rash, pruritus
Dosage:	75–100 mg PO qid (prosthetic valve); 150–400 mg/d (thromboembolic); 0.142 mg/kg/min IV over 4 min (imaging)
Contraindications:	NK
Drug Interactions:	$\uparrow$ Level of adenosine, $\uparrow$ anticoagulant effects of heparin, $\downarrow$ effects of cholinesterase inhibitors, aminophylline $\downarrow$ effects
Key Points:	Use with general anesthetic and major regional anesthetic techniques $\uparrow$ hypotension; check bleeding time before surgery and epidural block procedures

FENOLDOPAM

Trade Name:	**Corlopam**
Indications:	Severe (malignant) hypertension
Pharmacokinetics:	Onset: <1 min; peak: 2–3 min; duration: <30 min (after infusion); $T_{1/2}$ β: 5–10 min; hepatic metabolism, excreted in urine
Pharmacodynamics:	Rapid-acting vasodilator (R-isomer), agonist at D_1-like dopamergic receptors and α_2-adrenoreceptors
CNS:	Headache, $\uparrow$ IOP
CV:	$\uparrow$ HR, $\downarrow$ BP, arrhythmias
Other:	Hypokalemia, $\uparrow$ BUN/Cr
Dosage:	0.025–1.6 µg/kg/min IV infusion
Contraindications:	Pregnancy, breast-feeding, allergic to sulfites
Drug Interactions:	Use with antihypertensives $\uparrow$ hypotension
Key Points:	$\uparrow$ Vasodilation produced by propofol and volatile anesthetics $\uparrow$ hypotension

HYDRALAZINE

Trade Name:	**Apresoline**
Indications:	Hypertension, controlled hypotension during anesthesia, CHF

HYDRALAZINE *continued*

Pharmacokinetics:	Onset: 10–15 min (IV), 20–30 min (oral); peak: 30–60 min; protein binding: 82%; duration: 2–6 h (IV), 4–6 h (oral); $T_{1/2}$ β: 3–7 h; metabolized in GI mucosa and liver, excreted in urine
Pharmacodynamics:	Direct vasodilating effect on vascular smooth muscle
CNS:	↑ ICP, headache, dizziness, peripheral neuritis (paresthesia)
CV:	Orthostatic hypotension (due to ↓ SVR), ↑ HR, ↑ CO, angina
GI:	Anorexia, nausea, vomiting, diarrhea, ↑ LFTs
Pulmonary:	↓ PVR, ↓ PCWP, ↑ pulmonary V̇/Q̇ mismatch
Other:	Blood dyscrasias, ↑ renin activity, Na^+ and H_2O retention, pedal edema, lacrimation, muscle spasms, lupus-like syndrome, rash
Dosage:	5–20 mg IV boluses; 10–50 mg PO qid
Contraindications:	SLE, CAD, rheumatic valvular heart disease
Drug Interactions:	↑ Hypotensive effects of other antihypertensive drugs; ↓ bioavailability in rapid acetylators; ↓ effect of epinephrine
Key Points:	Use with general anesthesia and central neuroaxis blockade ↑ hypotension; neurological exam required prior to major peripheral nerve blocks

MECAMYLAMINE

Trade Name:	**Inversine**
Indications:	Hypertension
Pharmacokinetics:	Onset: <30 min; peak 1–2 h; duration: 6–12 h; crosses blood-brain and placental barriers; excreted unchanged in urine
Pharmacodynamics:	Ganglionic-blocking drug
CNS:	Drowsiness, hallucinations, tremor, dizziness, blurred vision
CV:	Orthostatic hypotension (↓ SVR), ↓ cardiac output, syncope
GI:	Dry mouth, constipation, nausea, vomiting, anorexia
Other:	Impotence, glaucoma, interstitial pulmonary fibrosis, urinary retention
Dosage:	5–25 mg/d PO in divided doses
Drug Interactions:	↓ Effect of neostigmine and pyridostigmine in myasthenia gravis; low urine pH ↑ excretion, high urine pH ↓ excretion
Contraindications:	Acute MI, uremia, glaucoma, pyloric stenosis

MECAMYLAMINE *continued*

Key Points: ↑ Hypotensive effect of volatile anesthetics and spinal
                          anesthesia if volume-depleted

MINOXIDIL

Trade Name: **Loniten**

Indications: Hypertension, hair-growth stimulant (topical)

Pharmacokinetics: Onset: 0.5 h; peak: 1 h; duration: 24 h; $T_{1/2}$ β: 2–3 h;
                          metabolized in liver, excreted in urine

Pharmacodynamics: Direct vasodilating effect on vascular smooth muscle
  CV: ↓ BP (due to ↓ SVR), ↑ HR, ↑ CO, ↑ CBF, angina,
                          pedal edema
  CV: Headache, paresthesias
  GI: Nausea, vomiting
  GU: Na^+ and H_2O retention, ↑ renin secretion
  Pulmonary: Pulmonary hypertension
  Other: Hypertrichosis, rash, Stevens-Johnson syndrome, glucose
                          intolerance, thrombocytopenia, breast tenderness

Dosage: 2.5–40 mg/d PO in divided doses

Contraindications: Pheochromocytoma, dissecting aortic aneurysm, acute MI

Drug Interactions: Diuretics prevent fluid retention; nitrates and
                          antihypertensive drugs ↑ hypotensive effect;
                          guanethidine ↑ orthostatic hypotension

Key Points: Use before general anesthesia (or spinal block) can
                          cause marked intraoperative hypotensive responses
                          in volume-depleted patients

MILRINONE

Trade Name: **Primacor**

Indications: CHF

Pharmacokinetics: Onset: 5–15 min; peak: 1–2 h; protein binding: 70%;
                          duration: 3–6 h; Vd: 0.38 L/kg; $T_{1/2}$ β: 2–3 h; excreted
                          unchanged in urine

Pharmacodynamics: Selective inhibition of cAMP phosphodiesterase
                          (peak III inhibitor) and vasodilation
  CNS: Headaches, tremor
  CV: ↓ BP, (+) inotrope, ↓ PCWP, angina, SVT
  Other: Pulmonary vasodilator, thrombocytopenia, ↓ K^+

Dosage: 50 µg/kg (slowly over 10 min), maintenance infusion of
                          0.4–0.75 µg/kg/min (max. 1.1 mg/kg/d)

MILRINONE *continued*

Drug Interactions: Furosemide precipitates when injected with milrinone

Key Points: If used for >48 h without improvement in CHF symptoms, ↑ risk of death

NICARDIPINE

Trade Name: Cardene

See Chapter 19, "Calcium Channel Blockers"

NITRIC OXIDE

Other Name: NO

Indications: Pulmonary hypertension (after cardiac surgery), ARDS, COPD, pulmonary embolism, lung transplantation

Pharmacokinetics: Inhaled NO becomes nitrates and nitrite, excreted in urine

Pharmacodynamics: EDRF activates guanylate cyclase in lung (↑ cGMP), relaxing vascular smooth muscle
CV: ↑ LV filling pressure, ↓ PAP, ↓ PVR, ↓ CVP
Pulmonary: Pulmonary vasodilation, rebound hypoxemia
Other: ↑ Bleeding time, H_2O intoxication, methemoglobinemia

Dosage: 6–20 ppm

Contraindications: Severe heart failure

Drug Interactions: Phosphodiesterase inhibitors (e.g., dipyridamole) ↑ sensitivity

Key Points: Invasive cardiovascular monitoring and determination of met-Hb levels are necessary to prevent side effects during treatment

NITROGLYCERIN (NTG)

Trade Names: Tridil, Nitrogard, Nitroglyn, Transderm-Nitro, Nitro-Bid

Indications: Angina, MI, hypertension, CHF, "controlled" hypotension

Pharmacokinetics: Onset: 1 min (IV); 1–3 min (SL), 30 min (ointment), 25–45 min (oral ER); duration: 3–5 min (IV), 30–60 min (sublingual), 4–8 h (ointment); 8–12 h (oral ER); metabolized in liver and plasma (oral undergoes 1st-pass metabolism), excreted in urine

Pharmacodynamics: Peripheral vasodilator, relaxes vascular smooth muscle
CNS: ↑ ICP, headache, dizziness

NITROGLYCERIN (NTG) *continued*

CV:	Orthostatic hypotension ($\downarrow$ SVR), $\uparrow$ HR (reflex), flushing
GU:	Impotence, dysuria
Pulmonary:	$\downarrow$ PVR, $\downarrow$ PCWP, $\uparrow$ pulmonary $\dot{V}/\dot{Q}$ mismatch
Other:	Methemoglobinemia, rash, nausea, vomiting
Dosage:	0.5–10 µg/kg/min infusion; 1.3–6.5 mg PO ER q 12 h; 0.15–0.6 mg SL, repeat q 5–10 min; 15–30 mg 2% ointment (0.6 mg/h)
Contraindications:	Severe hypovolemia, allergic to organic nitrates, acute MI, severe anemia, $\uparrow$ ICP, angle-closure glaucoma, restrictive cardiomyopathy
Drug Interactions:	$\uparrow$ Hypotensive effects of anesthetic drugs, alcohol and antihypertensives; $\downarrow$ effect of heparin; ergot alkaloids $\uparrow$ angina
Key Points:	Use with general or spinal anesthesia and uncompensated blood loss can produce severe hypotension (shock)

NITROPRUSSIDE

Trade Names:	**Nipride, Nitropress**
Indications:	Hypertensive emergencies, acute CHF, "controlled" hypotension
Pharmacokinetics:	Onset: 0.5–1 min; peak: 2–3 min; duration: 5–10 min; metabolized rapidly to cyanide, which is converted to thiocyanate in liver, excreted in urine
Pharmacodynamics:	Peripheral vasodilation via direct vascular smooth muscle relaxation
CNS:	$\uparrow$ CBF, $\uparrow$ ICP, headache, dizziness
CV:	$\downarrow$ SVR, $\downarrow$ BP, $\uparrow$ HR (reflex), rebound $\uparrow$ BP, flushing
Pulmonary:	$\downarrow$ PVR, $\downarrow$ PCWP, $\uparrow$ pulmonary $\dot{V}/\dot{Q}$ mismatch
Other:	Acidosis, methemoglobinemia, hypothyroidism, cyanide toxicity, "pink" color, rash, diaphoresis, muscle twitching
Dosage:	0.5–5 µg/kg/min (max. 10 µg/kg/min)
Contraindications:	Congenital (Leber's) optic atrophy, amblyopia, compensatory hypertension (with coarctation or AV shunting), severe hypovolemia
Drug Interactions:	$\uparrow$ Hypotensive effect with antihypertensive drugs
Key Points:	Use with general or spinal anesthesia $\uparrow$ intraoperative hypotension; treat overdosage (toxicity) by giving nitrites to induce methemoglobin formation; protect from UV light

PAPAVERINE

Trade Names:	**Pavabid, Pavagen**
Indications:	Peripheral vascular disease, angina, cerebral ischemia, arteriospasm, impotence
Pharmacokinetics:	Onset: 1–2 h; bioavailability: 54%; peak: 1–2 h; protein binding: 90%; duration: 6–12 h; $T_{1/2}$ β: 12–24 h; metabolized by liver, excreted in urine
Pharmacodynamics:	Relaxes smooth muscle by inhibiting phosphodiesterase
CNS:	Headache, drowsiness, vertigo, sedation
CV:	↑ HR, ↑ BP, ↓ intraventricular conduction, arrhythmias
GI:	Nausea, anorexia, jaundice, ↑ LFTs
Other:	Eosinophilia, rash, diaphoresis, flushing, priapism
Dosage:	150–300 mg PO q 8–12 h, or 30–120 mg IM/IV q 3 h 6 mg/kg/d (children)
Contraindications:	Parkinson's disease, advanced heart block
Drug Interactions:	CNS depressants ↑ CV effects; heavy smoking ↓ therapeutic effect; droperidol and physostigmine ↑ risk of Parkinson's syndrome
Key Points:	↑ CNS depressant effects of anesthetics and opioid analgesics; volatile or spinal anesthesia ↑ intraoperative hypotension

SILDENAFIL

Trade Name:	**Viagra**
	See Chapter 33, "Miscellaneous Compounds"

TADALAFIL

Trade Name:	**Cialis**
	See Chapter 33, "Miscellaneous Compounds"

TRIMETHAPHAN

Trade Name:	**Arfonad**
Indications:	Intraoperative blood pressure control, controlled hypotension
Pharmacokinetics:	Onset: 1–3 min; peak: 3–5 min; duration: 10 min; urinary excretion

TRIMETHAPHAN *continued*

Pharmacodynamics:	Ganglionic blocker
CV:	Orthostatic hypotension (↓ SVR), ↓ CO, ↑ HR, angina
GI:	Dry mouth, constipation/ileus, nausea, vomiting, anorexia
Other:	Urinary retention, cycloplegia, pruritus, urticaria
Dosage:	0.5–6.0 mg/min infusion
Contraindications:	Severe arteriosclerotic cardiovascular disease
Drug Interactions:	Inhibits plasma pseudocholinesterase, prolongs clinical effects of plasma esterase metabolized drugs
Key Points:	Prolongs muscle paralysis with succinylcholine and mivacurium, ↑ hypotensive effects of anesthetic and analgesic drugs

VARDENAFIL

Trade Name:	**Levitra**
	See Chapter 33, "Miscellaneous Compounds"

40

Vitamins

ASCORBIC ACID (VITAMIN C)

Trade Names:	**Ascorbicap, Cecon, Cendate, Cetane, Cevalin, Flavorcee**
Indications:	Scurvy, malnutrition (e.g., alcoholism, ileal resection, gastrectomy), adjunctive therapy for idiopathic methemoglobinemia, common cold prophylaxis
Pharmacokinetics:	Rapidly absorbed (jejunum); hepatic metabolism, excreted in urine
Pharmacodynamics:	Collagen formation, tissue repair, ↑ cellular metabolism
CNS:	Dizziness, fatigue, headache
GI:	Diarrhea, nausea, vomiting, cramps
GU:	Acid urine, oxaluria, renal calculi
Dosage:	50–250 mg/d PO; 35–45 mg/d (children)
Contraindications:	NK
Drug Interactions:	↑ Tubular reabsorption of acidic medications; ↓ GI absorption of anticoagulants (↓ PT); ↑ iron toxicity (deferoxamine), ↓ effect of basic drugs (e.g., amphetamines, TCAs); smoking ↓ drug level
Key Points:	Check coagulation status if concurrent use with coumadin products

BETA-CAROTENE

Trade Name:	**Solatene**
Indications:	Photosensitivity reactions, retinal adaptation to darkness, bone growth; testicular and ovarian function
Pharmacokinetics:	Absorption, dependent on presence of dietary fat and bile in GI tract; metabolized to retinaldehyde (converted to retinol), conversion inversely related to intake of β-carotene; elimination in feces
Pharmacodynamics:	Precursor to vitamin A
Dermatologic:	Yellow skin (carotene dermia)
Other:	Arthralgia, diarrhea, dizziness
Dosage:	25–50,000 IU/d PO
Contraindications:	NK
Drug Interactions:	Neomycin ↓ absorption; vitamin E ↑ absorption
Key Points:	No known interactions with anesthetic drugs

BIOTIN (VITAMIN H)

Trade Name:	**Biotin Forte**
Indications:	Inadequate nutrition or intestinal malabsorption (e.g., dermatitis, alopecia, hypercholesterolemia, arrhythmias)
Pharmacokinetics:	Absorption 50%; highly protein bound; urinary excretion
Pharmacodynamics:	Gluconeogenesis, lipogenesis, fatty acid biosynthesis
Dosage:	30–100 mg/d PO
Contraindications:	NK
Drug Interactions:	NK
Key Points:	No known anesthetic drug interactions

CALCIFEDIOL, CALCITRIOL (VITAMIN D), DIHYDROTACHYSTEROL (DHT)

Trade Names:	**Calcijex, Calderol, Drisdol, Hytakerol, Rocaltrol**
Indications:	Chronic hypocalcemia, hypophosphatemia, osteodystrophy/malacia (rickets), tetany, vitamin D deficiency (due to inadequate nutrition, intestinal malabsorption, or lack of sunlight), psoriasis
Pharmacokinetics:	Onset: 2–3 h; peak: 4–12 h; ergocalciferol requires bile salts; highly protein bound to α-globulins; duration: 2 d–6 mo; $T_{1/2}$ β: (calcifediol) 16 d, (calcitriol) 3–6 h, (ergocalciferol) 19–48 h; metabolism in kidney, excreted in bile and urine
Pharmacodynamics:	$\uparrow$ Absorption of Ca^{2+} and phosphate from small intestine, $\uparrow$ mobilization of Ca^{2+} from bone, $\uparrow$ Ca^{2+}-binding protein in intestinal mucosa and $\uparrow$ reabsorption of Ca^{2+} in distal renal tubule
CNS:	Headache, lethargy
CV:	$\uparrow$ BP, arrhythmias
GI:	Constipation, nausea, vomiting, dry mouth, anorexia
GU:	Urinary frequency, azotemia, polyuria, albuminuria, $\downarrow$ libido
Metabolic:	Hypercalcemia, hyperthermia, weight loss
Other:	Bone and muscle pain, pruritus, soft tissue calcification
Dosage:	0.5–12.5 mg/d PO; 0.5–5 mg/d (children)
Drug Interactions:	Mg^{+2}-containing antacids lead to hypermagnesemia with CRF; anticonvulsants $\uparrow$ metabolism; hypercalcemia with thiazide diuretics
Key Points:	Cardiac glycosides $\uparrow$ arrhythmias due to hypercalcemia

CYANOCOBALAMIN, HYDROXOCOBALAMIN (VITAMIN B$_{12}$)

Trade Names:	**Alphamin, Cobex, Crystamine, Crysti-12, Cyanoject, Cyomin, Hydrobexan, Hydro-Cobex, Hydro-Crysti-12**
Indications:	Pernicious anemia, vitamin B$_{12}$ deficiency (macrocytic and megaloblastic anemia), neurologic disorders in elderly
Pharmacokinetics:	Onset: <70 min; peak levels: 60 min; protein binding: >90%; T$_{1/2}$ β: 6 d; rapid absorption (8–12 h) in distal ileum as a vitamin B$_{12}$–IF complex; enterohepatic recirculation; metabolized in liver, excreted in feces
Pharmacodynamics:	Coenzyme for fat and carbohydrate metabolism, protein synthesis, cell replication, hematopoiesis, synthesis of nucleoprotein/myelin
CV:	Peripheral vascular thrombosis
GI:	Diarrhea
Other:	Pruritus, polycythemia vera, anaphylaxis
Dosage:	1–25 µg/d PO; 0.1–0.3 mg/d IM/SC for 1–2 wk, follow with 0.1–0.2 mg/mo; 0.3 µg/d PO for 1–2 wk, then 0.1 mg/mo (children)
Contraindications:	Leber's disease
Drug Interactions:	Aminoglycosides, aminosalicylic acid, anticonvulsants, colchicine ↓ ascorbic acid; alcohol ↓ absorption
Key Points:	N$_2$O oxidizes vitamin B$_{12}$, ↓ activity of methionine synthetase; lack of gastric secretion of IF ↓ absorption of vitamin B$_{12}$

FOLIC ACID (VITAMIN B$_9$, VITAMIN M)

Trade Names:	**Apo-Folic, Novo-Folacid**
Indications:	Folate deficiencies (due to alcoholism; hemolytic, megaloblastic, macrocytic anemia; after gastrectomy; malabsorption syndromes [e.g., tropical sprue]), chronic hemodialysis, pregnancy
Pharmacokinetics:	Onset: 5 min (IV), 10–20 min (IM), 20–30 min (oral); peak: 30–60 min; rapidly absorbed (upper duodenum); metabolized in liver, metabolically active form, excreted in urine
Pharmacodynamics:	Maintains erythropoiesis, purine and thymidylate synthesis, amino acid metabolism after conversion to tetrahydrofolic acid
CNS:	Malaise

FOLIC ACID (VITAMIN B₉, VITAMIN M) *continued*

Pulmonary:	Bronchospasm (rare)
Other:	Rash, pruritus, erythema, fever
Dosage:	0.4–1 mg/d PO; 0.05–0.3 mg/d (children)
Contraindications:	NK
Drug Interactions:	↓ Phenobarbital and phenytoin levels; ↓ pyrimethamine effect; methotrexate, pyrimethamine, sulfasalazine, trimethoprim ↓ folic acid
Key Points:	Reverses adverse effects of N_2O on bone marrow

LEUCOVORIN (CIVTROVORUM FACTOR/FOLINIC ACID)

Trade Name:	Wellcovorin
Indications:	Megaloblastic anemia (due to methotrexate [MTX], pyrimethamine, or trimethoprim), colorectal cancer, folic acid antagonists
Pharmacokinetics:	Onset: 5 min (IV), 10–20 min (IM), 20–30 min (oral); peak: 10 min (IV), <1 h (IM), 2–3 h (oral); duration: 3–6 hr; metabolized in liver, excreted in urine
Pharmacodynamics:	Derivative of tetrahydrofolic acid, cofactor in biosynthesis of purines and pyrimidines, antidote for folic acid antagonists
Other:	Urticaria, anaphylactoid reactions, seizures (with chemotherapy)
Dosage:	10–20 mg/m^2 IV/PO, then 10 mg/m^2 q 6 h, 1 mg/d PO (folate-deficient); 4–8 mg IM (MTX toxicity)
Contraindications:	Pernicious anemia
Drug Interactions:	↑ Fluorouracil toxicity, ↓ effect of phenobarbital and phenytoin
Key Points:	No known adverse interaction with anesthetic drugs

MULTIPLE VITAMINS

Trade Names:	Poly-Vi-Flor, Tri-Vi-Flor, Vi-Daylin
Indications:	Vitamin replenisher, dental caries prophylaxis
Pharmacokinetics:	Rapid and complete absorption from GI tract
Pharmacodynamics:	Remineralization of decalcified tooth enamel
Other:	Hypocalcemia, mucous membrane ulceration, bone pain
Dosage:	0.6–1.0 mL/d PO (fluoride: 0.25–0.5 mg/d)

MULTIPLE VITAMINS *continued*

Contraindications:	NK
Drug Interactions:	NK
Key Points:	No known interactions with anesthetic drugs

NIACIN, NICOTINIC ACID (VITAMIN B₃)

Trade Names:	**Endur-Acin, Nia-Bid, Niacor, Niacels, Nico-400, Nicobid, Nicolar, Nicotinex, Slo-Niacin, Tega-Span**
Indications:	Nutritional deficiency or malabsorption (pellagra); 1° hyperlipidemia; peripheral vascular disease; Hartnup's disease
Pharmacokinetics:	Peak: 45 min (slow onset of action); $T_{1/2}$ β: 45 min; dietary tryptophan converted by intestinal bacteria to niacin and then to niacinamide; hepatic metabolism, excreted in urine
Pharmacodynamics:	Niacinamide is a component of two coenzymes, NAP and NADP
CNS:	↑ Glaucoma, amblyopia, headache
CV:	Orthostatic arrhythmias
GI:	Peptic ulceration, nausea, vomiting, diarrhea, ↑ LFTs
Hepatic:	Hepatotoxicity, cholestasis
Other:	Impaired glucose tolerance, hyperuricemia, skin rash, pruritus
Dosage:	125–500 mg/d (dietary replacement); 1 g PO tid, max. 6 g/d (hyperlipidemia)
Contraindications:	Hepatic impairment, active peptic ulcer, severe hypotension
Drug Interactions:	Aspirin ↓ clearance; β-blockers ↑ hypotension
Key Points:	Use sympatholytic drugs (e.g., β-blockers, α-antagonists) with caution during anesthesia to avoid CV instability

PANTOTHENIC ACID (VITAMIN B₅)

Trade Name:	**None**
Indications:	Dietary deficiency; malabsorption due to tropical sprue, celiac disease, or regional enteritis
Pharmacokinetics:	Readily absorbed; not metabolized, excreted in urine
Pharmacodynamics:	Precursor of coenzyme
CNS:	Sensory and motor neuropathy

PANTOTHENIC ACID
(VITAMIN B₅) *continued*

Dosage:	25–100 mg/d (max. 100 mg/d)
Contraindications:	NK
Drug Interactions:	NK
Key Points:	Assess neurological status before regional nerve blocks

PHYTONADIONE (VITAMIN K)

Trade Names:	**AquaMephyton, Mephyton**
Indications:	Malabsorption or drug-induced hypoprothrombinemia/antihemorrhagic effects, abetalipoproteinemia, TPN therapy, hemorrhagic disease (neonates)
Pharmacokinetics:	Onset: 1–2 h (IV/IM), 6–12 h (oral); rapid absorption (duodenum) in presence of bile salts; metabolized by liver, excreted in urine and bile
Pharmacodynamics:	Promotes formation of prothrombin, proconvertin, thromboplastin component (or Christmas factor), Stuart factor (Factor X)
CNS:	Headaches, dizziness, anorexia
CV:	↓ BP (transient), arrhythmias, flushing
Pulmonary:	Dyspnea, bronchospasm
Other:	Hemolytic anemia, kernicterus, ↑ bilirubin, diaphoresis, ↓ PT
Dosage:	2–25 mg/d PO; 2–10 mg/d (children)
Contraindications:	NK
Drug Interactions:	Broad-spectrum antibiotics (e.g., cefoperazone, cefotetan); ↓ effect (↑ PT); ↓ oral anticoagulants (↓ PT); mineral oil ↓ GI absorption
Key Points:	Check PT before surgery in patients receiving coumadin therapy

PYRIDOXINE (VITAMIN B₆)

Trade Names:	**Rodex, Aminoxin, Nestrex**
Indications:	Inadequate nutrition, intestinal malabsorption (e.g., axanthurenic aciduria, sideroblastic anemia, seborrheic dermatitis, cheilosis), isoniazid overdose, premenstrual syndrome
Pharmacokinetics:	Pyridoxal phosphate bound to plasma proteins; $T_{1/2}$ β: 15–20 d; readily absorbed (jejunum); hepatic metabolism, excreted in urine

PYRIDOXINE
(VITAMIN B_6) *continued*

Pharmacodynamics:	Converted in erythrocytes to coenzyme pyridoxal phosphate
CNS:	Sensory neuropathy
Dosage:	30–600 mg/d PO; 10–100 mg/d (children)
Contraindications:	NK
Drug Interactions:	↑ Excretion of cycloserine and isoniazide, penicillamine is antagonist, ↓ levels of phenobarbital and phenytoin
Key Points:	Assess neurologic status prior to nerve block procedures

RIBOFLAVIN (VITAMIN B_2)

Trade Name:	**None**
Indications:	Deficiency (ariboflavinosis) due to intestinal malabsorption (e.g., angular stomatitis, cheilosis, corneal vascularization, dermatoses)
Pharmacokinetics:	Rapid absorption; $T_{1/2} \beta$: 66–84 min; hepatic metabolism, excreted in urine
Pharmacodynamics:	Riboflavin is converted to two coenzymes, FMN and FAD
GU:	Yellow urine (with high doses)
Dosage:	5–30 mg/d PO, then 1–4 mg/d; 3–10 mg/d, then 0.6–1.2 mg/d (children)
Contraindications:	NK
Drug Interactions:	↑ Dosage requirements with probenecid, hormonal contraceptives, phenothiazines; alcohol ↓ intestinal absorption
Key Points:	No known adverse interaction with anesthetic drugs

THIAMINE (VITAMIN B_1)

Trade Name:	**Thiamilate**
Indications:	Deficiency due to diet or malabsorption (beri-beri, Wernicke's encephalopathy), anemia (due to thiamine deficiency); polyneuritis due to alcoholism, pregnancy, or pellagra
Pharmacokinetics:	Rapidly absorbed (duodenum); hepatic metabolism, excreted in urine
Pharmacodynamics:	Regulation of carbohydrate metabolism
CNS:	Restlessness

THIAMINE (VITAMIN B₁) *continued*

CV:	↓ BP
Other:	Hemorrhage, angioedema (anaphylaxis)
Dosage:	5–10 mg PO tid; 20–100 mg/d IM/IV (×14 d); 10 mg/d (children)
Contraindications:	NK
Drug Interactions:	Incompatible with carbonates, sulfites, citrates, bicarbonate solutions
Key Points:	↑ Effects of neuromuscular blockers, ↑ residual muscle paralysis

α-TOCOPHEROL (VITAMIN E)

Trade Names:	**Aquasol E, Eprolin, Aquavit-E**
Indications:	Vitamin E deficiency (low birth weight), premature infants with retrolental fibroplasia and bronchopulmonary dysplasia; peripheral neuropathy; ophthalmoplegia, necrotizing myopathy
Pharmacokinetics:	Binding to plasma betalipoproteins, ↓ absorption in presence of fat and bile salts, hepatic metabolism, excreted in feces and urine
Pharmacodynamics:	Antioxidant effect with selenium protects against free radicals, protects RBCs against hemolysis
CNS:	Blurred vision, headache, dizziness, weakness, fatigue
GI:	Diarrhea, nausea, cramps
Other:	Breast enlargement, flulike symptoms
Dosage:	30–75 U/d PO; 1 U/kg/d (children)
Contraindications:	NK
Drug Interactions:	Coumarin ↑ hypoprothrombinemic response (↑ bleeding); impaired hematologic response to iron supplements; cholestyramine, colestipol, mineral oil, sucralfate ↑ absorption
Key Points:	Check coagulation panel if patient is receiving anticoagulants

VITAMIN A (RETINOL)

Trade Names:	**Aquasol A, Palmitate-A, Del-Vi-A**
Indications:	Deficiency due to diet or intestinal malabsorption (keratomalacia, xerophthalmia, night blindness), bone growth, testicular and ovarian function, regulation of growth of epithelial tissues

VITAMIN A *continued*

Pharmacokinetics: Rapid absorption with bile salts, pancreatic lipase,
                         protein, dietary fat (water miscible > oil solution);
                         metabolized in liver, eliminated in feces and urine

Pharmacodynamics: Retinol combines with opsin to form rhodopsin
  CNS: Headache, confusion, double vision
  GI: Diarrhea, vomiting, ↑ LFTs
  Other: Dry skin/lips, alopecia, photosensitive, arthralgia,
                         bleeding

Dosage: 50–100,000 U/d for 3 d, then 25–50,000 U/d × 14 d;
                         10,000 U/kg/d for 5 d, then 5–10,000 U/d × 14 d

Contraindications: Malabsorption, hypervitaminosis A

Drug Interactions: ↑ Ca^{2+} with Ca^{2+} supplements; ↓ absorption with
                         cholestyramine, colestipol, mineral oil, neomycin,
                         and fat malabsorption; hormonal contraceptives
                         ↑ levels; ↓ anticoagulant effect of warfarin

Key Points: Check coagulation status in patients receiving coumadin

Oral Analgesic Drug Combinations

A. NONOPIOID ANALGESIC COMBINATIONS

Trade Names	Generic Names (Drug Dosage)
Actifed Cold & Sinus, Comtrex Allergy-Sinus, Sine-Off Sinus Medicine Caplets, Sinutab Sinus Maximum Strength	Acetaminophen (500 mg) + pseudoephedrine (30 mg) + chlorpheniramine (2 mg)
Alka-Seltzer Plus Cold & Sinus Liqui-Gels, Coldrine, Omex No Drowsiness Caplets, Sinutab Sinus	Acetaminophen (325 mg) + pseudoephedrine (30 mg)
Anacin, P-A-C	Aspirin (400 mg) + caffeine (32 mg)
Ascriptin, Magnaprin	Aspirin (325 mg) + magnesium (50 mg)/aluminum hydroxide (50 mg) + calcium carbonate (50 mg)
Ascriptin A/D, Magnaprin Arthritis Strength Caplets	Aspirin (325 mg) + magnesium (75 mg)/aluminum hydroxide (75 mg) + calcium carbonate (75 mg)
Aspirin-free Anacin PM, Excedrine PM, Extra Strength Tylenol PM, Sominex Pain Relief	Acetaminophen (500 mg) + diphehydramine (25 mg)
Axocet, Bucet, Butex Forte, Phrenilin Forte, Tencon	Acetaminophen (650 mg) + butalbital (50 mg)
Bufferin AF Nite Time, Excedrine PM	Acetaminophen (500 mg) + diphenhydramine (38 mg)
Cama Arthritis Pain Reliever	Aspirin (500 mg) + magnesium oxide (150 mg) + aluminum hydroxide (125 mg)
Dristan Cold Maximum Strength Caplets Non-Drowsy, Sudafed Sinus Headache Non-Drowsy, Tavist Sinus Maximum Strength, Sine-Off Maximum Strength No Drowsiness Formula	Acetaminophen (500 mg) + pseudoephedrine (30 mg)
Esgic, Floricet, Margesic, Medigesic, Repan, Triad	Acetaminophen (325 mg) + caffeine (40 mg) + butalbital (50 mg)
Esgic Plus	Acetaminophen (500 mg) + caffeine (40 mg) + butalbital (50 mg)
Excedrin Extra Strength, Excedrin Migraine	Aspirin (250 mg) + acetaminophen (250 mg) + caffeine(65 mg)
Florinal, Flortal	Aspirin (325 mg) + caffeine (40 mg) + butalbital (50 mg)

Trade Names	Generic Names (Drug Dosage)
Isocom, Isopap, Midchlor, Midrin, Migratine	Acetaminophen (325 mg) + dichloralphenazone (100 mg) + isometheptene mucate (65 mg)
Marten-Tab, Phrenilin	Acetaminophen (325 mg) + butalbital (50 mg)
Vanquish	Aspirin (227 mg) + acetaminophen (194 mg) + caffeine (33 mg) + aluminum hydroxide (25 mg) + magnesium hydroxide (50 mg)

B. OPIOID-CONTAINING ANALGESIC COMBINATIONS

Trade Names	Generic Names (Drug Dosage)
Aceta with Codeine, Tylenol with Codeine #3	Acetaminophen (300 mg) + codeine (30 mg)
Alor 5/500, Damason-P, Lortab ASA	Aspirin (500 mg) + hydrocodone bitartrate (5 mg)
Anexsia 7.5/650, Lorcet Plus	Acetaminophen (650 mg) + hydrocodone (7.5 mg)
Capital with Codeine, Tylenol with Codeine Elixir	Acetaminophen (120 mg) + codeine (12 mg/5 mL)
Darvocet-N 50	Acetamiophen (325 mg) + propoxyphene (50 mg)
Darvocet-N 100, Propacet 100	Acetaminophen (650 mg) + propoxyphene (100 mg)
Empirin with Codeine No. 3	Aspirin (325 mg) + codeine (30 mg)
Empirin with Codeine No. 4	Aspirin (325 mg) + codeine (60 mg)
Floricet with Codeine	Acetaminophen (325 mg) + butalbital (50 mg) + caffeine (40 mg) + codeine (30 mg)
Florinal with Codeine	Aspirin (325 mg) + butalbital (50 mg) + caffeine (40 mg) + codeine (30 mg)
Lorcet 10/650	Acetaminophen (650 mg) + hydrocodone (10 mg)
Lortab 2.5/500	Acetaminophen (500 mg) + hydrocodone (2.5 mg)
Lortab 5/500, Vicodin	Acetaminophen (500 mg) + hydrocodone (5 mg)
Lortab 7.5/500	Acetaminophen (500 mg) + hydrocodone (7.5 mg)
Lortab 10/500	Acetaminophen (500 mg) + hydrocodone (10 mg)
Maxidone	Acetaminophen (750 mg) + hydrocodone (10 mg)
Norco	Acetaminophen (325 mg) + hydrocodone (5–10 mg)
Percocet 2.5/325	Acetaminophen (325 mg) + oxycodone (2.5 mg)
Percocet 5/325, Roxicet	Acetaminophen (325 mg) + oxycodone (5 mg)
Percocet 7.5/500	Acetaminophen (500 mg) + oxycodone (7.5 mg)
Percocet 10/650	Acetaminophen (650 mg) + oxycodone (10 mg)
Percodan-Demi	Aspirin (325 mg) + oxycodone (2.25 mg) + oxycodone terephthalate (0.19 mg)
Percodan, Roxiprin	Aspirin (325 mg) + oxycodone (4.5 mg) + oxycodone terephthalate (0.38 mg)
Roxicet 5/500, Roxilox	Acetaminophen (500 mg) + oxycodone (5 mg)

Trade Names	Generic Names (Drug Dosage)
Roxicet Oral Solution	Acetaminophen (65 mg/mL) + oxycodone (1 mg/mL)
Talacen	Acetaminophen (650 mg) + pentazocine (25 mg)
Talwin	Aspirin (325 mg) + pentazocine (12.5 mg)
Tylenol with Codeine No. 2	Acetaminophen (300 mg) + codeine (15 mg)
Tylenol with Codeine No. 4	Acetaminophen (300 mg) + codeine (60 mg)
Tylox	Acetaminophen (500 mg) + oxycodone (5 mg)
Vicodin ES	Acetaminophen (750 mg) + hydrocodone (7.5 mg)
Vicodin HP	Acetaminophen (660 mg) + hydrocodone (10 mg)
Wygesic	Acetaminophen (650 mg) + propoxyphene (65 mg)
Vicoprofen	Ibuprofen (200 mg) + hydrocodone (7.5 mg)
Zydone	Acetaminophen (400 mg) + hydrocodone (10 mg)

Factors Altering Drug Metabolism by Cytochrome P$_{450}$ Isoenzymes

Cytochrome (CYP) Isoenzymes	Metabolized Drugs	Increases Metabolism	Decreases Metabolism
CYP 1A2	Amitriptyline, caffeine, chlordiazepoxide, clomipramine, clozapine, cyclobenzaprine, desipramine, diazepam, haloperidol, imipramine, olanzapine, tacrine, theophylline, warfarin, zileuton	Cigarette smoking, phenobarbital, phenytoin, primidone, rifampin, ritonavir	Ciprofloxacin, cimetidine, clarithromycin, enoxacin, erythromycin, fluvoxamine, grapefruit juice, isoniazid, ketoconazole, levofloxacin, mexiletine, norethindone, norfloxacin, omeprazole, paroxetine, tacrine, zileuton
CYP 2C9	Amitriptyline, carvedilol, clomipramine, dapsone, diazepam, diclofenac, flurbiprofen, fluvastatin, glimepiride, ibuprofen, imipramine, indomethacin, losartan, mirtazapine, naproxen, omeprazole, phenytoin, piroxicam, ritonavir, sildenafil, tolbutamide, torsemide, S-warfarin, zafirlukast, zileuton	Carbamazepine, phenobarbital, phenytoin, primidone, rifampin	Amiodarone, chloramphenicol, cimetidine, co-trimoxazole, disulfiram, fluconazole, fluoxetine, fluvastatin, fluvoxamine, isoniazid, itraconazole, ketoconazole, metronidazole, omeprazole, ritonavir, sulfinpyrazone, ticlopidine, zafirlukast
CYP 2C19	Amitroptyline, cariosprodol, clomipramine, diazepam, imipramine, lansoprazole, mephenytoin, omeprazole, pentamidine, R-warfarin	None known	Felbamate, fluconazole, fluoxetine, fluvoxamine, omeprazole, ticlopidine

Cytochrome (CYP) Isoenzymes	Metabolized Drugs	Increases Metabolism	Decreases Metabolism
CYP 2D6	Amitriptyline, chlorpromazine, carvedilol, chlorpheniramine, clomipramine, clozapine, codeine, cyclobenzaprine, desipramine, dextromethorphan, donepezil, doxepin, fentanyl, flecainide, fluoxetine, fluphenazine, fluvoxamine, haloperidol, hydrocodone, imipramine, loratidine, maprotiline, meperidine, methadone, metoprolol, mexiletine, morphine, methamphetamine, nortriptyline, oxycodone, paroxetine, perphenazine, propafenone, propoxyphene, propranolol, risperidone, thioridazine, timolol, tramadol, trazodone, venlafixine	Carbamazepine, phenobarbital, phenytoin, primidone	Amiodarone, chloroquine, cimetidine, fluxetine, fluphenazine, fluvoxamine, haloperidol, paroxetine, perphenazine, propafenone, propoxyphene, quinidine, ritonavir, sertraline, thioridazine
CYP 3A4	Alfentanil, alprazolam, amiodarone, amitriptyline, amlodipine, atorvastatin, bromocriptine, buspirone, carbamazepine, clarithromycin, clomipramine, clonazepam, cocaine, corticosteroids, cyclophosphamide, cyclosporine, dapsone, delavirdine, doxorubicin, dexamethasone, diazepam, diltiazem, disopyramide, ergotamine, erythromycin, ethosuximide, etoposide, felodipine, fentanyl, fexofenadine, finasteride, flutamide, fluvastatin, ifosfamide, imipramine, indinavir, isradipine, itraconazole, ketoconazole, lidocaine, loratidine, losartan, lovastatin, midazolam, methadone, methylprednisolone, miconazole, nefazodone, nicardipine, nifedipine, nimodipine, nisoldipine, paclitaxel, pravastatin, prednisone, quinidine, quinine, rifabutin, ritonavir, saquinavir, sertraline, sildenafil, simvastatin, tacrolimus, tamoxifen, teniposide, testosterone, triazolam, troleandomycin, verapamil, vinca alkaloids, warfarin, zileuton, zolpidem	Barbiturates, carbamazepine, glucocorticoids, griseofulvin, nafcillin, phenytoin, primidone, rifabutin, rifampin	Clarithromycin, cyclosporine, danazol, de:avirdine, diltiazem, erythromycin, fluconazole, fluoxetine, fluvoxamine, grapefruit juice, indinavir, isoniazid, itraconazole, ketoconazole, metronidazole, miconazole, nefazodone, nelfinavir, nicardipine, nifedipine, norflaxacin, omeprazole, prednisone, quinidine, quinine, rifabutin, ritonavir, saquinavir, sertraline, troleandomycin, verapamil, zafirlukast

Glossary

a.c. before meals
ACE angiotensin-converting enzyme
ACh acetylcholine
ACLS advanced cardiac life support
ACTH adrenocorticotropic hormone
ADH antidiuretic hormone
ADP adenosine diphosphate
AF atrial fibrillation
AHA American Heart Association
AHF antihemophilic factor
AIDS acquired immunodeficiency syndrome
AIP acute intermittent porphyria
Al aluminum
ALL acute lymphocytic leukemia
ALT alanine aminotransferase
AML acute myelocytic leukemia
ANA antinuclear antibody
APD action potential duration
a-PTT activated partial thromboplastin time
ARDS adult respiratory distress syndrome
ARF acute respiratory failure
ASA acetylsalicylic acid
ASCVD atherosclerotic cardiovascular disease
AST aspartate aminotransferase
ATP adenosine triphosphate
AUL acute undifferentiated leukemia
AV atrioventricular
AVB atrioventricular block
AVM "arteriovenous" malformation
bid twice a day
BP blood pressure
BPH benign prostatic hypertrophy
BUN blood urea nitrogen
BUN/CR blood urea nitrogen/creatine
Ca^{2+} calcium

CaCO$_3$ calcium carbonate
CAD coronary artery disease
cAMP cyclic adenosine monophosphate
CBF cerebral blood flow
CCB calcium channel blocker
cGMP cyclic guanosine monophosphate
CHF congestive heart failure
Cl^{-1} chloride
CLL chronic lymphocytic leukemia
CMRO$_2$ cerebral metabolic rate of oxygen
CMV cytomegalovirus
CNS central nervous system
CO carbon monoxide
CO$_2$ carbon dioxide
COMT catechol-o-methyltransferase
COPD chronic obstructive pulmonary disease
CPB cardiopulmonary bypass
CPR cardiopulmonary resuscitation
CrCl creatinine clearance
CRF chronic renal failure
CSF cerebrospinal fluid
CTZ chemoreceptor trigger zone
CV cardiovascular
CVA cerebrovascular accidents
CVP central venous pressure
CVR cerebral vascular resistance
CVS cardiovascular system
CYP cytochrome P$_{450}$
DI diabetes insipidus
DIC disseminated intravascular coagulation
DM diabetes mellitus
DTs delirium tremons
DVT deep venous thrombosis
D$_5$W 5% dextrose in water
EBV Epstein-Barr virus
ECG electrocardiogram

ED   effective dose

EDRF   endothelium-derived relaxing factor

EEG   electroencephalogram

ENL   erythema nodosum leprosum

ER   emergency room

ERP   effective refractory period

ESR   erythrocyte sedimentation rate

FDA   Food and Drug Administration

FSH   follicle-stimulating hormone

FU   fluorouracil

G-6-PD   glucose-6-phosphate dehydrogenase

GABA   gamma-aminobutyric acid

G-CSF   granulocyte colony–stimulating factor

GERD   gastroesophageal reflux disease

GFR   glomerular filtration rate

GI   gastrointestinal

GMP   guanosine monophosphate

GTF   glucose tolerance factor

GU   genitourinary

GVHD   graft-versus-host disease

H_2   histamine type-2 receptor

hCG   human chorionic gonadotropin

HDL   high-density lipoprotein

HIV   human immunodeficiency virus

HMG CoA   3-hydroxy-3-methylglutaryl coenzyme A

HR   heart rate

hs   at bedtime

HSV   herpes simplex virus

I^-   iodine

IA   intra-articular

ICP   intracranial pressure

ICU   intensive care unit

IF   intrinsic factor

IgE   immunoglobulin E

IGF   insulin-like growth factor

IHSS   idiopathic hypertrophic subaortic stenosis

IL   interleukin

IM   intramuscular

INR   International Normalized Ratio

IOP   intraocular pressure

IV   intravenous

K^+   potassium

LDL   low-density lipoprotein

LFT   liver function test

LH   luteinizing hormone

LPE   lipoprotein electrophoresis

LV   left ventricular

MAC   minimal alveolar concentration

MAO   monoamine oxidase

MAOI   monoamine oxidase inhibitor

MAP   mean arterial pressure

max   maximum

Mg^{2+}   magnesium

MH   malignant hyperthermia

MI   myocardial infarction

MOPP   mustard oncovin procarbazine and prednisone

MP   mercaptopurine

MS   multiple sclerosis

MTX   methotrexate

MVO_2   myocardial oxygen consumption

MW   molecular weight

NA   not applicable

Na^{2+}   sodium

NE   norepinephrine

NG   nasogastric

NK   not known

NMDA N-methyl-D-aspartate

NMS   neuroleptic malignant syndrome

NO   nitric oxide

N_2O   nitrous oxide

NSAID   nonsteroidal anti-inflammatory drug

O_2   oxygen

OCD   obsessive-compulsive disorder

OCP   oral contraceptive pill

PABA   para-aminobenzoic acid

PAC   premature atrial contraction

PAT   paroxysmal atrial tachycardia

PCA   patient-controlled analgesia

PCV   packed cell volume

PCWP   pulmonary capillary wedge pressure

PE   pulmonary embolism

PGE_1   prostaglandin E_1

PID   pelvic inflammatory disease

PKU   phenylketonuria

PO   orally

PONV postoperative nausea and vomiting

PPARγ peroxisome proliferator–activated receptor-gamma

PR ECG interval

pr rectally

prn as needed

PSVT paroxysmal supraventricular tachycardia

PT prothrombin time

PTCA percutaneous transluminal coronary angioplasty

PTSD post-traumatic stress disorder

PTT partial thromboplastin time

PUD peptic ulcer disease

PVC premature ventricular contraction

PVR peripheral vascular resistance

q every

qd once a day

qid four times a day

RA rheumatoid arthritis

RBC red blood cell

RBF renal blood flow

RDS respiratory distress syndrome

RES reticuloendothelial system

RR respiratory rate

RSV respiratory syncytial virus

SBP systolic blood pressure

SC subcutaneous

SGPT serum glutamate pyruvate transaminase

SIADH syndrome of inappropriate antidiuretic hormone secretion

SLE systemic lupus erythematosus

SOB shortness of breath

SpO$_2$ pulse oximetry

SR sustained release

SRS-A slow-reacting substance of anaphylaxis

SSRI selective serotonin release inhibitor

sup suppository

SV stroke volume

SVR systemic vascular resistance

SVT supraventricular tachycardia

T$_{1/2}$ half-life

T$_3$ triiodothyronine

T$_4$ thyroxine

TCA tricyclic antidepressant

TIA transient ischemic attack

tid three times a day

TNS transient neuropathic symptoms

TPN total parenteral nutrition

TTP thrombotic thrombocytopenic purpura

TTS transdermal drug delivery

TURP transurethral prostatectomy

TV tidal volume

URI upper respiratory infection

UROD ultra-rapid opioid detoxification

UTI urinary tract infection

UV ultraviolet

Vc volume of distribution of the central compartment

Vd volume of distribution

Vd$_{ss}$ volume of distribution at steady-state

VF ventricular fibrillation

VLDL very–low density lipoprotein

$\dot{V}/\dot{Q}$ ventilation-perfusion ratio

VT tidal volume

Index